# Cavernomas of the CNS

Ondřej Bradáč • Vladimír Beneš

Editors

# Cavernomas of the CNS

## Basic Science to Clinical Practice

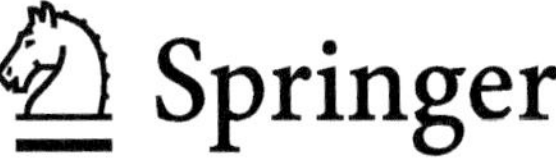 Springer

*Editors*
Ondřej Bradáč
Department of Neurosurgery and
Neurooncology, First Medical Faculty
Military University Hospital and
Charles University
Prague
Czech Republic

Vladimír Beneš
Department of Neurosurgery and
Neurooncology, First Medical Faculty
Military University Hospital and
Charles University
Prague
Czech Republic

ISBN 978-3-030-49408-7     ISBN 978-3-030-49406-3   (eBook)
https://doi.org/10.1007/978-3-030-49406-3



This Springer imprint is published by the registered company Springer Nature Switzerland AG
The registered company address is: Gewerbestrasse 11, 6330 Cham, Switzerland

# Introduction

Dear reader

Cavernomas (also known as cavernous malformations, cavernous hemangiomas, or cavernous angiomas) are vascular hamartomas made up of thin-walled, grossly dilated blood vessels lined with endothelium. There is no smooth muscle within the blood vessel walls, and there is a lack of intervening brain parenchyma. Although the brain is the most common site for these lesions, cavernomas may occur virtually in any organ. The prevalence within the population is approximately 0.6 per 100,000, which puts them among the most common vascular malformations of the brain. In recent years, significant contributions to the pathophysiology, biology, and genetics of these lesions have been made. Although there has also been significant development in the neuroimaging and active treatment techniques, especially surgical resection, observation alone is still a useful management strategy for some cavernomas. The decision to perform surgical treatment in each individual case depends on many features of a particular lesion, namely its anatomical location, eloquence of adjacent brain tissue, and type of presentation. Moreover, the natural history of the disease must be taken into account and compared to the possible benefits of surgical treatment.

In this book, we present a complete up-to-date description of cavernoma disease together with its known biology and genetics, presentation, and treatment options together with decision-making algorithms in indication of surgical treatment. All chapters in this book are written by respected neurosurgeons with huge experience in vascular neurosurgery.

The main features of this book, common to the separately authored chapters, are the following:

- Garaphic documentation of all aspects of cavernomas, which improves the reader's understanding of the pathological nuances under consideration.
- Introductions consisting of each author's key guiding principles, including their philosophy of treatment decisions.
- Presentation of each author's patient data, which helps readers understand what is really achievable in cavernoma treatment.

– Thorough discussion of particular cases, which helps readers understand decision making in cavernoma treatment.

We feel that a book covering all aspects of cavernomas with up-to-date information from well-known contributors would be suitable for all practicing neurosurgeons and vascular neurologists and will be a valuable source of information for
neurosurgical residents in preparations for their exams.

We are deeply indebted to Mrs. Lenka Bernardová for her help with literature
search and Miss Helen Whitley for her valuable help with English editing.

Last but not least, we are deeply indebted to our wives Eva and Lenka for their
patience with us during the editing of this book.

Prague, Czech Republic                                              Ondřej Bradáč
January 2020                                                       Vladimír Beneš

# Contents

# Chapter 1
# Brief History of Cavernous Malformations

Petr Skalický, Vladimír Beneš, and Ondřej Bradáč

The first description of cavernous malformation was made by pioneer dermatologist Joseph Jakob Plenck in 1776. Although the cavernous malformation was described previously with varying degrees of credibility and probability to actually be the cavernous malformation under the terms: Labii tuberculum atrum cruentum (M.A. Severinus), Telangiectasis (C.F. Graefe), Aneurysm by anastomosin (J. Bell), fungus haematodes (W. Hey), tumeurs érectiles (Dupuytren), substantia cavernosa (Boyer), tumeurs fongueses sanguines, Aftermilzen, placenta-like tissue, etc. [1] it was Carl Freiherr von Rokitansky (Karel Rokytanský) to be the first who presented a detailed pathological description of cavernous malformation (*"Cavernöse Geschwulst"*) in his *Handbook of special pathological anatomy* (*"Handbuch der speciellen patologischen Anatomie"*) published in 1844 [2]. Between 1851 and 1854 Robert Ludwig Carl Virchow defined differences between vascular lesions [1] and in 1863 he presented the first complex classification of vascular malformations [3]. In 1854 Hubert von Luschka published a first comprehensive report of brain cavernoma which was found in the brain of a man who committed suicide with such a detailed description that there can be no doubt that it was indeed a cavernoma [4]. The first case report with successful surgical removal of brain cavernoma was introduced by Bremer and Carson in 1890 [5]. The first pathological description of a man with multiple cavernous angioma was reported by Ohlmacher in Gallipolis, Ohio in 1899 [6]. The first overview was presented by Dandy in 1928 in which he described 5 of his own cases and collected 44 previously published cases that described the typical pathological features of the disease. He identified basic clinical signs such as predisposition to bleed causing focal neurological deficits and epilepsy as a major clinical manifestation and also described basic technical aspects of cavernoma removal, concluding that: "the cavernous angiomas… should be treated surgically

P. Skalický · V. Beneš · O. Bradáč (✉)
Department of Neurosurgery and Neurooncology, First Medical Faculty, Military University Hospital and Charles University, Prague, Czech Republic
e-mail: ondrej.bradac@uvn.cz

© Springer Nature Switzerland AG 2020
O. Bradáč, V. Beneš (eds.), *Cavernomas of the CNS*,
https://doi.org/10.1007/978-3-030-49406-3_1

by complete removal of the solid tumor together with a margin of contiguous brain tissue." [7]. Also in 1928 Cushing and Bailey published their book *Tumors Arising from Blood Vessels of the Brain* and classified cavernous malformations as a solid subtype of hemangioblastomas [8].

Over this period number of detected cavernous malformations remained low due to insufficient diagnostic possibilities. Angiography was introduced by Moniz in 1927. This huge discovery for the diagnostics of vascular lesions however did not bring much in the cases of cavernoma patients because they are typically not seen on cerebral angiogram [9, 10]. The interest in surgical removal of these lesions continued in the following years (Evans and Courville, Noran, Penfield and Ward, Bodin and Heller, Manuelidis, et al.) [11]. The discrepancy in the classification lasted until 1966 when McCormick presented a modern pathological classification that became widely accepted [11].

In 1957 Yasargil and Krayenbuhl described 82 cases of cerebral cavernomas collected from the literature [12]. Almost 20 years later, in 1976, Yasargil and Voigt published their comprehensive review of 164 well-documented cases together with one of their own patients being successfully operated by Yasargil. They described the pathological appearance, clinical presentation, incidence and diagnosis. They also stressed the difficulty of establishing a diagnosis of brain cavernoma during life. Only 24 cases had been surgically treated and 140 had been diagnosed at autopsy [13]. The essential novelties for the management of cavernoma patients have to be the introduction of operating microscope with establishment of microsurgical operating techniques in the late 1960s together with the development of imaging diagnostic procedures—CT (1970s) and MRI (1980s). Since the start of the use of these techniques, cavernomas have been becoming increasingly recognized and the number of surgically treated cases has exponentially grown [14]. During the 1990s, the natural history of cavernous malformations has been gradually elucidated [15–17], radiosurgery began to find its place in the treatment by the groups from Pittsburgh and the Mayo Clinic [18, 19] and the identification of genes which play role in familial cases started with CCM1 in 1999 [20], CCM2 in 2003 [21] and CCM3 in 2005 [22].

# References


1. Pfeiffer G, Vv B. Über Telangiectasie und cavernöse Blutgeschwulst: eine Inaugural-Abhandlung. Tübingen: Heinrich Laupp; 1854.
2. Rokitansky CV. Handbuch der pathologischen Anatomie, vol. 1. Wien: Braunmüller und Seidel; 1844.
3. Virchow RLC. Die krankhaften Geschwülste: dreissig Vorlesungen, gehalten während des Wintersemesters 1862-1863 an der Universität zu Berlin vol 3. Berlin: Hirschwald, Friedrich-Wilhelms-Universität; 1863.
4. Luschka HV. Cavernöse Blutgeschwulst des Gehirnes. In: Reimer G, Virchow RLC, editors. Archiv für pathologische Anatomie und Physiologie und für klinische Medicin, vol. 6. Berlin: Springer; 1854.

5.  Bremer L, Carson NB. A case of brain tumor (angioma cavernosum), causing spastic paralysis and attacks of tonic spasms, operation. Am J Med Sci. 1890;100:219–42.
6.  Ohlmacher AP. Multiple cavernous angioma, fibroendothelioma, osteoma and hematomyelia of the central nervous system in a case of secondary epilepsy. J Nerv Ment Dis. 1899;26:395–423.
7.  Dandy WE. Venous abnormalities and angiomas of the brain. Arch Surg. 1928;17:715. https://doi.org/10.1001/archsurg.1928.01140110002001.
8.  Cushing H, Bailey P. Tumors arising from the blood-vessels of the brain: angiomatous malformations and hemangioblastomas. Springfield, IL: C.C. Thomas; 1928.
9.  Crawford JV, Russell DS. Cryptic arteriovenous and venous hamartomas of the brain. J Neurol Neurosurg Psychiatry. 1956;19:1–11. https://doi.org/10.1136/jnnp.19.1.1.
10. Radvany MG, Rigamonti D, Gailloud P. Angiographic detection of cerebral cavernous malformations with C-arm cone beam CT imaging in three patients. BMJ Case Rep. 2013; https://doi.org/10.1136/bcr-2013-010650.
11. McCormick WF. The pathology of vascular ("Arteriovenous") malformations. J Neurosurg. 1966;24:807–16. https://doi.org/10.3171/jns.1966.24.4.0807.
12. Krayenbuhl H, Yasargil MG. Die vaskulären Erkrankungen im Gebiet der Arteria vertebralis und Arteria basilaris. Stuttgart: Thieme-Verlag; 1957. p. 458–70.
13. Voigt K, Yaşargil M. Cerebral cavernous haemangiomas or cavernomas. Minim Invasive Neurosurg. 1976;19:59–68. https://doi.org/10.1055/s-0028-1090391.
14. Houtteville JP. The surgery of cavernomas both supra-tentorial and infra-tentorial. Adv Tech Stand Neurosurg. 1995;22:185–259.
15. Del Curling O, Kelly DL, Elster AD, Craven TE. An analysis of the natural history of cavernous angiomas. J Neurosurg. 1991;75:702–8. https://doi.org/10.3171/jns.1991.75.5.0702.
16. Kim D-S, Park Y-G, Choi J-U, Chung S-S, Lee K-C. An analysis of the natural history of cavernous malformations. Surg Neurol. 1997;48:9–17. discussion 17-18.
17. Porter PJ, Willinsky RA, Harper W, Wallace MC. Cerebral cavernous malformations: natural history and prognosis after clinical deterioration with or without hemorrhage. J Neurosurg. 1997;87:190–7. https://doi.org/10.3171/jns.1997.87.2.0190.
18. Coffey RJ, Lunsford LD. Radiosurgery of cavernous malformations and other angiographically occult vascular malformations. In: Cavernous malformations. Park Ridge, IL: AANS; 1993. p. 187–200.
19. Kondziolka D, Lunsford LD, Flickinger JC, Kestle JRW. Reduction of hemorrhage risk after stereotactic radiosurgery for cavernous malformations. J Neurosurg. 1995;83:825–31. https://doi.org/10.3171/jns.1995.83.5.0825.
20. Sahoo T, Johnson EW, Thomas JW, Kuehl PM, Jones TL, Dokken CG, Touchman JW, Gallione CJ, Lee-Lin S-Q, Kosofsky B. Mutations in the gene encoding KRIT1, a Krev-1/rap1a binding protein, cause cerebral cavernous malformations (CCM1). Hum Mol Genet. 1999;8:2325–33.
21. Liquori CL, Berg MJ, Siegel AM, Huang E, Zawistowski JS, Stoffer TP, Verlaan D, Balogun F, Hughes L, Leedom TP. Mutations in a gene encoding a novel protein containing a phosphotyrosine-binding domain cause type 2 cerebral cavernous malformations. Am J Hum Genet. 2003;73:1459–64.
22. Bergametti F, Denier C, Labauge P, Arnoult M, Boetto S, Clanet M, Coubes P, Echenne B, Ibrahim R, Irthum B. Mutations within the programmed cell death 10 gene cause cerebral cavernous malformations. Am J Hum Genet. 2005;76:42–51.

# Chapter 2
# Definition and Structure of Cerebral Cavernous Malformations

Michihiro Tanaka

## 2.1 Definition and Terminology

Cavernomas have various different names. Cerebral cavernoma, cerebral cavernous malformation (CCM), cryptic angioma, cavernous hemangioma, and cavernous angioma are well used and sometimes confused in terms of nomenclature. As these lesions are not neoplastic, it has been argued that the terms 'hemangioma' and 'cavernoma' should be avoided. Additionally, it is important to note that according to newer nomenclature (ISSVA classification of vascular anomalies), these lesions are known as slow flow venous malformations [1]. It is probably helpful in reports to include the word 'cavernous' as this term is ubiquitous in the literature and most familiar to many clinicians. Therefore, the term 'cerebral cavernous malformations (CCMs)' are recommended and used in this chapter [1–6].

## 2.2 Structure

CCMs are abnormally formed blood vessels and consists of clusters of thin walled cavernous vessels without intervening stroma (Fig. 2.1).

They belong to the group of low-flow vascular malformations and occur in the venous-capillary vascular bed. CCMs consist of a mulberry- or raspberry-like cluster of enlarged endothelial channels (caverns) surrounded by a thick, segmental

---

The authors affirm that this manuscript has been approved by all authors; the manuscript does not infringe or violate any private, personal, or property right; and this manuscript has not been previously published in whole or in part and is not being submitted or considered for publication elsewhere in any language.

---

M. Tanaka (✉)
Department of Neuroendovascular Surgery, Kameda Medical Center, Kamogawa City, Chiba, Japan

© Springer Nature Switzerland AG 2020
O. Bradáč, V. Beneš (eds.), *Cavernomas of the CNS*,
https://doi.org/10.1007/978-3-030-49406-3_2

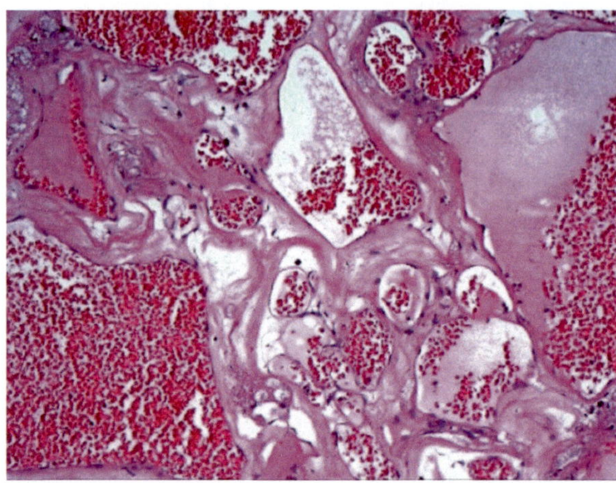

**Fig. 2.1** Microscopic findings of CCM with 20 × magnification. This section shows a nidus of small caliber vascular channels which is sharply demarcated from surrounding white matter. Vessels have a back-to-back arrangement with no intervening brain parenchyma. The vessel walls are composed of collagen with no smooth muscle or elastic tissue identified

layered basal membrane. The vascular channels are generally arranged in a back-to-back pattern with little or no intervening brain parenchyma and are often surrounded by gliotic tissue. The cells that line these caverns sometimes ooze small amounts of blood into surrounding brain tissue and produce the hemosiderin in the parenchyma. This deposition of hemosiderin sometimes results in symptoms like seizure. CCMs can grow in size, but this growth is not cancerous, and they do not spread to other areas of the body [7–10].

## 2.3 CCMs Associated with Developmental Venous Anomalies (DVAs)

The association between developmental venous anomalies (DVAs) and CCMs has been well recognized. CCMs are known to occur in 8–33% of the DVAs [11–13]. The coexistence of a CCM and an associated DVA is the most common mixed vascular malformation. Patients with CCM associated with DVA are more likely to have lesions in the posterior fossa. The most prone site for the development of CCMs is the central portion of DVA where abnormal small branches of tributaries of medullary vein converged (Fig. 2.2).

The anatomical complexities of the DVAs may create certain anatomical angio-architectural factors responsible for the occurrence of CCMs in its territory [11–15].

## 2.4 Demography and Genetic Factors

CCMs affect approximately 0.4%–0.6% of the population [16]. Approximately 20% of CCMs are familial, autosomal dominant, and the rest are sporadic. Familial CCMs tend to be multiple. Up to half of patients with CCMs, more in some studies,

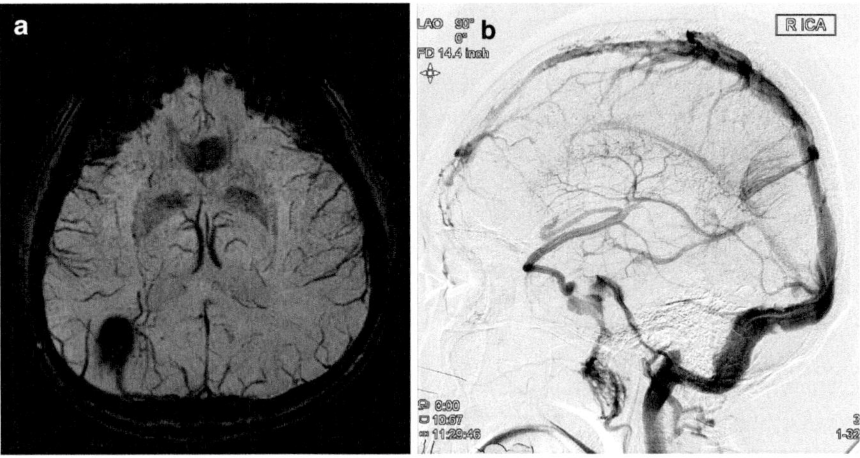


**Fig. 2.2** (a) SWI showed the CCM associated with DVA. (b) Venous phase of angiography of the same patient demonstrates the typical appearance of DVA adjacent to the CCM. CCMs are always occult angiographically

remain asymptomatic through their lives. The rest have seizures, focal neurologic deficits, headaches, and cerebral bleeds. Symptoms usually develop between the second to fifth decade of life. Recent studies showed that CCMs are caused by mutations of three genes. The three genes associated with CCM disease encode the proteins KRIT1/CCM1 (Krev interaction trapped 1/cerebral cavernous malformations), CCM2/Malcavernin/OSM (cerebral cavernous malformations 2, osmosensing scaffold for MEKK3), and CCM3/PDCD10 (cerebral cavernous malformations 3/programmed cell death 10) [3, 4].

KRIT1 (CCM1) is a disease gene responsible for CCMs, a major cerebrovascular disease of proven genetic origin affecting 0.3–0.5% of the population. Mutations in the KRIT1 gene account for up to 50 percent of all familial CCM cases [3, 9]. One particular mutation is responsible for up to 70 percent of cases in people of Hispanic heritage. It is possible that CCMs are all caused by genetic defects in KRIT1 and related genes encoding proteins that lie in a single signal transduction pathway. This pathway may be important in the normal formation and function of microvasculature. Formation of competent cerebral microvasculature relies on appropriate signaling between adjacent endothelial cells and between endothelial cells, pericytes, astrocytes, and the extracellular matrix. These mutations place a premature stop signal in the instructions for making the KRIT1 protein, preventing adequate KRIT1 protein production [3, 8–10]. A shortage of this protein likely impairs the function of the complex. As a result, RhoA-GTPase signaling is turned on abnormally, weakening cellular junctions and increasing the permeability of blood vessel walls. The increased leakage into the brain can cause health problems such as headaches, seizures, and bleeding in the brain (cerebral hemorrhage) in some people with cerebral cavernous malformations [3, 4, 6, 8–10].

## 2.5 Neuroradiology of CCMs

CCMs tend to be supratentorial and more than 80% cases of CCMs are locating in the parenchyma of supratentorial telencephalon, but they can be found anywhere including the brainstem. They are usually solitary, although up to one-third of patients with sporadic lesions have more than one [17, 18].

**CT** Unless large, these lesions are difficult to see on CT. They do not enhance. If it would be large, then a region of hyperdensity can be seen. If there has been a recent bleeding, then it is more conspicuous and may be surrounded by a mantle of edema [19].

**MRI** MRI sequences sensitive to the magnetic susceptibility artefact of iron (such as gradient echo and susceptibility-weighting) have been found to be more sensitive for the detection of multiple CCM in comparison to conventional spin echo in studies undertaken in families with inherited CCM.

The CCMs can be defined by the MRIs' appearance, if they had more than two of the following findings:

1. a central core of reticulated mixed signal blood containing locules with "popcorn ball or raspberry like appearance"
2. a surrounding rim of low-signal intensity on T2-weighted image
3. minimal or no enhancement on SPGR (Spoiled Gradient-echo sequence) image

The developmental venous anomalies (DVAs) are defined on MRIs by typical stellate or tubular vascular lesions which converged on collecting vein and drained into dural or ependymal sinus and caput medusa appearance on SPGR image [12, 15, 20].

MRI is the best modality of choice, demonstrating a characteristic "popcorn" or "berry" appearance with a rim of signal loss due to hemosiderin, which demonstrates prominent blooming on susceptibility weighted sequences. T1 and T2 weighted images are varied internally depending on the age of the blood products and small fluid-fluid levels may be evident. Gradient echo or T2* sequences are able to delineate these lesions better than T1 or T2 weighted images. In patients with familial or multiple cavernous angiomas GRE T2* sequences are very important in identifying the number of lesions missed by conventional Spin echo sequences. Susceptibility weighted imaging (SWI) may have sensitivity equal to that of GRE in detecting these capillary telangiectasias in the brain. SWI is also highly sensitive in detecting calcification as compared to T1 and T2 images [17, 19].

If a recent bleed has occurred, the surrounding edema can usually be presented.

The lesions generally do not enhance, although enhancement is possible.

CCMs can be grouped into four types based on MRI appearances using the Zabramski classification [21] (Table 2.1).

This classification of cerebral cavernomas has been proposed as a way of classifying cerebral cavernous malformations, and although not used in clinical practice it is useful in scientific publications that seek to study cavernous malformations.

**Table 2.1** Zabramski's classification based on the MRI findings (1994)

| Type I: Subacute hemorrhage |
| --- |
| T1: Hyperintense |
| T2: Hypo or hyperintense |
| Type II: Most common type - classic "popcorn" lesion |
| T1: Mixed signal intensity centrally |
| T2: Mixed signal intensity centrally |
| T2*: Low signal rim with blooming |
| Type III: Chronic hemorrhage |
| T1: Hypointense to isointense centrally |
| T2: Hypointense centrally |
| T2*: Low signal rim with blooming |
| Type IV: Multiple punctate microhemorrhages |
| T1: Difficult to identify |
| T2: Difficult to identify |
| T2* gradient Echo: "Black dots" with blooming |
| Difficult to distinguish from small capillary telangiectasias |

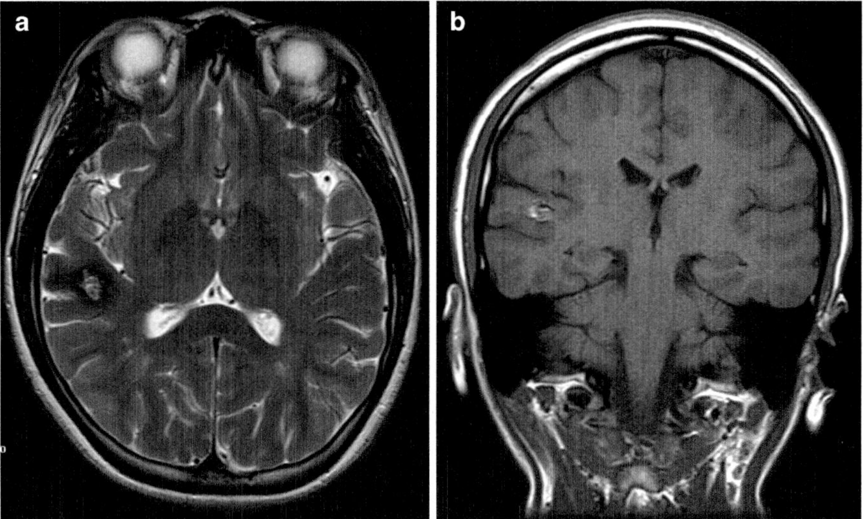

**Fig. 2.3** (**a**) T2 weighted image: A mixed signal intensity lesion is seen centrally in the right superior temporal gyrus. (**b**) T1 weighted image: a classic "popcorn" lesion is seen

According to Zabramski classification, Type I lesions are characterized by hyperintensity on both T1- and T2-weighted images (depending on the state of methemoglobin) which is consistent with subacute hemorrhage. Type II malformations, loculated regions of hemorrhage are surrounded by gliosis and hemosiderin-stained brain parenchyma (Fig. 2.3).

Type III lesions demonstrate a core that is iso- or hypointense on T1-weighted sequences and hypointense on T2-weighted sequences as well as a rim that is hypointense on T2-weighted sequences, compatible with chronic resolved hemorrhage or hemosiderin within and surrounding the lesion. Pathologically, Type 4 lesions may represent capillary telangiectasias or early stage CCMs seen frequently in the familial form.

**Angiography** The internal channel of CCM consists of numerous caverns. The mean transit time of the blood flow through the internal channels is so slow that the cerebral angiography does not show the opacification of the CCM itself even with the superselective angiography. Therefore, CCMs are angiographically occult and do not demonstrate any arteriovenous shunting. However, CCMs are often concurrent with DVAs, therefore the appearance of DVAs can be a clue to suggest the existing of CCM [11–13, 15, 22].

## 2.6 Differential Diagnosis

The differential, when cavernous venous malformations are numerous, is that of other causes of cerebral microhemorrhages, including Parry-Romberg syndrome [23–25]:

- Cerebral amyloid angiopathy: usually numerous small foci
- Chronic hypertensive encephalopathy: more common in the basal ganglia
- Diffuse axonal injury (DAI)
- Cerebral vasculitis
- Radiation-induced vasculopathy
- Hemorrhagic metastases
- Parry-Romberg syndrome

  Larger lesions can mimic:

- Hemorrhagic cerebral metastases
- Hemorrhagic primary brain tumors (e.g. ependymoma, glioblastoma)

  Calcified lesions, such as old neurocysticercosis, or other infections (e.g. tuberculoma) should also be considered [26].

## 2.7 Summary

The pathogenesis of CCMs remains to date unknown. Especially the familial form of CCMs is a dynamic disease. Therefore, patients with familial CCMs require careful follow-up monitoring with serial MRI. If DVAs would be observed on the MRI or the other modality of imaging, coexisting CCMs should be considered. Molecular targeted therapy or further specific pharmacological strategies are required for preventing the de novo formation of CCM lesions and counteracting disease progression and severity in susceptible individuals, including CCM gene mutation carriers. If some established experimental model of the system would show the role of endothelial cells and associated molecular biology, the pathomechanism of CCMs will be clarified near future.

**Conflict of interest**  Authors declare no conflict of interest.

# References


1. Wassef M, Blei F, Adams D, et al. Vascular anomalies classification: recommendations from the International Society for the Study of Vascular Anomalies. Pediatrics. 2015;136:e203–14.
2. Boukobza M, Enjolras O, Guichard JP, Gelbert F, Herbreteau D, Reizine D, Merland JJ. Cerebral developmental venous anomalies associated with head and neck venous malformations. AJNR Am J Neuroradiol. 1996;17:987–94.
3. Fischer A, Zalvide J, Faurobert E, Albiges-Rizo C, Tournier-Lasserve E. Cerebral cavernous malformations: from CCM genes to endothelial cell homeostasis. Trends Mol Med. 2013;19:302–8.
4. Haasdijk RA, Cheng C, Maat-Kievit AJ, Duckers HJ. Cerebral cavernous malformations: from molecular pathogenesis to genetic counselling and clinical management. Eur J Hum Genet. 2012;20:134–40.
5. Calonje E, Fletcher CD. Sinusoidal hemangioma. A distinctive benign vascular neoplasm within the group of cavernous hemangiomas. Am J Surg Pathol. 1991;15:1130–5.
6. Li X, Fisher OS, Boggon TJ. The cerebral cavernous malformations proteins. Oncotarget. 2015;6:32279–80.
7. Zhao Y, Tan Y-Z, Zhou L-F, Wang H-J, Mao Y. Morphological observation and in vitro angiogenesis assay of endothelial cells isolated from human cerebral cavernous malformations. Stroke. 2007;38:1313–9.
8. Marchi S, Corricelli M, Trapani E, et al. Defective autophagy is a key feature of cerebral cavernous malformations. EMBO Mol Med. 2015;7:1403–17.
9. Revencu N, Vikkula M. Cerebral cavernous malformation: new molecular and clinical insights. J Med Genet. 2006;43:716–21.
10. Clatterbuck RE, Eberhart CG, Crain BJ, Rigamonti D. Ultrastructural and immunocytochemical evidence that an incompetent blood-brain barrier is related to the pathophysiology of cavernous malformations. J Neurol Neurosurg Psychiatry. 2001;71:188–92.
11. Zhang P, Liu L, Cao Y, Wang S, Zhao J. Cerebellar cavernous malformations with and without associated developmental venous anomalies. BMC Neurol. 2013;13:134.
12. Hong YJ, Chung T-S, Suh SH, Park CH, Tomar G, Seo KD, Kim KS, Park IK. The angioarchitectural factors of the cerebral developmental venous anomaly; can they be the causes of concurrent sporadic cavernous malformation? Neuroradiology. 2010;52:883–91.
13. Pereira VM, Geibprasert S, Krings T, Aurboonyawat T, Ozanne A, Toulgoat F, Pongpech S, Lasjaunias PL. Pathomechanisms of symptomatic developmental venous anomalies. Stroke. 2008;39:3201–15.
14. Abdulrauf SI, Kaynar MY, Awad IA. A comparison of the clinical profile of cavernous malformations with and without associated venous malformations. Neurosurgery. 1999; 44:41–6. discussion 46-7.
15. Gökçe E, Acu B, Beyhan M, Celikyay F, Celikyay R. Magnetic resonance imaging findings of developmental venous anomalies. Clin Neuroradiol. 2014;24:135–43.
16. Gross BA, Du R. The natural history of cerebral dural arteriovenous fistulae. Neurosurgery. 2012;71:594–602.

17. Moran NF, Fish DR, Kitchen N, Shorvon S, Kendall BE, Stevens JM. Supratentorial cavernous haemangiomas and epilepsy: a review of the literature and case series. J Neurol Neurosurg Psychiatry. 1999;66:561–8.
18. Gross BA, Lin N, Du R, Day AL. The natural history of intracranial cavernous malformations. Neurosurg Focus. 2011;30:E24.
19. Hagiwara N, Yahikozawa H. Multiple cavernous haemangioma showing marked calcification on cranial radiography. J Neurol Neurosurg Psychiatry. 2002;72:410.
20. Campbell PG, Jabbour P, Yadla S, Awad IA. Emerging clinical imaging techniques for cerebral cavernous malformations: a systematic review. Neurosurg Focus. 2010;29:E6.
21. Zabramski JM, Wascher TM, Spetzler RF, Johnson B, Golfinos J, Drayer BP, Brown B, Rigamonti D, Brown G. The natural history of familial cavernous malformations: results of an ongoing study. J Neurosurg. 1994;80:422–32.
22. Dammann P, Wrede KH, Maderwald S, et al. The venous angioarchitecture of sporadic cerebral cavernous malformations: a susceptibility weighted imaging study at 7 T MRI. J Neurol Neurosurg Psychiatry. 2013;84:194–200.
23. Wong M, Phillips CD, Hagiwara M, Shatzkes DR. Parry Romberg syndrome: 7 cases and literature review. AJNR Am J Neuroradiol. 2015;36:1355–61.
24. Mespreuve M, Vanhoenacker F, Lemmerling M. Familial multiple cavernous malformation syndrome: MR features in this uncommon but silent threat. J Belg Soc Radiol. 2016;100:1–12.
25. Jain R, Robertson PL, Gandhi D, Gujar SK, Muraszko KM, Gebarski S. Radiation-induced cavernomas of the brain. AJNR Am J Neuroradiol. 2005;26:1158–62.
26. Gasparetto EL, Alves-Leon S, Domingues FS, Frossard JT, Lopes SP, de Souza JM. Neurocysticercosis, familial cerebral cavernomas and intracranial calcifications: differential diagnosis for adequate management. Arq Neuropsiquiatr. 2016;74:495–500.

# Chapter 3
# Molecular Biology of CCM

Arnošt Mládek, Petr Skalický, Vladimír Beneš, and Ondřej Bradáč

## 3.1   Introduction

Cerebral cavernous malformations (CCMs, OMIM: 116860), also known as cavernous angiomas or cavernomas, are common vascular malformations that consist of clusters of irregular and enlarged endothelial channels forming a densely packed sinusoids embedded in a collagen matrix with little or no intervening brain parenchyma [1–3]. Due to the lack of the elastic fibers and smooth muscle the lesions are characterized by thin and leaky vessel walls, intact basal lamina and absence of a sub-endothelial support. Further investigation of CCM neurovasculature ultrastructural features using transmission and scanning electron microscopy revealed a decreased number and damaged architecture of pericytes as well as frequent ruptures in the luminal endothelium [4]. CCMs belong to the slow-flow anomalies and are normally found in the venous-capillary vascular bed. The capillary channels, arranged in a back-to-back pattern and lined by rare sub-endothelial cells and thin endothelium may be filled with blood at various stages of thrombosis creating a mulberry- or raspberry-like cluster. Cavernous malformations can occur anywhere in the body, but usually produce serious signs and symptoms only in the brain and spinal cord.

The exact prevalence of CCMs is unknown because many patients are asymptomatic. Autopsy studies estimate the prevalence of CCM to be between 0.2% and 0.5% of the population and account for 5%–15% of all vascular malformations [1, 2, 5–9]. However, autopsy studies may suffer from sampling limitations, referral and selection bias, and limited or no clinical information. In addition to this, there may be significant differences in inter-observer variation depending on the level of scrutiny for particular lesions between pathologists [5]. CCMs are predominantly

A. Mládek · P. Skalický · V. Beneš · O. Bradáč (✉)
Department of Neurosurgery and Neurooncology, First Medical Faculty, Military University Hospital and Charles University, Prague, Czech Republic
e-mail: ondrej.bradac@uvn.cz

© Springer Nature Switzerland AG 2020
O. Bradáč, V. Beneš (eds.), *Cavernomas of the CNS*,
https://doi.org/10.1007/978-3-030-49406-3_3

found in the central nervous system (CNS; brain, retina, spinal cord) vasculature where they elevate the risk of seizures, strokes and neurological focal deficits [1, 2, 10]. Approximately 25% of individuals with CCM never experience any related health problems. CCM may occur sporadically, but most of the time it has an autosomal dominant inheritance pattern with variable expression and incomplete penetrance [11–15].

## 3.2 Identification of Genetic Loci: CCM Genes

### 3.2.1 *CCM1/KRIT1 Gene*

The first and unsuccessful attempt at mapping of the CCM genes was carried out in 1982 using serological and biochemical markers [16]. Twelve years later a study using short tandem repeat polymorphism and linkage analysis has shown that the respective gene causing familial cavernoma lies on the long arm of chromosome 7 in the q11-q12 region [17]. At the same time a gene for this disorder had been mapped in two families [18], one of Italian-American origin and one of Mexican-American origin, to markers on proximal 7q. Haplotype analysis of these families placed the locus harboring the gene of interest between markers D7S502 proximally and D7S515 distally, an interval of approximately 41 cM. After 1 year the group of Rich reported a large white kindred with familial CCM and confirmed the mapping to q11-q22 on chromosome 7 [19]. Using recombination between several markers it has been suggested that the candidate CCM region is distal to D7S804, and in combination with the previously published date, the results clearly indicated that the gene is likely to reside within a 15 cM region bounded by markers D7S660 and D7S558/D7S1789. Günel at el [20] applied a general multipoint linkage approach in two extended cavernous malformation kindreds, identified a linkage of the CCM disease and chromosome 7q11.2-q21 (locus D7S669) and further bracketed the interval to 7 cM region. Owing to the rapid development of molecular biology techniques, the prospective DNA region of the human chromosome 7 q21-q22 containing the CCM1 gene was further refined down to a 4 cM fragment, approximately 2 Mb long. The critical region was likely contained within this fragment and bounded by D7S698 and D7S2410 loci [2, 21–24]. Of note is the fact that the 21–22 locus of chromosome's 7 long arm is often amplified or even deleted in many malignant tumors [25, 26]. Finally Sahoo et al. [27] applied a genomic sequence-based positional cloning strategy and determined the disease KRIT1 or CCM1 gene—a sequence encoding a protein interacting with the Rap1A/Krev1 tumor suppressor and a member of the RAS family GTPases, which plays a key role in angiogenesis and cerebrovascular disease transduction pathways. Further verification was delivered by Couteulx et al. [28] who reported a physical and transcriptional map of the D7S2410-D7S689 interval showing that the CCM1 gene whose product, KRIT1/CCM1 protein, interacts with Rap1A GTPase, is mutated in CCM1 families [2, 28].

In 2001 Eerola et al. [29] proposed that the overall genomic structure of the human CCM1 gene comprises 20 exons spanning 3343 base pairs and suggested that these exons are likely to contain mutations in the families in which no CCM1 mutation had been identified, yet CCM1 linkage had been established. In line with those findings other groups have also reported the CCM1 gene to contain 20 coding segments [30–32].

**CCM1 Mutation Analyses**  Over 100 CCM1 gene mutations have been identified so far in families with CCM. Virtually all of the identified mutations induce premature stop signal in the transcription. This results in loss of function via generation of unstable mRNA, or truncated KRIT1 protein, partially or completely devoid of the putative Rap1A-interaction domain. At the onset of mutation analyses studies seven different germline mutations have been discovered: two single base transitions (splice site mutations), two single base transversions, two single base deletions leading to a frameshift, and one transition leading to a nonsense codon and premature termination [2]. As a result, RhoA-GTPase signaling is turned on abnormally, weakening cellular junctions and increasing the permeability of blood vessel walls. In 2001, ten new CCM1 gene mutations were identified by screening 29 families and 5 seemingly sporadic cases of CCM. The mutations predicted truncation of the KRIT1 mRNA encoded by CCM1, supporting the contention that CCM result from loss of KRIT1 protein function and the possibility that this protein acts as a tumor suppressor [33]. Subsequent genomic mapping analyses [30, 34] reported point mutations in various CCM1 regions each of which leads to diverse protein products. Verlaan et al. [34] discovered two point mutations in CCM1 leading to changes in amino acids (D137G and Q210E) both of which activate cryptic splice-donor sites, causing aberrant splicing and leading to a frameshift and protein truncation. Cavé-Riant et al. [30] screened CCM1 gene in 121 consecutively recruited and unrelated CCM probands having at least one affected relative and/or showing multiple lesions on cerebral MRI. Approximately 43% of the probands were shown to harbor a CCM1 mutation, 52 distinct mutations were identified including six recurrent ones. Nearly 75% of these mutations, which are predicted to lead to a premature stop codon, were located in the C-terminal region, mostly within exons 13, 15 and 17 [30]. Further progress in understanding CCM molecular biology has been enabled by Multiplex Ligation-dependent Probe Amplification (MLPA) method. This recently developed technique is designed to detect variations in the copy number of studied human genes. Due to this ability, MLPA can be applied in the molecular diagnosis of genetic diseases whose pathogenesis is related to the presence of deletions or duplications of specific genes [35, 36]. MLPA analyses done by Gaetzner et al. [37] detected a massive deletion involving the entire CCM1 coding region in the proband and were first to report a CCM1 gene deletion. Moreover MLPA data, corroborated by analyses of single nucleotide polymorphisms within the CCM1 gene, confirmed a loss-of-function mutation mechanism and demonstrated that MLPA has the clear potential to improve CCM mutation detection rate, which is crucial for predictive testing of at-risk relatives [37]. The large CCM1 deletions revealed by MLPA have been confirmed by examination of Italian and American cohorts [38–40]. The authors suggested [40] that there are elements within the CCM genes that predispose them to large deletion/duplication events but that the common deletion spanning respective CCM exons appears to be specific to the US population due to a founder effect.

Davenport et al. [33] provided evidence that the high frequency of KRIT1 loss-of-function mutations in CCM1 leading to an mRNA decay of the mutated allele was compatible with previous suggestions made by Sahoo et al. [27] and Laberge-le Couteulx [28] that the CCM1 gene function similarly to a tumor suppressor where somatic mutations leading to loss of the balancing wild-type allele predispose to loss of formation of a tumor and growth control. As a result and along with the fact that the presence of a solitary CCM lesion in most of the sporadic cases, but multiple CCM lesions in the majority of inherited forms has led to the assumption that biallelic mutations of the same gene are prerequisite for CCMs formation [12, 13, 41]. The so-called two-hit Knudsen [42] mechanism, which might explain CCM formation has been backed up by the observation that slowly enlarging CCMs may evolve as late sequelae of cranial radiation therapy within fields of prior irradiation [41, 43]. Other studies claiming the biallelic nature of the CCM1 germline mutations also support the two-hit model mechanism [2, 41, 44].

### 3.2.2 CCM2/MGC4607 and CCM3/PDCD10 Genes

Identification, localization and mutation assessment of the CCM1 gene has led to an undeniable progress in the understanding of the Mendelian model of CCM as an autosomal dominant trait with incomplete penetrance. CCM lesions of virtually all examined Italian- and Mexican-Americans could be associated with any of the founder CCM1 mutations. Yet, genetic screening of some non-Hispanic families harboring familial CCM without linkage to CCM1 indicated that there might be at least one additional CCM locus involved [2, 45]. In order to locate additional CCM loci Craig et al. [45] conducted a genome-wide linkage search, genotyping in total over 300 highly polymorphic marker loci scattered across all 22 autosomes in seven non-Hispanic families without linkage to the CCM1 locus. The data from all seven families combined showed that CCM transmission cannot be explained by linkage to one particular locus, suggesting that at least mutations in two separate loci may rationalize CCM transmission among these families. The evaluation of three separate non-Hispanic kindreds yielded the following linkages: (i) in one family to a segment on chromosome 7 short arm (7p, labeled as CCM2), and (ii) in the remaining two families to a small interval on chromosome 3 long arm (3q, labeled as CCM3). The LOD score of the subsequent multilocus linkage analysis of the three-locus model was 14.11 with 40% of families linked to CCM1 on 7q, 20% to CCM2 on 7p and 40% to CCM3 on 3q. The significance of linkage to these two additional loci was determined by comparison with the LOD score of the null hypothesis assuming linkage to only CCM1 with locus heterogeneity. The three-locus model was supported with an odds ratio of $1.6 \cdot 10^9 : 1$ over the single-locus model, providing clear evidence of CCM linkage to more than one locus [45]. The inferior LOD score of a four-locus model ruling out a prospective fourth CCM locus [45] led to a broadly recognized assumption that CCM is attributable to mutations in either of the three CCM1-3 loci.

Craig et al. [45] assigned the CCM2 gene locus to chromosome 7p15-p13 region bounded by D7S2846-D7S1818 markers. Five years later Liquori et al. [46] sequenced positional candidate genes in the 7p domain for mutations in CCM2. Eight potential genes out of a total 55 spanning the 11 cM region were determined for further consideration. One of these genes tagged as MGC4607, was selected as its translation product protein encodes a putative phosphotyrosine-binding (PTB) domain. PTB was predicted to interact with KRIT1 since the same domain is found in ICAP-1α, a binding partner of the CCM1 gene. In a panel of 27 probands without CCM linked to a CCM1 mutation, Liquori et al. [46] recognized eight different CCM2 gene mutations. These findings regarding CCM2 were supported and extended by Denier et al. [47] who identified the MGC4607 or the CCM2 gene as a new player in vessel development and/or maturation. An in-depth genetic linkage analysis was used to reduce the previously reported size of the CCM2 interval from 22 cM down to 7.5 cM. Denier et al. [47] proposed that large deletions involving at least exon 1, all resulting in loss of function, might be associated with the CCM disorder as reported in other hamartomatous conditions, such as neurofibromatosis or tuberous sclerosis [2, 47]. In 2007 Liquori et al. [38] noted an apparent discrepancy in the reported 45 relative frequencies of mutations in the three CCM genes between the values obtained by DNA sequence-analysis screens and the values originally predicted by Craig et al. [45] using linkage in families. DNA sequence analysis 38 of the known CCM genes in a cohort of 63 CCM-affected families revealed that 40% of these lacked any identifiable mutation. MLPA assay, exploited to screen 25 CCM1-3 mutation–negative probands for potential duplications or deletions within all three CCM genes, identified a total of 15 deletions: 1 in the CCM1 gene, 0 in the CCM3 gene, and 14 in the CCM2 gene yielding the following disease-gene frequencies: 40% for CCM1, 38% for CCM2, 6% for CCM3, and 16% with no mutation detected [38]. The calculated frequencies demonstrate that the prevalence of the CCM2 form is actually close to that of the CCM1 form and significantly exceeds what had been previously expected. Moreover, the data indicate that large genomic deletions in the CCM2 gene represent a major component of the CCM disease. Liquori et al. [38] hypothesized that these intragenic deletions are likely catalyzed by a hypermutable as a result of surrounding repetitive sequence elements.

The third CCM locus labeled as CCM3 was identified on the long arm of chromosome 3 (3q25.2-27) within a 22 cM interval bounded by D3S1763 and D3S1262 [45]. Bergametti et al. [48] have performed a high-density microsatellite genotyping of the respective 22 cM interval to search for putative null alleles, as identified in CCM2 [47], in 20 potentially informative families suffering from the familial form of CCM but lacking any known mutations within the CCM1 and CCM2 loci. A de novo deletion within a 4 Mb interval flanked by markers D3S3668 and D3S1614 and encompassing D3S1763, the centromeric boundary of the CCM3 interval, has been identified in one subject. This finding suggests that the CCM3 gene lies within a 970 kb interval bracketed by D3S1763 and D3S1614. Deleterious mutations within the programmed cell death 10 gene (PDCD10) have been identified in seven unrelated families. It should be noted that PDCD10 is one of the five known genes that have been mapped to this interval (FLJ33620, GOLPH4, LOC389174, PDCD10, SERPINI1) [48]. Experimental data from Bergametti et al. [48] suggest that PDCD10, a gene that is highly conserved in both invertebrates and vertebrates, is a likely candidate due to its putative role in the vessel maturation, development and apoptosis. The frequency of CCM3 mutations has been reported to be rather low in extensive studies assessing kindreds who lack CCM1 and CCM2 mutations. This is in contrast with an expected frequency of nearly 40% in inherited cases [2, 38, 39, 48, 49]. Moreover the frequency of affected members per family is higher in CCM1 and CCM2 families as compared to families harboring CCM3 [2, 49].

## 3.3   CCM Proteins

Hereditary CCM is known to be associated with a heterozygous germ-line loss-of-function mutation in any of the three CCM genes and the malformation development seems to be operative in the case of a local second hit knocking out the remaining wild-type copy of the respective CCM gene [1, 2, 41, 50–52]. There are, however, a number of other factors in the neurovasculature microenvironment which are potentially involved in lesion formation [1, 51, 53]. The fact that CCMs are related to loss-of-function mutations in whichever CCM gene and that all the CCM proteins can be found in the same complex within a cell indicates that there is a joint fundamental pathway involving all the respective CCM gene products [52]. In recent years we have witnessed advances in determining CCM protein structures at the atomic level and conformational behavior, in identifying protein-protein interaction patterns and in studying CCM-knockout animals. Yet, insight into the molecular mechanisms through which the loss of function of each of these proteins leads to CCM formation remains limited. In the following paragraphs a brief overview of the CCM proteins structure, functions and interactions is provided.

### 3.3.1   *The KRIT1/CCM1 Protein*

KRIT1 or CCM1 consisting of 736 amino acids is the largest of the three CCM proteins and the most common CCM gene mutated [54, 55]. From N-terminal to C-terminal direction, KRIT1 protein contains a NUDIX domain followed by a stretch of three intrinsically disordered NPxY/F motifs, an ankyrin repeat domain (ARD), and a C-terminal FERM domain including F1-F3 subdomains (Fig. 3.1) [56–58]. The conformational organization of KRIT1 seems to be correlated with its subcellular localization.

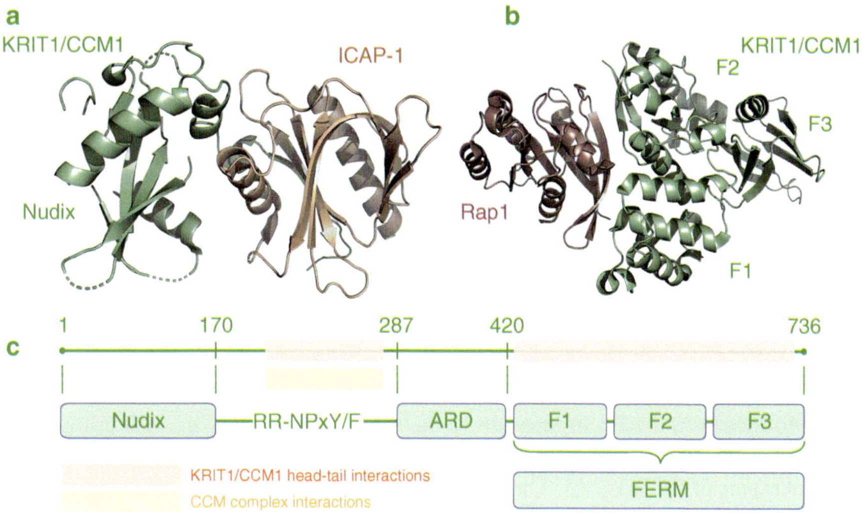



**Fig. 3.1** (**a**) Overall structure of KRIT1/CCM1 in complex with ICAP-1. ICAP-1 is shown in orange and KRIT1/CCM1 in green. Dashed lines indicate unstructured loops. PDB ID: 4DX8 [56]. (**b**) Ribbon diagram showing the crystal structure of KRIT1/CCM1 in complex with Rap1. KRIT1/CCM1 is shown in green and Rap1 in purple. PDB ID: 4HDQ [57]. (**c**) Domain schematic of KRIT1/CCM1 containing an N-terminal Nudix domain (1–170) followed by the bidentate ICAP-1-binding region; sites RR and NPxY. In the C-terminal direction to this there are two intrinsically disordered NPxF motifs (to 287), an ankyrin repeat domain (ARD, 288–420) and a FERM domain (421–736) that includes F1, F2, and F3 subdomains. KRIT1/CCM1 head-tail interaction region is highlighted by transparent pink boxes, CCM complex interaction domain in the orange box [1]

The NUDIX domain (residues 1–170) is found in the N-terminus of KRIT1 and is composed of a stretch of a polybasic sequence of residues that potentially interact with cellular microtubules, the mode of interaction is not yet well understood [1, 59]. NUDIX domains are usually embedded in hydrolase enzymes which bind to a variety of substrates. The NUDIX fold in KRIT1 is a centrally positioned β-sheet with flanking α-helices [60]. Despite various similarities, superposition of the X-ray crystal structure of the NUDIX domain with known substrates revealed no potential binding partners and thus the function of the NUDIX domain remains unclear [56]. A sequence analysis has revealed the presence of several known sequences such as potential tubulin binding sequence [59] and a nuclear localization sequence (NLS) [61] within the NUDIX domain.

The following three NPxY/F motifs (NPAY: residues 192–195; NPLF: residues 231–234, and NPYF: residues 250–253) in the central part of KRIT1 provide important interactions with phosphotyrosine binding (PTB), PH, as well as FERM domains. The first motif, which is the only one that can be phosphorylated, has a remarkably strong binding affinity to ICAP-1 [32, 62]. The second and the third NPcY motif can only bind to DAB-like PTB domains, including CCM2 [60, 63]. The ankyrin repeat domain (ARD) (residues 288–420) in KRIT1 is formed by four subsequent ankyrin repeats. From a conformational viewpoint ARD packs onto the

N-terminal end of the FERM-embedded F1 subdomain with each repeat being identical and composed of two α-helices joined by a β-hairpin. The ankyrin repeats are stacked vertically forming an "L"-shaped fold. According to structural x-ray diffraction data ARD is tightly bound to the adjacent FERM domain via a highly conserved interaction, which is particularly mediated by the convex surfaces of two ankyrin repeats in ARD domain and the β2 strand and α2 helix in F1 subdomain. It should be noted that the CCM1 ankyrin domain is rather distinctive due to its inability to interact with β-tubulin. Even though CCM1 was claimed to be a protein with tubulin binding activity, both binding assays and structural studies give no evidence that ARD takes part in this particular interaction [60, 64, 65]. Heretofore no CCM1 ankyrin domain binding partners have been revealed [60].

The FERM domain (residues 420–736) in the C-terminus consists of three subdomains tagged as F1, F2, and F3. While the F1 subdomain folds into an ubiquitin-like conformation, the F2 subdomain folds into an acyl-Coenzyme A binding fold. There are a number of proteins which have been identified to interact with this particular part of CCM1 [66]. The last FERM subdomain labeled as F3 is known to interact with the stretch of the three NPxY motifs of KRIT1 [60, 63, 67, 68]. Through the FERM domain KRIT1 also localizes to intercellular junctions or endothelial cell boundaries [1, 69, 70].

KRIT1 is ubiquitously expressed in early embryogenesis with pronounced endothelial expression in large vessels [1, 71]. While KRIT1 is deemed to communicate via its binding partners, no intrinsic catalytic activity has been detected. Due to various intramolecular binding sites and head-to-tail interactions, e.g. between the FERM domain and NPxY/F motif [59, 67], the KRIT1 structural ensemble consists of 'open' and 'closed' conformations [68]. The conformational changes likely regulate KRIT1 localization, consistent with the observation that KRIT1 is found in various locations within a cell and can be shuttled between the nucleus and the cytoplasm [70]. The presumed 'open' and 'closed' KRIT1 conformation corresponds to the ICAP-1 and microtubule binding, respectively [1, 59, 67].

**KRIT1 Interaction with Rap1** KRIT1 was resolved to be a Rap1-binding protein utilizing its FERM domain by means of yeast two-hybrid (Fig. 3.1) [72]. Rap1 is a small GTPase securing various cellular functions such as integrin-mediated cell adhesion or maintaining cell-cell contacts [60, 73]. A crystallographic analysis [57, 60, 74] uncovered an interaction mode between FERM domain of KRIT1 and Rap1, which localizes KRIT1 to the periphery of the cell to facilitate signaling and stabilization of the cell-cell junctions. The Rap1-induced relocalization of KRIT1 is made possible by the inhibition of KRIT1-microtubule interaction [59]. It should be noted, however, that the exact mechanism of the molecular process controlling the subcellular KRIT1 localization has not been resolved. KRIT1 features a great affinity towards the activated form of Rap1, which is induced to adapt the respective conformation via various GTPase-activating proteins [75]. Additionally, KRIT1 interacts via its FERM domain with the heart of glass 1 (HEG1) membrane anchor protein, which is responsible for KRIT1 junction localization [1]. Several cardiovascular development defects have been identified to be linked with KRIT1 mutations leading to the inability to bind either HEG1 or Rap1 proteins [1, 58, 75].

**KRIT1 Interaction with ICAP-1** The release of KRIT1 from the plasma membrane is established through the bidentate interaction of the highly-conserved RR region and the first of the three NPxY motifs of KRIT1 with ICAP-1 (integrin cytoplasmatic domain associated protein-1), another essential KRIT1 binding partner. ICAP-1 is a serine/threonine-rich protein that binds to the cytoplasmic tail domains of $\beta$1 integrins in a highly specific manner, binding to a NPxY sequence motif on $\beta$1 integrins and negatively regulating their activation [1, 56, 76, 77]. The cytoplasmic domains of integrins are essential for cell adhesion, and the fact that phosphorylation of ICAP-1 occurs by interaction with the cell-matrix implies an important role of ICAP-1 during integrin-dependent cell adhesion [77]. The interaction of KRIT1 and ICAP-1 yields a molecular complex (Fig. 3.1), which is localized to the nucleus [60, 70]. Since ICAP-1 interacts with both the cytoplasmic domain of $\beta$1 integrin and KRIT1 protein using the same binding NPxY motif, integrin activation cannot be inhibited when ICAP-1 is bound to KRIT1. In endothelial cells ICAP-1 is likely stabilized by KRIT1 and hence KRIT1 loss leads to decreased ICAP-1 levels and as a result to decreased $\beta$1 integrin inhibition [1, 78].

**KRIT1 Involvement in Signaling Pathways** KRIT1 is known to be involved in several other cellular signal transduction pathways, for example in Notch and KLF4/KLF2 signaling pathways. While cells with increased KRIT1 activity feature overexpression of two essential players in Notch signaling: HEY1 and DLL4 proteins, the KRIT1 knocked-out cells show diminished Notch signaling [60, 79]. Notch signaling activates the phosphoinositol 3-kinase (PI3K)/AKT pathway and the phosphorylated AKT in turn suppresses ERK1/2 (extracellular signal-regulated kinases) by dephosphorylation. In line with this, KRIT1-deficient endothelial cells as well as CCM lesions display elevated levels of ERK1/2 phosphorylation [79]. Phosphorylation of AKT is critical in the expression of SOD2, a reactive oxygen species (ROS)-scavenging enzyme. SOD2 is known to be up-regulated as a response to the increase of ROS concentration through AKT activation. Therefore loss of KRIT1 leads to the elevation of the steady state ROS levels and thus oxidative damage in the cell [80–82]. Moreover KRIT1 is also an inducer of SOD2 through interaction with the long isoform of Nd1 (Nd1-L), an important actin cytoskeleton-stabilizing protein. KRIT1 thus plays a key role in various collateral pathways preventing cell death [1, 60, 83].

### 3.3.2 The CCM2/MGC4607/Malcaverin Protein

CCM2 (also named as MGC4607 or Malcaverin) scaffolding protein consists of 444 amino acids, making it the second largest of the three CCM proteins with no enzymatic activity (Fig. 3.2). At its N-terminus, CCM2 contains a predicted PTB

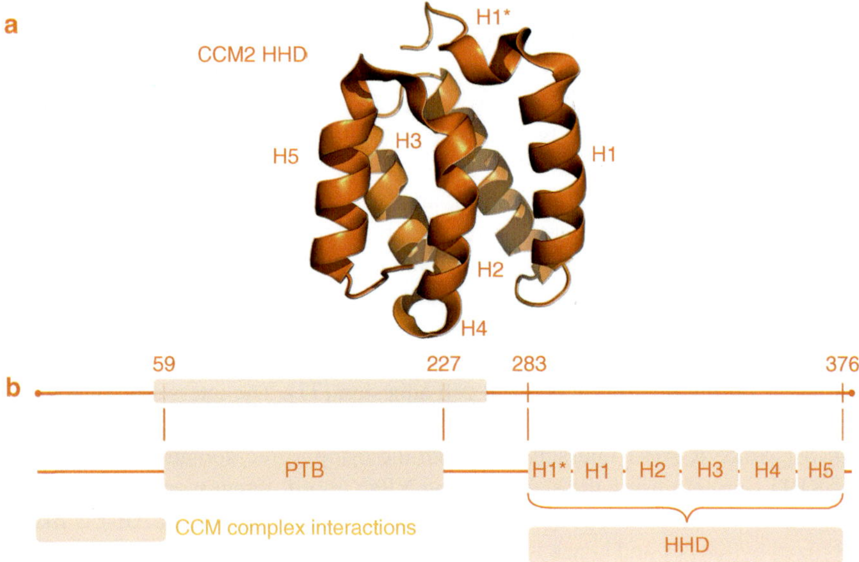



**Fig. 3.2** (**a**) Cartoon diagram of the CCM2 HH domain (HHD) with helices labeled. PDB ID: 4FQN [10]. (**b**) Domain schematic of CCM2 containing an N-terminal phosphotyrosine binding PTB domain (59–227) followed by a harmonin-homology (HH) domain (283–376) containing H1*, H1, H2, H3, H4, and H5 helices. The CCM complex interaction domain is highlighted in orange [1]

domain [46] and a helical harmonin homology (HH) domain [10]. It has been estimated that approximately 20% of all congenital CCM originate from CCM2 mutations [84, 85], however, the CCM2 mutation penetrance was reported to be as high as 100% [11, 60]. The expression pattern of CCM2 resembles that of KRIT1, including the arterial endothelial cells of various tissues [1, 86, 87]. Despite the lack of a signature nuclear localization (NLS) and export (NES) sequence, CCM2 is found throughout the cell and can shuttle between nucleus and cytoplasm due to its interaction with KRIT1 [88, 89]. CCM2 can be regarded as a scaffold of the CCM signaling complex as it simultaneously binds both KRIT1 and PDCD10 proteins along with other signaling peptides [1, 90]. It has been suggested that the localization of CCM2 to the endothelial cell-cell junctions is regulated through its in-membrane interaction with KRIT1. It has been shown that CCM2 mutant with altered PTB domain (CCM2-F217A) does not localize to cell-cell junctions as it is unable to bind to one of the KRIT1 NPxY/F motifs. Similar behavior was observed in the absence of functional KRIT1, in which case CCM2 did not localize to the cell junctions. The localization was recovered with the addition of wild-type KRIT1, rendering it a key factor for CCM2 localization [91].

The predicted PTB domain lies at the N-terminus of CCM2 and contains seven β strands arranged into two β-sheets and capping α-helices. Besides the aforementioned interaction with KRIT1 NPxY/F motif, PTB domain was speculated to bind membrane phospholipids, however no conclusive data have been put forward [10,

63, 92]. In 2009 Harel et al. [93] demonstrated that PTB domain also binds the juxtamembrane region of TrkA, a receptor tyrosine kinase crucial for differentiation and survival of nerve-growth-factor-dependent neurons, and mediates TrkA-induced death in neuroblastoma or medulloblastoma cells. Affinity proteomics experiments [94] have identified the germinal center kinase class III (GCKIII) serine/threonine kinases STK24 and STK25 as novel CCM2 interactors. Down-modulation of STK25 rescued medulloblastoma cells from NGF-induced TrkA-dependent cell death, suggesting that STK25 is part of the death-signaling pathway initiated by TrkA and CCM2 [94].

The HH domain at the CCM2 C-terminus (Fig. 3.2, residues 283-376) consists of six packed α-helices labeled as H1*, H1-H5 in the N- to C-terminal direction, is stabilized by number of intramolecular electrostatic and hydrophobic interactions and bears structural similarity to harmonin protein. The upstream H1* is a one turn-long α-helix, H4 is a $3_{10}$ helix containing 13 residues. Despite the structural correspondence HHD does not bind to PDCD10. There are two stable conformations of HH domain—monomeric and dimeric with the latter featuring higher propensity for dimerization [60, 66]. HH domain is also known to provide CCM2 the binding affinity for the mitogen-activated protein kinase (MAPK), MEKK3 [70, 95]. This is required for hyperosmolar-induced p38 MAPK activation, and upon osmotic shock a significant percentage of CCM2 relocalizes to membrane ruffles where CCM2 is thought to scaffold RAC1 and MEKK3 in the p38 MAPK cascade [1, 70, 95]. Zhou et al. [96] proposed that the response of the CCM2-RAC1 signaling pathway upon osmotic perturbation might proceed through phospholipase C (PLC)γ1, while Whitehead et al. [97] reported that CCM2 knock-out rather affects MAPK kinase and JNK instead of p38 MAPK pathway. It should be noted that the complexity of the MAPK signaling pathways significantly aggravates investigation of the CCM2 involvement, which is still not fully understood.

### 3.3.3  The CCM3/PDCD10 Protein

CCM3 (also named as programmed cell death 10 or PDCD10) is the smallest of the three CCM proteins and ubiquitously expressed. Under physiological conditions PDCD10 forms a homodimeric structure (Fig. 3.3). Each monomer unit is composed of 212 amino acid residues folded into a V-shaped conformation with two separate domains joined by a flexible hinge region [98]. Even though KRIT1 and CCM2 are predominantly found in vertebrates [98, 99], studies of *C. elegans* analogs have revealed PDCD10 to be the most evolutionary conserved of the CCM proteins [100, 101].

At its N-terminus PDCD10 contains a dimerization domain (residues 6–69) [98, 102], a short flexible linker (residues 71–84), and a focal adhesion targeting (FAT)-homology domain (residues 98–212) [98]. The dimerization domain is made up of four α-helices (αA-αD) which interlock with the corresponding dimerization domain of the opposite PDCD10 monomer [90, 103]. Through the dimerization

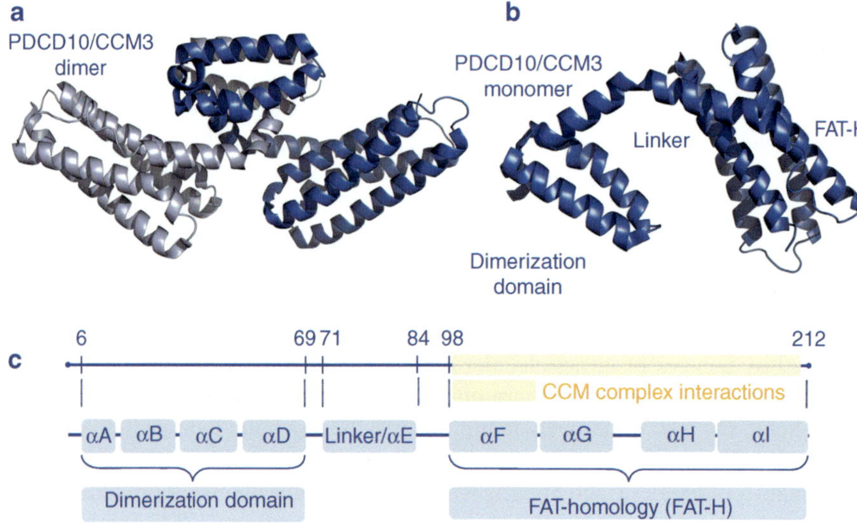



**Fig. 3.3** (**a**) Scheme representation of the PDCD10/CCM3 dimer [98]. (**b**) Backbone trace for three monomer domains: N-terminal dimerization domain composed of A, B, C, D α-helices, a linker domain composed of α-helix E followed by an EF loop, and a C-terminal focal adhesion targeting (FAT)-homology domain. (**c**) Domain schematic of PDCD10/CCM3 monomer. The CCM complex interaction domain is highlighted in orange [1]

domain CCM3 can also heterodimerize with GCKIII serine/threonine kinases (e.g. MST4/MASK, STK24/MST3, and STK25/YSK1/SOK1) [104] in a manner structurally resembling the CCM3 homodimerization with the linker domain-GCKIII interaction being the controling factor effectively shifting the equilibrium between PDCD10-PDCD10 homodimer and PDCD10-GCKIII heterodimer [60, 66, 105–107]. It has been shown [102] that the PDCD10-GCKIII supramolecular assembly localizes to the cis face of the Golgi complex due to a mutually exclusive GCKIII-GOLGA2 interaction. Fidalgo et al. [106] demonstrated that cells depleted of PDCD10 exhibit a Golgi apparatus disassembly. Furthermore, in wound-healing assays, PDCD10-depleted cells could not reposition the Golgi apparatus and centrosome properly and demonstrated impaired migration. Conversely, a significant rise in cell migration was reported in the case of overexpression of PDCP10 [105]. Note that the impaired cell migration prevents normal blood vessel formation and may lead to the vascular malformations [1]. Since PDCD10 was also reported to be involved in exocytosis [108], there might be a potential link between the loss of PDCD10 and defective tubular morphology observed in CCM lesions [1].

The C-terminus of PDCD10 harbors a FAT-homology domain commonly found in various tyrosine kinases like FAK or Pyk2. The FAT-homology domain is composed of a vertically aligned four-α-helical bundle (αF-αI) able to bind a large variety of proteins and compounds including CCM2 [90, 98, 103], phosphatidylinositol-3,4,5-trisphosphates (PtdIns(3,4,5)P3) [109], paxillin [110], striatin [102, 111], etc. Through the biding CCM2 via the FAT-homology domain,

PDCD10 is the third component in the heterotrimeric KRIT1-CCM2-PDCD10 structure, however its function within the CCM complex is still under study [90]. Even though PDCD10 is certainly involved in cell death, hence its name, its specific role remains to be determined as both the pro-survival and pro-apoptotic effects have been reported. The maintenance of the endothelial integrity, defective in CCM lesions, requires a proper cell death control in which PDCD10 plays a key role. He et al. [112] reported that mice with global or endothelial cell-specific deletion of PDCD10 exhibited defects in embryonic angiogenesis and died at an early embryonic stage due to the PDCD10 deletion-induced reduction of vascular endothelial growth factor receptor 2 (VEGFR2) signaling. It was shown that in response to VEGF stimulation, PDCD10 is recruited to and stabilizes VEGFR2 through its carboxyl-terminal domain, demonstrating that PDCD10 promotes VEGFR2 signaling during vascular development and cell survival [112, 113]. On the other hand PDCD10 expression has also been associated with apoptosis boosting, while PDCD10 knock-outs demonstrate increased cellular proliferation and survival, possibly through the enhanced VEGF or ERK activity or reduced Notch signaling [114–118].

## 3.4  Conclusions

Cerebral cavernous malformation is a major cerebrovascular disease with a distinctive appearance on magnetic resonance imaging. CCM affects approximately 0.3–0.5% of the population and is characterized by slow-flow vascular malformations, enlarged and leaky capillaries that predispose to seizures, focal neurological deficits, and fatal intracerebral hemorrhages. CCM is a genetic disease that may arise either sporadically or be inherited as an autosomal dominant condition with incomplete penetrance and variable expressivity. To date, causative germline loss-of-function mutations have been identified in three genes, KRIT1 (also known as CCM1), CCM2 (also known as MGC4607), and PDCD10 (also known as CCM3), which occur in both familial and sporadic forms. CCM genes encode for three interacting proteins involved in various cellular pathways contributing to correct angiogenesis, regulation of intercellular junctions, apoptosis, and response to stress. Even though the role of the three CCM genes in the formation of the intracranial vascular lesions has been known since the 1990s, additional studies have further elucidated the mechanisms at the molecular level, namely the exact mutations in the CCM genes and the interactions of the resultant aberrant proteins, leading to the formation of CCMs. CCM proteins interact with each other and form a trimeric complex, however, each component protein is capable of interacting on its own with a number of other signaling and cytoskeletal molecules, allowing for a diverse range of functions in cellular signaling pathways via unique protein-protein interactions. Despite significant progress in revealing the genetics and architecture of respective protein products, the complete molecular biology picture of CCM is far from being complete.

## 3.5 Key Points

- CCM can occur either sporadically or as a familial autosomal disorder caused by germline mutation with variable clinical and neuroradiological penetrance.
- Loss-of-functions mutations in the genes KRIT1, CCM2, and PDCD10 are known to result in the formation of cerebral cavernous malformations.
- CCM proteins can exist in a trimeric complex, the significance of which remains controversial. Each of these multi-domain proteins also interacts with a range of cytoskeletal, signaling and adaptor proteins.
- CCM proteins have many roles in a range of basic cellular processes including apoptosis, cell adhesion, migration, and polarity.

## References


1. Draheim KM, Fisher OS, Boggon TJ, Calderwood DA. Cerebral cavernous malformation proteins at a glance. J Cell Sci. 2014;127:701–7. https://doi.org/10.1242/jcs.138388.
2. Cavalcanti DD, Kalani MYS, Martirosyan NL, Eales J, Spetzler RF, Preul MC. Cerebral cavernous malformations: from genes to proteins to disease. J Neurosurg. 2012;116:122–32. https://doi.org/10.3171/2011.8.JNS101241.
3. Fischer A, Zalvide J, Faurobert E, Albiges-Rizo C, Tournier-Lasserve E. Cerebral cavernous malformations: from CCM genes to endothelial cell homeostasis. Trends Mol Med. 2013;19:302–8. https://doi.org/10.1016/j.molmed.2013.02.004.
4. Tanriover G, Sozen B, Seker A, Kilic T, Gunel M, Demir N. Ultrastructural analysis of vascular features in cerebral cavernous malformations. Clin Neurol Neurosurg. 2013;115:438–44. https://doi.org/10.1016/j.clineuro.2012.06.023.
5. Flemming KD, Graff-Radford J, Aakre J, Kantarci K, Lanzino G, Brown RD, Mielke MM, Roberts RO, Kremers W, Knopman DS, Petersen RC, Jack CR. Population-based prevalence of cerebral cavernous malformations in older adults: Mayo Clinic Study of Aging. JAMA Neurol. 2017;74:801–5. https://doi.org/10.1001/jamaneurol.2017.0439.
6. Rocco CD, Iannelli A, Tamburrini G. Cavernous angiomas of the brain stem in children. Pediatr Neurosurg. 1997;27:92–9. https://doi.org/10.1159/000121233.
7. Giombini S, Morello G. Cavernous angiomas of the brain. Account of fourteen personal cases and review of the literature. Acta Neurochir. 1978;40:61–82.
8. Lonjon M, Roche JL, George B, Mourier KL, Paquis P, Lot G, Grellier P. Intracranial cavernoma. 30 cases. Presse Med. 1993;22:990–4.
9. Moriarity N, Wetzel N, Clatterbuck N, Javedan N, Sheppard N, Hoenig-Rigamonti N, Crone N, Breiter N, Lee N, Rigamonti N. The natural history of cavernous malformations: a prospective study of 68 patients. Neurosurgery. 1999;44:1166–71.. discussion 1172–1173
10. Fisher OS, Zhang R, Li X, Murphy JW, Demeler B, Boggon TJ. Structural studies of cerebral cavernous malformations 2 (CCM2) reveal a folded helical domain at its C-terminus. FEBS Lett. 2013;587:272–7. https://doi.org/10.1016/j.febslet.2012.12.011.
11. Haasdijk RA, Cheng C, Maat-Kievit AJ, Duckers HJ. Cerebral cavernous malformations: from molecular pathogenesis to genetic counselling and clinical management. Eur J Hum Genet. 2012;20:134–40. https://doi.org/10.1038/ejhg.2011.155.
12. Labauge P, Denier C, Bergametti F, Tournier-Lasserve E. Genetics of cavernous angiomas. Lancet Neurol. 2007;6:237–44. https://doi.org/10.1016/S1474-4422(07)70053-4.
13. Revencu N, Vikkula M. Cerebral cavernous malformation: new molecular and clinical insights. J Med Genet. 2006;43:716–21. https://doi.org/10.1136/jmg.2006.041079.

14. Dashti SR, Hoffer A, Hu YC, Selman WR. Molecular genetics of familial cerebral cavernous malformations. Neurosurg Focus. 2006;21:e2.
15. Felbor U, Sure U, Grimm T, Bertalanffy H. Genetics of cerebral cavernous angioma. Zentralblatt Fur Neurochirurgie. 2006;67:110–6. https://doi.org/10.1055/s-2006-933537.
16. Dubovsky J, Zabramski JM, Kurth J, Spetzier RF, Rich SS, Orr HT, Weber JL. A gene responsible for cavernous malformations of the brain maps to chromosome 7q. Hum Mol Genet. 1995;4:453–8. https://doi.org/10.1093/hmg/4.3.453.
17. Kurth JH, Zabramski JM, Dubovsky J. Genetic linkage of the familial cavernous malformation (CM) gene to chromosome 7q. Am J Hum Genet. 1994;55:211–20.
18. Marchuk DA, Gallione CJ, Morrison LA, Clericuzio CL, Hart BL, Kosofsky BE, Louis DN, Gusella JF, Davis LE, Prenger VL. A locus for cerebral cavernous malformations maps to chromosome 7q in two families. Genomics. 1995;28:311–4.
19. Gil-Nagel A, Dubovsky J, Wilcox KJ, Stewart JM, Anderson VE, Leppik IE, Orr HT, Johnson EW, Weber JL, Rich SS. Familial cerebral cavernous angioma: a gene localized to a 15-cM interval on chromosome 7q. Ann Neurol. 1996;39:807–10. https://doi.org/10.1002/ana.410390619.
20. Gaijnel M, Awad IA, Anson J, Lifton RP. Mapping a gene causing cerebral cavernous malformation to 7q11.2-q21. Proc Natl Acad Sci U S A. 1995;92:6620–4.
21. Green ED, Green P. Sequence-tagged site (STS) content mapping of human chromosomes: theoretical considerations and early experiences. PCR Methods Appl. 1991;1:77–90.
22. Green ED, Braden VV, Fulton RS, Lim R, Ueltzen MS, Peluso DC, Mohr-Tidwell RM, Idol JR, Smith LM, Chumakov I. A human chromosome 7 yeast artificial chromosome (YAC) resource: construction, characterization, and screening. Genomics. 1995;25:170–83.
23. Johnson EW, Iyer LM, Rich SS, Orr HT, Gil-Nagel A, Kurth JH, Zabramski JM, Marchuk DA, Weissenbach J, Clericuzio CL, Davis LE, Hart BL, Gusella JF, Kosofsky BE, Louis DN, Morrison LA, Green ED, Weber JL. Refined localization of the cerebral cavernous malformation gene (CCM1) to a 4-cM interval of chromosome 7q contained in a well-defined YAC contig. Genome Res. 1995;5:368–80.
24. Bouffard GG, Idol JR, Braden VV, Iyer LM, Cunningham AF, Weintraub LA, Touchman JW, Mohr-Tidwell RM, Peluso DC, Fulton RS, Ueltzen MS, Weis-senbach J, Magness CL, Green ED. A physical map of human chromosome 7: an integrated YAC contig map with average STS spacing of 79 kb. Genome Res. 1997;7:673–92.
25. Kere J, Ruutu T, Davies KA, Roninson IB, Watkins PC, Winqvist R, de la Chapelle A. Chromosome 7 long arm deletion in myeloid disorders: a narrow breakpoint region in 7q22 defined by molecular mapping. Blood. 1989;73:230–4.
26. Nibert M, Heim S. Uterine leiomyoma cytogenetics. Genes Chromosom Cancer. 1990;2:3–13.
27. Sahoo T, Johnson EW, Thomas JW, Kuehl PM, Jones TL, Dokken CG, Touch-man JW, Gallione CJ, Lee-Lin SQ, Kosofsky B, Kurth JH, Louis DN, Mettler G, Morrison L, Gil-Nagel A, Rich SS, Zabramski JM, Boguski MS, Green ED, Marchuk DA. Mutations in the gene encoding KRIT1, a Krev-1/rap1a binding protein, cause cerebral cavernous malformations (CCM1). Hum Mol Genet. 1999;8:2325–33.
28. Laberge-le Couteulx S, Jung HH, Labauge P, Houtteville JP, Lescoat C, Cecillon M, Marechal E, Joutel A, Bach JF, Tournier-Lasserve E. Truncating mutations in CCM1, encoding KRIT1, cause hereditary cavernous angiomas. Nat Genet. 1999;23:189–93. https://doi.org/10.1038/13815.
29. Eerola I, McIntyre B, Vikkula M. Identification of eight novel 5′-exons in cerebral capillary malformation gene-1 (CCM1) encoding KRIT1. Biochim Biophys Acta. 2001;1517:464–7.
30. Cavai-Riant F, Denier C, Labauge P, Caicillon M, Maciazek J, Joutel A, Laberge-Le Couteulx S, Tournier-Lasserve E. Spectrum and expression analysis of KRIT1 mutations in 121 consecutive and unrelated patients with cerebral cavernous malformations. Eur J Hum Genet. 2002;10:733–40. https://doi.org/10.1038/sj.ejhg.5200870.
31. Sahoo T, Goenaga-Diaz E, Serebriiskii IG, Thomas JW, Kotova E, Cuellar JG, Peloquin JM, Golemis E, Beitinjaneh F, Green ED, Johnson EW, Marchuk DA. Computational and experimental analyses reveal previously undetected coding exons of the KRIT1 (CCM1) gene. Genomics. 2001;71:123–6. https://doi.org/10.1006/geno.2000.6426.

32. Zhang J, Clatterbuck RE, Rigamonti D, Chang DD, Dietz HC. Interaction between krit1 and icap1alpha infers perturbation of integrin beta1-mediated angiogenesis in the pathogenesis of cerebral cavernous malformation. Hum Mol Genet. 2001;10:2953–60.

33. Davenport WJ, Siegel AM, Dichgans J, Drigo P, Mammi I, Pereda P, Wood NW, Rouleau GA. CCM1 gene mutations in families segregating cerebral cavernous malformations. Neurology. 2001;56:540–3.

34. Verlaan DJ, Siegel AM, Rouleau GA. Krit1 missense mutations Lead to splicing errors in cerebral cavernous malformation. Am J Hum Genet. 2002;70:1564–7.

35. Stuppia L, Antonucci I, Palka G, Gatta V. Use of the MLPA assay in the molecular diagnosis of gene copy number alterations in human genetic diseases. Int J Mol Sci. 2012;13:3245–76. https://doi.org/10.3390/ijms13033245.

36. Schouten JP, McElgunn CJ, Waaijer R, Zwijnenburg D, Diepvens F, Pals G. Relative quantification of 40 nucleic acid sequences by multiplex ligation-dependent probe amplification. Nucleic Acids Res. 2002;30:e57.

37. Gaetzner S, Stahl S, Saijraijcaij O, Schaafhausen A, Halliger-Keller B, Bertalanffy H, Sure U, Felbor U. CCM1 gene deletion identified by MLPA in cerebral cavernous malformation. Neurosurg Rev. 2007;30:155–9. https://doi.org/10.1007/s10143-006-0057-1.. discussion 159–160

38. Liquori CL, Berg MJ, Squitieri F, Leedom TP, Ptacek L, Johnson EW, Marchuk DA. Deletions in CCM2 are a common cause of cerebral cavernous malformations. Am J Hum Genet. 2007;80:69–75. https://doi.org/10.1086/510439.

39. Liquori CL, Berg MJ, Squitieri F, Ottenbacher M, Sorlie M, Leedom TP, Cannella M, Maglione V, Ptacek L, Johnson EW, Marchuk DA. Low frequency of PDCD10 mutations in a panel of CCM3 probands: potential for a fourth CCM locus. Hum Mutat. 2006;27:118. https://doi.org/10.1002/humu.9389.

40. Liquori CL, Penco S, Gault J, Leedom TP, Tassi L, Esposito T, Awad IA, Frati L, Johnson EW, Squitieri F, Marchuk DA, Gianfrancesco F. Different spectra of genomic deletions within the CCM genes between Italian and American CCM patient cohorts. Neurogenetics. 2008;9:25–31. https://doi.org/10.1007/s10048-007-0109-x.

41. Pagenstecher A, Stahl S, Sure U, Felbor U. A two-hit mechanism causes cerebral cavernous malformations: complete inactivation of CCM1, CCM2 or CCM3 in affected endothelial cells. Hum Mol Genet. 2009;18:911–8. https://doi.org/10.1093/hmg/ddn420.

42. Knudson AG. Two genetic hits (more or less) to cancer. Nat Rev Cancer. 2001;1:157–62. https://doi.org/10.1038/35101031.

43. Strenger V, Sovinz P, Lackner H, Dornbusch HJ, Lingitz H, Eder HG, Moser A, Urban C. Intracerebral cavernous hemangioma after cranial irradiation in childhood. Incidence and risk factors. Strahlentherapie Und Onkologie: Organ Der Deutschen Rontgengesellschaft. 2008;184:276–80. https://doi.org/10.1007/s00066-008-1817-3.

44. Gault J, Shenkar R, Recksiek P, Awad IA. Biallelic somatic and germ line CCM1 trun-cating mutations in a cerebral cavernous malformation lesion. Stroke. 2005;36:872–4. https://doi.org/10.1161/01.STR.0000157586.20479.fd.

45. Craig HD, GÃijnel M, Cepeda O, Johnson EW, Ptacek L, Steinberg GK, Ogilvy CS, Berg MJ, Crawford SC, Scott RM, Steichen-Gersdorf E, Sabroe R, Kennedy CTC, Mettler G, Beis MJ, Fryer A, Awad IA, Lifton RP. Multilocus linkage identifies two new loci for a mendelian form of stroke, cerebral cavernous malformation, at 7p15âÃß13 and 3q25.2âÃβ27. Hum Mol Genet. 1998;7:1851–8. https://doi.org/10.1093/hmg/7.12.1851.

46. Liquori CL, Berg MJ, Siegel AM, Huang E, Zawistowski JS, Stoffer T, Verlaan D, Balogun F, Hughes L, Leedom TP, Plummer NW, Cannella M, Maglione V, Squitieri F, Johnson EW, Rouleau GA, Ptacek L, Marchuk DA. Mutations in a gene encoding a novel protein containing a phosphotyrosine-binding domain cause type 2 cerebral cavernous malformations. Am J Hum Genet. 2003;73:1459–64. https://doi.org/10.1086/380314.

47. Denier C, Goutagny S, Labauge P, Krivosic V, Arnoult M, Cousin A, Benabid A, Comoy J, Frerebeau P, Gilbert B, Houtteville J, Jan M, Lapierre F, Loiseau H, Menei P, Mercier P, Moreau J, Nivelon-Chevallier A, Parker F, Redondo A, Scara-bin J, Tremoulet M, Zerah M,

Maciazek J, Tournier-Lasserve E. Mutations within the MGC4607 gene cause cerebral cavernous malformations. Am J Hum Genet. 2004;74:326–37. https://doi.org/10.1086/381718.

48. Bergametti F, Denier C, Labauge P, Arnoult M, Boetto S, Clanet M, Coubes P, Echenne B, Ibrahim R, Irthum B, Jacquet G, Lonjon M, Moreau JJ, Neau JP, Parker F, Tremoulet M, Tournier-Lasserve E. SociÃĺtÃĺ FranÃğaise de Neurochirurgie, mutations within the programmed cell death 10 gene cause cerebral cavernous malformations. Am J Hum Genet. 2005;76:42–51. https://doi.org/10.1086/426952.

49. Denier C, Labauge P, Bergametti F, Marchelli F, Riant F, Arnoult M, Maciazek J, Vicaut E, Brunereau L, Tournier-Lasserve E. Sociatat Franangaise de Neurochirurgie, genotype-phenotype correlations in cerebral cavernous malformations patients. Ann Neurol. 2006;60:550–6. https://doi.org/10.1002/ana.20947.

50. Akers AL, Johnson E, Steinberg GK, Zabramski JM, Marchuk DA. Biallelic somatic and germline mutations in cerebral cavernous malformations (CCMs): evidence for a two-hit mechanism of CCM pathogenesis. Hum Mol Genet. 2009;18:919–30. https://doi.org/10.1093/hmg/ddn430.

51. Dammann P, Hehr U, Weidensee S, Zhu Y, Gerlach R, Sure U. Two-hit mechanism in cerebral cavernous malformation? A case of monozygotic twins with a CCM1/KRIT1 germline mutation. Neurosurg Rev. 2013;36:483–6. https://doi.org/10.1007/s10143-013-0456-z.

52. Stahl S, Gaetzner S, Voss K, Brackertz B, Schleider E, SÃijrÃijcÃij O, Kunze E, Netzer C, Korenke C, Finckh U, Habek M, Poljakovic Z, Elbracht M, Rudnik-SchÃűneborn S, Bertalanffy H, Sure U, Felbor U. Novel CCM1, CCM2, and CCM3 mutations in patients with cerebral cavernous malformations: in-frame deletion in CCM2 prevents formation of a CCM1/CCM2/CCM3 protein complex. Hum Mutat. 2008;29:709–17. https://doi.org/10.1002/humu.20712.

53. Boulday G, BlÃ́con A, Petit N, Chareyre F, Garcia LA, Niwa-Kawakita M, Giovan-nini M, Tournier-Lasserve E. Tissue-specific conditional CCM2 knockout mice establish the essential role of endothelial CCM2 in angiogenesis: implications for human cerebral cavernous malformations. Dis Model Mech. 2009;2:168–77. https://doi.org/10.1242/dmm.001263.

54. Zhang J, Clatterbuck RE, Rigamonti D, Dietz HC. Mutations in KRIT1 in familial cerebral cavernous malformations. Neurosurgery. 2000;46:1272–7;. discussion 1277–1279. https://doi.org/10.1097/00006123-200005000-00064.

55. Gunel M, Awad IA, Finberg K, Anson JA, Steinberg GK, Batjer HH, Kopitnik TA, Morrison L, Giannotta SL, Nelson-Williams C, Lifton RP. A founder mutation as a cause of cerebral cavernous malformation in Hispanic Americans. N Engl J Med. 1996;334:946–51. https://doi.org/10.1056/NEJM199604113341503.

56. Liu W, Draheim KM, Zhang R, Calderwood DA, Boggon TJ. Mechanism for KRIT1 release of ICAP1-mediated suppression of integrin activation. Mol Cell. 2013;49:719–29. https://doi.org/10.1016/j.molcel.2012.12.005.

57. Li X, Zhang R, Draheim KM, Liu W, Calderwood DA, Boggon TJ. Structural basis for small G protein effector interaction of Ras-related protein 1 (Rap1) and adaptor protein Krev interaction trapped 1 (KRIT1). J Biol Chem. 2012;287:22317–27. https://doi.org/10.1074/jbc.M112.361295.

58. Gingras AR, Liu JJ, Ginsberg MH. Structural basis of the junctional anchorage of the cerebral cavernous malformations complex. J Cell Biol. 2012;199:39–48. https://doi.org/10.1083/jcb.201205109.

59. Bairaud-Dufour S, Gautier R, Albiges-Rizo C, Chardin P, Faurobert E. Krit 1 interactions with microtubules and membranes are regulated by Rap1 and integrin cytoplasmic domain associated protein-1. FEBS J. 2007;274:5518–32. https://doi.org/10.1111/j.1742-4658.2007.06068.x.

60. Padarti A, Zhang J. Recent advances in cerebral cavernous malformation research. Vessel Plus. 2018;2:1–23. https://doi.org/10.20517/2574-1209.2018.34.

61. Zhang J, Clatterbuck RE, Rigamonti D, Dietz HC. Cloning of the murine Krit1 cDNA reveals novel mammalian 5′ coding exons. Genomics. 2000;70:392–5. https://doi.org/10.1006/geno.2000.6410.

62. Zhang J, Basu S, Rigamonti D, Dietz HC, Clatterbuck RE. Krit1 modulates beta 1-integrin-mediated endothelial cell proliferation. Neurosurgery. 2008;63:571–8;. discussion 578. https://doi.org/10.1227/01.NEU.0000325255.30268.B0.
63. Zhang J, Dubey P, Padarti A, Zhang A, Patel R, Patel V, Cistola D, Badr A. Novel functions of CCM1 delimit the relationship of PTB/PH domains. Biochim Biophys Acta, Proteins Proteomics. 2017;1865:1274–86. https://doi.org/10.1016/j.bbapap.2017.07.002.
64. Pecqueur L, Duellberg C, Dreier B, Jiang Q, Wang C, PlÃijckthun A, Surrey T, Gigant B, Knossow M. A designed ankyrin repeat protein selected to bind to tubulin caps the microtubule plus end. Proc Natl Acad Sci U S A. 2012;109:12011–6. https://doi.org/10.1073/pnas.1204129109.
65. Zhang R, Li X, Boggon TJ. Structural analysis of the KRIT1 ankyrin repeat and FERM domains reveals a conformationally stable ARD-FERM interface. J Struct Biol. 2015;192:449–56. https://doi.org/10.1016/j.jsb.2015.10.006.
66. Fisher OS, Boggon TJ. Signaling pathways and the cerebral cavernous malformations proteins: lessons from structural biology. Cell Mol Life Sci. 2014;71:1881–92. https://doi.org/10.1007/s00018-013-1532-9.
67. Francalanci F, Avolio M, De Luca E, Longo D, Menchise V, Guazzi P, SgrÃš F, Marino M, Goitre L, Balzac F, Trabalzini L, Retta SF. Structural and functional differences between KRIT1A and KRIT1B isoforms: a framework for understanding CCM pathogenesis. Exp Cell Res. 2009;315:285–303. https://doi.org/10.1016/j.yexcr.2008.10.006.
68. Faurobert E, Albiges-Rizo C. Recent insights into cerebral cavernous malformations: a complex jigsaw puzzle under construction. FEBS J. 2010;277:1084–96. https://doi.org/10.1111/j.1742-4658.2009.07537.x.
69. Glading A, Han J, Stockton RA, Ginsberg MH. KRIT-1/CCM1 is a Rap1 effector that regulates endothelial cellâĂßcell junctions. J Cell Biol. 2007;179:247–54. https://doi.org/10.1083/jcb.200705175.
70. Zawistowski JS, Stalheim L, Uhlik MT, Abell AN, Ancrile BB, Johnson GL, Marchuk DA. CCM1 and CCM2 protein interactions in cell signaling: implications for cerebral cavernous malformations pathogenesis. Hum Mol Genet. 2005;14:2521–31. https://doi.org/10.1093/hmg/ddi256.
71. Guzeloglu-Kayisli O, Amankulor NM, Voorhees J, Luleci G, Lifton RP, Gunel M. KRIT1/cerebral cavernous malformation 1 protein localizes to vascular endothelium, astrocytes, and pyramidal cells of the adult human cerebral cortex. Neurosurgery. 2004;54:943–9. https://doi.org/10.1227/01.NEU.0000114512.59624.A5.
72. Serebriiskii I, Estojak J, Sonoda G, Testa JR, Golemis EA. Association of Krev-1/Rap1a with Krit1, a novel ankyrin repeat-containing protein encoded by a gene mapping to 7q21-22. Oncogene. 1997;15:1043–9. https://doi.org/10.1038/sj.onc.1201268.
73. Frische EW, Zwartkruis FJT. Rap1, a mercenary among the Ras-like GTPases. Dev Biol. 2010;340:1–9. https://doi.org/10.1016/j.ydbio.2009.12.043.
74. Gingras AR, Puzon-McLaughlin W, Ginsberg MH. The structure of the ternary complex of Krev interaction trapped 1 (KRIT1) bound to both the Rap1 GTPase and the heart of glass (HEG1) cytoplasmic tail. J Biol Chem. 2013;288:23639–49. https://doi.org/10.1074/jbc.M113.462911.
75. Liu JJ, Stockton RA, Gingras AR, Ablooglu AJ, Han J, Bobkov AA, Ginsberg MH. A mechanism of Rap1-induced stabilization of endothelial cell–cell junctions. Mol Biol Cell. 2011;22:2509–19. https://doi.org/10.1091/mbc.E11-02-0157.
76. Millon-Fraumillon A, Bouvard D, Grichine A, Manet-DupÃľ S, Block MR, Albiges-Rizo C. Cell adaptive response to extracellular matrix density is controlled by ICAP-1âĂßdependent Îš1-integrin affinity. J Cell Biol. 2008;180:427–41. https://doi.org/10.1083/jcb.200707142.
77. Chang DD, Wong C, Smith H, Liu J. ICAP-1, a novel beta1 integrin cytoplasmic domain-associated protein, binds to a conserved and functionally important NPXY sequence motif of beta1 integrin. J Cell Biol. 1997;138:1149–57. https://doi.org/10.1083/jcb.138.5.1149.
78. Faurobert E, Rome C, Lisowska J, Manet-Dupai S, Boulday G, Malbouyres M, Bal-land M, Bouin A-P, KÃľramidas M, Bouvard D, Coll J-L, Ruggiero F, Tournier-Lasserve E, Albiges-Rizo C. CCM1âĂßICAP-1 complex controls Îš1 integrinâĂßdependent endothelial con-

tractility and fibronectin remodeling. J Cell Biol. 2013;202:545–61. https://doi.org/10.1083/jcb.201303044.

79. Wãijstehube J, Bartol A, Liebler SS, BrÃijtsch R, Zhu Y, Felbor U, Sure U, Au-gustin HG, Fischer A. Cerebral cavernous malformation protein CCM1 inhibits sprouting angiogenesis by activating DELTA-NOTCH signaling. Proc Natl Acad Sci U S A. 2010;107:12640–5. https://doi.org/10.1073/pnas.1000132107.

80. Liu H, Rigamonti D, Badr A, Zhang J. Ccm1 regulates microvascular morphogenesis during angiogenesis. J Vasc Res. 2011;48:130–40. https://doi.org/10.1159/000316851.

81. Liu H, Rigamonti D, Badr A, Zhang J. Ccm1 assures microvascular integrity during angiogenesis. Transl Stroke Res. 2010;1:146–53. https://doi.org/10.1007/s12975-010-0010-z.

82. Goitre L, Balzac F, Degani S, Degan P, Marchi S, Pinton P, Retta SF. KRIT1 regulates the homeostasis of intracellular reactive oxygen species. PLoS One. 2010;5:e11786. https://doi.org/10.1371/journal.pone.0011786.

83. Guazzi P, Goitre L, Ferro E, Cutano V, Martino C, Trabalzini L, Retta SF. Identification of the Kelch family protein Nd1-L as a novel molecular interactor of KRIT1. PLoS One. 2012;7:e44705. https://doi.org/10.1371/journal.pone.0044705.

84. Choquet H, Pawlikowska L, Lawton MT, Kim H. Genetics of cerebral cavernous mal-formations: current status and future prospects. J Neurosurg Sci. 2015;59:211–20.

85. Riant F, Bergametti F, Ayrignac X, Boulday G, Tournier-Lasserve E. Recent insights into cere-bral cavernous malformations: the molecular genetics of CCM. FEBS J. 2010;277:1070–5. https://doi.org/10.1111/j.1742-4658.2009.07535.x.

86. Petit N, Baicon A, Denier C, Tournier-Lasserve E. Patterns of expression of the three cerebral cavernous malformation (CCM) genes during embryonic and postnatal brain development. Gene Expr Patterns. 2006;6:495–503. https://doi.org/10.1016/j.modgep.2005.11.001.

87. Seker A, Pricola KL, Guclu B, Ozturk AK, Louvi A, Gunel M. CCM2 expression parallels that of CCM1. Stroke. 2006;37:518–23. https://doi.org/10.1161/01.STR.0000198835.49387.25.

88. Zhang J, Rigamonti D, Dietz HC, Clatterbuck RE. Interaction between krit1 and malcavernin: implications for the pathogenesis of cerebral cavernous malforma-tions. Neurosurgery. 2007;60:353–9;. discussion 359. https://doi.org/10.1227/01.NEU.0000249268.11074.83.

89. Zhang J, Carr C, Badr A. The cardiovascular triad of dysfunctional angiogenesis. Transl Stroke Res. 2011;2:339–45. https://doi.org/10.1007/s12975-011-0065-5.

90. Hilder TL, Malone MH, Bencharit S, Colicelli J, Haystead TA, Johnson GL, Wu CC. Proteomic identification of the cerebral cavernous malformation signaling complex. J Proteome Res. 2007;6:4343–55. https://doi.org/10.1021/pr0704276.

91. Stockton RA, Shenkar R, Awad IA, Ginsberg MH. Cerebral cavernous malformations pro-teins inhibit rho kinase to stabilize vascular integrity. J Exp Med. 2010;207:881–96. https://doi.org/10.1084/jem.20091258.

92. Uhlik MT, Temple B, Bencharit S, Kimple AJ, Siderovski DP, Johnson GL. Structural and evolutionary division of phosphotyrosine binding (PTB) domains. J Mol Biol. 2005;345:1–20. https://doi.org/10.1016/j.jmb.2004.10.038.

93. Harel L, Costa B, Tcherpakov M, Zapatka M, Oberthuer A, Hansford LM, Vojvodic M, Levy Z, Chen Z-Y, Lee FS, Avigad S, Yaniv I, Shi L, Eils R, Fischer M, Brors B, Kaplan DR, Fainzilber M. CCM2 mediates death signaling by the TrkA receptor tyrosine kinase. Neuron. 2009;63:585–91. https://doi.org/10.1016/j.neuron.2009.08.020.

94. Costa B, Kean MJ, Ast V, Knight JDR, Mett A, Levy Z, Ceccarelli DF, Badillo BG, Eils R, Kaunig R, Gingras A-C, Fainzilber M. STK25 protein mediates TrkA and CCM2 protein-dependent death in pediatric tumor cells of neural origin. J Biol Chem. 2012;287:29285–9. https://doi.org/10.1074/jbc.C112.345397.

95. Uhlik MT, Abell AN, Johnson NL, Sun W, Cuevas BD, Lobel-Rice KE, Horne EA, Dell'Acqua ML, Johnson GL. Rac–MEKK3–MKK3 scaffolding for p38 MAPK activation during hyper-osmotic shock. Nat Cell Biol. 2003;5:1104–10. https://doi.org/10.1038/ncb1071.

96. Zhou X, Izumi Y, Burg MB, Ferraris JD. Rac1/osmosensing scaffold for MEKK3 contributes via phospholipase C-δ1 to activation of the osmoprotective transcription factor NFAT5. Proc Natl Acad Sci. 2011;108:12155–60. https://doi.org/10.1073/pnas.1108107108.

97. Whitehead KJ, Chan AC, Navankasattusas S, Koh W, London NR, Ling J, Mayo AH, Drakos SG, Jones CA, Zhu W, Marchuk DA, Davis GE, Li DY. The cerebral cavernous malformation signaling pathway promotes vascular integrity via rho GTPases. Nat Med. 2009;15:177–84. https://doi.org/10.1038/nm.1911.

98. Li X, Zhang R, Zhang H, He Y, Ji W, Min W, Boggon TJ. Crystal structure of CCM3, a cerebral cavernous malformation protein critical for vascular integrity. J Biol Chem. 2010;285:24099–107. https://doi.org/10.1074/jbc.M110.128470.

99. Berman JR, Kenyon C. Germ-cell loss extends *C. elegans* life span through regula-tion of DAF-16 by kri-1 and lipophilic-hormone signaling. Cell. 2006;124:1055–68. https://doi.org/10.1016/j.cell.2006.01.039.

100. Lant B, Pal S, Chapman EM, Yu B, Witvliet D, Choi S, Zhao L, Albiges-Rizo C, Faurobert E, Derry WB. Interrogating the ccm-3 Gene Network. Cell Rep. 2018;24:2857–2868.e4. https://doi.org/10.1016/j.celrep.2018.08.039.

101. Rehain-Bell K, Love A, Werner ME, MacLeod I, Yates JR, Maddox AS. A sterile 20 family kinase and its co-factor CCM-3 regulate contractile ring proteins on germline inter-cellular bridges. Curr Biol. 2017;27:860–7. https://doi.org/10.1016/j.cub.2017.01.058.

102. Kean MJ, Ceccarelli DF, Goudreault M, Sanches M, Tate S, Larsen B, Gibson LCD, Derry WB, Scott IC, Pelletier L, Baillie GS, Sicheri F, Gingras A-C. Structure-function analysis of core Stripak proteins a signaling complex implicated in Golgi polarization. J Biol Chem. 2011;286:25065–75. https://doi.org/10.1074/jbc.M110.214486.

103. Voss K, Stahl S, Schleider E, Ullrich S, Nickel J, Mueller TD, Felbor U. CCM3 inter-acts with CCM2 indicating common pathogenesis for cerebral cavernous malformations. Neurogenetics. 2007;8:249–56. https://doi.org/10.1007/s10048-007-0098-9.

104. Sugden PH, McGuffin LJ, Clerk A. SOcK, MiSTs, MASK and STicKs: the GCKIII (germinal Centre kinase III) kinases and their heterologous protein-protein interactions. Biochem J. 2013;454:13–30. https://doi.org/10.1042/BJ20130219.

105. Zhang M, Dong L, Shi Z, Jiao S, Zhang Z, Zhang W, Liu G, Chen C, Feng M, Hao Q, Wang W, Yin M, Zhao Y, Zhang L, Zhou Z. Structural mechanism of CCM3 heterodimerization with GCKIII kinases. Structure. 2013;21:680–8. https://doi.org/10.1016/j.str.2013.02.015.

106. Fidalgo M, Fraile M, Pires A, Force T, Pombo C, Zalvide J. CCM3/PDCD10 stabilizes GCKIII proteins to promote Golgi assembly and cell orientation. J Cell Sci. 2010;123:1274–84. https://doi.org/10.1242/jcs.061341.

107. Xu X, Wang X, Zhang Y, Wang D-C, Ding J. Structural basis for the unique heterodimeric assembly between cerebral cavernous malformation 3 and germinal center kinase III. Structure. 2013;21:1059–66. https://doi.org/10.1016/j.str.2013.04.007.

108. Zhang Y, Tang W, Zhang H, Niu X, Xu Y, Zhang J, Gao K, Pan W, Boggon TJ, Toomre D, Min W, Wu D. A network of interactions enables CCM3 and STK24 to coordinate UNC13D-driven vesicle exocytosis in neutrophils. Dev Cell. 2013;27:215–26. https://doi.org/10.1016/j.devcel.2013.09.021.

109. Dibble CF, Horst JA, Malone MH, Park K, Temple B, Cheeseman H, Barbaro JR, Johnson GL, Bencharit S. Defining the functional domain of programmed cell death 10 through its interactions with phosphatidylinositol-3,4,5-trisphosphate. PLoS One. 2010;5:e11740. https://doi.org/10.1371/journal.pone.0011740.

110. Li X, Ji W, Zhang R, Folta-Stogniew E, Min W, Boggon TJ. Molecular recognition of leucine-aspartate repeat (LD) motifs by the focal adhesion targeting homology domain of cerebral cavernous malformation 3 (CCM3). J Biol Chem. 2011;286:26138–47. https://doi.org/10.1074/jbc.M110.211250.

111. Goudreault M, DAmbrosio LM, Kean MJ, Mullin MJ, Larsen BG, Sanchez A, Chaudhry S, Chen GI, Sicheri F, Nesvizhskii AI, Aebersold R, Raught B, Gingras A-C. A PP2A phosphatase high density interaction network identifies a novel Striatin-interacting phosphatase and kinase complex linked to the cerebral cavernous malformation 3 (CCM3) protein. Mol Cell Proteomics. 2009;8:157–71. https://doi.org/10.1074/mcp.M800266-MCP200.

112. He Y, Zhang H, Yu L, Gunel M, Boggon TJ, Chen H, Min W. Stabilization of VEGFR2 signaling by cerebral cavernous malformation 3 is critical for vascular development. Sci Signal. 2010;3:ra26. https://doi.org/10.1126/scisignal.2000722.

113. Fidalgo M, Guerrero A, Fraile M, Iglesias C, Pombo CM, Zalvide J. Adaptor protein cerebral cavernous malformation 3 (CCM3) mediates phosphorylation of the cytoskeletal proteins Ezrin/radixin/Moesin by mammalian Ste20-4 to protect cells from oxidative stress. J Biol Chem. 2012;287:11556–65. https://doi.org/10.1074/jbc.M111.320259.

114. Leiling C, Gamze T, Hiroko Y, Robert F, Angeliki L, Murat G. Apoptotic functions of PDCD10/CCM3, the gene mutated in cerebral cavernous malformation 3. Stroke. 2009;40:1474–81. https://doi.org/10.1161/STROKEAHA.108.527135.

115. Lin C, Meng S, Zhu T, Wang X. PDCD10/CCM3 acts downstream of Iδ-Protocadherins to regulate neuronal survival. J Biol Chem. 2010;285:41675–85. https://doi.org/10.1074/jbc.M110.179895.

116. Zhu Y, Wu Q, Xu J-F, Miller D, Sandalcioglu IE, Zhang J-M, Sure U. Differential angiogenesis function of CCM2 and CCM3 in cerebral cavernous malformations. Neurosurg Focus. 2010;29:E1. https://doi.org/10.3171/2010.5.FOCUS1090.

117. Louvi A, Chen L, Two AM, Zhang H, Min W, GÃijnel M. Loss of cerebral cavernous malformation 3 (Ccm3) in neuroglia leads to CCM and vascular pathology. Proc Natl Acad Sci. 2011;108:3737–42. https://doi.org/10.1073/pnas.1012617108.

118. You C, Sandalcioglu IE, Dammann P, Felbor U, Sure U, Zhu Y. Loss of CCM3 impairs DLL4-Notch signalling: implication in endothelial angiogenesis and in inherited cerebral cavernous malformations. J Cell Mol Med. 2013;17:407–18. https://doi.org/10.1111/jcmm.12022.

# Chapter 4
# Presentation

Martin Aichholzer and Andreas Gruber

## 4.1 Summary

The most common clinical manifestations of cerebral cavernous malformations [CCMs] include epileptic seizures [50%], symptomatic intracerebral hemorrhage [ICH, 25%], and non-hemorrhagic focal neurologic deficits [NH-FNDs, 25%]. A significant number of CCM patients [20%–50%] is asymptomatic. CCM related symptoms can be attributed to intralesional or extralesional hemorrhage, mass effect, or other mechanisms including perilesional hemosiderin deposition. Variations in assessment [imaging parameters and timing of MRI], clinical event definition [ICH vs. NH-FND vs. not otherwise specified-FND], study design [retrospective vs. prospective], CCM location [supratentorial vs. infratentorial] and clincial history [previous CCM bleeding] account for the range of published estimates of CCM hemorrhage rates. The most comprehensive information currently available indicates that the 5 year estimated risk of ICH during untreated follow up is around 3.8% for patients with non-brainstem CCMs presenting without ICH or NH-FND, around 8.0% forpatients with brainstem CCMs presenting without ICH or NH-FND, around 18.4% for patients with non-brainstem CCMs presenting with ICH or NH-FND, and around 30.8% for patients with brainstem CCMs presenting with ICH or NH-FND. The major predictors for future CCM hemorrhage are previous CCM bleeding and CCM location in the brainstem. CCM location influences the form of CCM related NH-FNDs. Small CCM hemorrhages into non-eloquent supratentorial parenchyma may be clinically silent. Reflecting the sensitivity of eloquent surrounding tissue, patients with thalamic and basal ganglia CCMs as well as those with infratentorial CCMs are more likely to present with NH-FNDs. Established risk factors for cavernoma related epilepsy [CRE] are supratentorial CCM location,

M. Aichholzer (✉) · A. Gruber
Department of Neurosurgery, Johannes Kepler University Linz, Kepler University Clinic/Neuromed Campus, Linz, Austria
e-mail: martin.aichholzer@kepleruniklinikum.at; andreas.gruber_1@kepleruniklinikum.at

© Springer Nature Switzerland AG 2020
O. Bradáč, V. Beneš (eds.), *Cavernomas of the CNS*,
https://doi.org/10.1007/978-3-030-49406-3_4

cortical CCM involvement, and archicortical/mesiotemporal CCM location. The risk to develop CRE varies between 1.5% and 2.4% per patient year. The risk of recurrent seizures is around 94%. The chance of achieving 2 year seizure freedom is around 47%. Patients with a first-ever CCM related seizure can be considered to have epilepsy according to the international League Against Epilepsy criteria.

## 4.2   Introduction

Cerebral cavernous malformations [CCMs] are angiographically occult neurovascular malformations with a characteristic radiographic and pathological appearance [1, 2]. CCMs are the second most common type of vascular lesions in the central nervous system and account for approximately 8% to 15% of all neurovascular malformations [3, 4]. Unlike arteriovenous malformations [AVMs], CCMs are low-pressure lesions and have no high-pressure arterial supply or distinct venous drainage [5]. Upon histological examination, CCMs are clusters of ectatic, endothelium lined sinusoidal channels without interposing neural or glial tissue embedded in a connective tissue matrix. There is no evidence of normally developed vessel layers and structures, e.g. intervening tight junctions, mural muscular fibres or elastic fibres. Since blood flow within these channels is stagnant, subsequent undulating episodes of thrombosis and recanalisation result in the characteristic MRI appearance of intralesional blood at various stages of thrombosis and organisation [3]. Although CCMs are not encapsulated, there is typically gliosis and hemosiderin deposition in the surrounding neural parenchyma. The periphery of the lesion may contain cavernous lobules invading adjacent brain. CCMs occur throughout the central nervous system in rough proportion to the volume of neural tissue, i.e. 80% supratentorial, 15% basal ganglia and infratentorial, and 5% in the spinal cord [3]. The prevalence of CCMs in the general population ranges from 0.16% [6] to 0.9% [7–10]. The population based annual detection rate of CCMs has increased from 0.17 per 100,000 per year in the USA from 1965 to 1992 [11] to 0.56 per 100.000 per year in Scotland from 1999 to 2000 [12], a development best explained by the increasing availability of MRI. CCMs occur in both sporadic and familiar forms. Heterozygous loss of function mutations in at least three different CCM genes, i.e. CCM 1 [KRIT 1], CCM 2 [MGC 4607], CCM 3 [PDCD 10], have been identified in both sporadic and familiar forms. Somatic mutations in CCM genes were identified in the endothelial cells of CCM lesion tissue, i.e. the endothelial cell is the primary site of CCM lesion pathogenesis. CCM lesion genesis is thought to follow a "two hit" mechanism, requiring biallelic germline and somatic mutations in one of the known CCM genes [13, 14]. Sporadic cases of CCMs are characterised by a lack of family history and usually the presence of only a single lesion on MRI. Familial CCMs mostly exhibit multiple lesions that show progression in both number and size over time. Familial CCMs follow and autosomal dominant inheritance heritance pattern with incomplete penetrance [15–18].

## 4.3 Clinical Presentation

A significant number of CCM patients [20%–50%] is asymptomatic and lesions are discovered incidentally due to an increasing utilization of MRI [3, 18–24]. The most common clinical manifestations of CCMs include epileptic seizures [50%], stroke due to symptomatic intracerebral hemorrhage [ICH, 25%], and focal neurologic deficits [FNDs] without evidence of of recent hemorrhage [25%] [18, 25, 26]. Although 6% to 65% of CCM patients can complain of headache, CCMs have not been proven to cause chronic headache disorders in recent case-control studies [27, 28]. Clinical CCM related symptoms can be attributed to intralesional or extralesional hemorrhage, mass effect, or other mechanisms including perilesional hemosiderin deposition.

### *4.3.1 CCM Hemorrhage*

Strokes due to symptomatic CCM hemorrhage must be discussed in context with the radiologic definitions of CCM hemorrhage and the CCM natural history data available.

The radiologic definitions of CCM hemorrhage are explained in detail in Chap. 5 and are here briefly referred to for the purpose of discussion of overall CCM hemorrhage rates. Variations in MRI assessment and clinical event definitions may in part account for the range of published estimates of CCM hemorrhage rates.

*CCM hemorrhage* [i.e. most frequently ICH] is standardized as "requiring acute or subacute onset symptoms [any of headache, epileptic seizure, impaired consciousness, or new/worsened FND referable to the anatomic location of the CCM] accompanied by radiological, pathological, surgical, or rarely only cerebrospinal fluid evidence of recent extra- or intralesional hemorrhage". The definition includes neither an increase in CCM diameter without other evidence of recent hemorrhage, nor the mere existence of a hemosiderin halo [27].

*Non-hemorrhagic focal neurologic deficit [NH-FND]* is defined as "a new or worsened focal neurological deficit referable to the anatomic location of the CCM, which may present with other clinical features of ICH, but without evidence of recent blood on timely brain imaging oth pathological examination, or examination of the cerebrospinal fluid. These cases may be accompanied by an increase in CCM diameter alone or edema on MRI" [27].

*Focal neurologic deficits that are not otherwise specified [NOS-FND]* are "identical to NH-FND, with the exception that the term NOS-FND is used when pathological investigations, cerebrospinal fluid examinations, or timely imaging have not been performed at all or at the correct time to establish whether hemorrhage, edema, or lesion growth underlie the clinical deterioration. Inevitably, some NOS-FNDs are missed hemorrhages." [27].

The distinctions and overlaps between ICH, NH-FND, and NOS-FND based on these definitions are given in Fig. 4.1. Surgery is indicated in cases of space-occupying extralesional CCM hemorrhage as demonstrated in illustrative case 1 (Fig. 4.2).

The natural history of CCMs is explained in detail in Chap. 6 and is here briefly referred to for the purpose of discussion of factors increasing the risks for CCM hemorrhage.

Variations in assessment [imaging parameters and timing of MRI], clinical event definition [ICH vs. NH-FND vs. NOS-FND], study design [retrospective vs. prospective], CCM location [supratentorial vs. infratentorial] and clincial history [history of CCM bleeding] account for the range of published estimates of CCM hemorrhage rates.

The prospective annual ICH rate in patients with CCMs has been estimated to be 0.4%–4.2% for sporadic CCMs [16, 27, 29] and 4.3%–6.5% for familiar CCMs [3, 23]. The most comprehensive information on the clinical course of untreated CCMs and on the factors increasing the CCM hemorrhage risk is provided in the meta-analysis by Horne MA et al. [26]. Therein, 204 of 1620 CCM patients experienced a symptomatic ICH during 5197 person years of follow up, equaling a 5 year bleeding risk of 15.8%. The authors concluded, that brainstem CCM location and

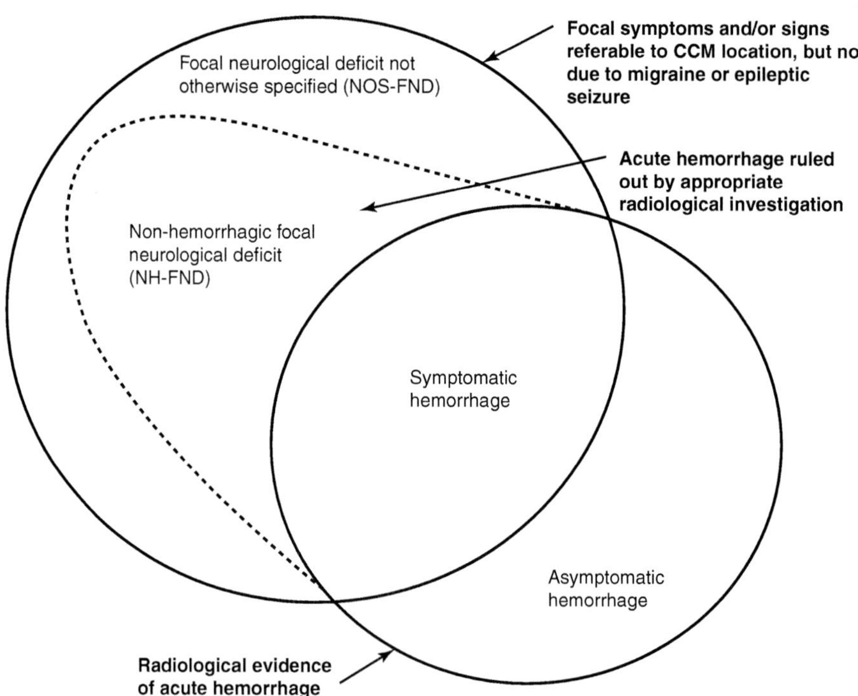


**Fig. 4.1** Radiological and clinical reporting standards on CCM presentation [ICH, NH-FND, NOS-FND]. Reprint with permission from: Al-Shahi R, Berg MJ, Morrison L, Awad IA. Hemorrhage from Cavernous Malformations of the Brain. Definition und Reporting Standards. Stroke 2008; 39:3222–3230 [27]

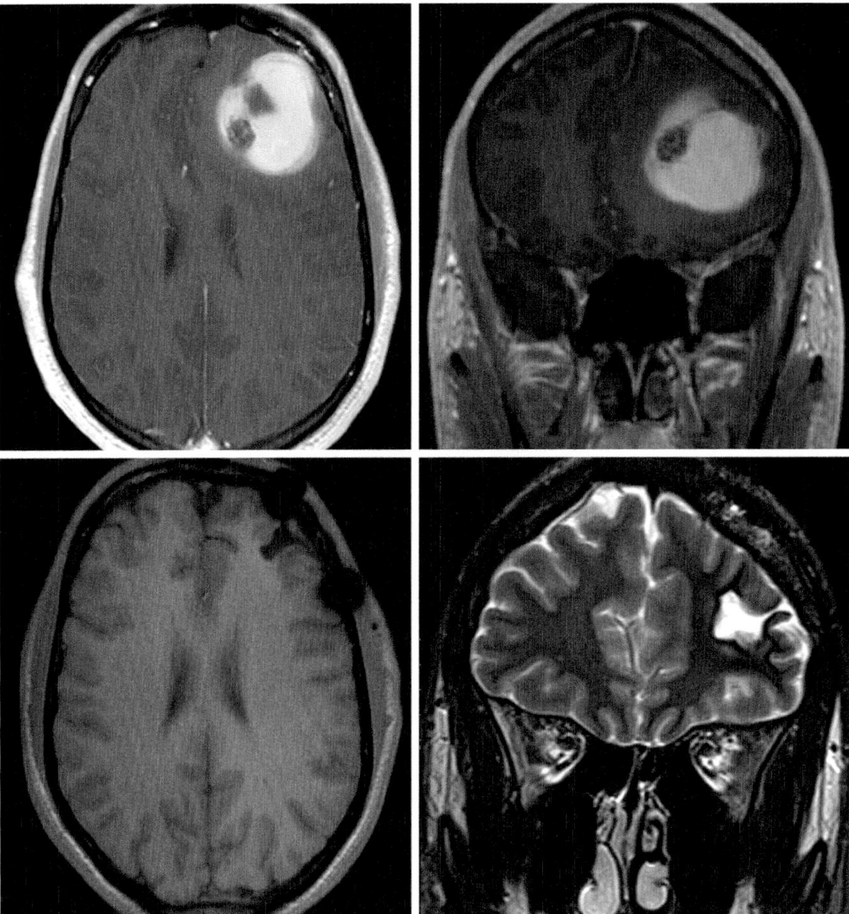

**Fig. 4.2** Illustrative case 1. Extralesional CCM related ICH. A 23 year old male patient was admitted to with a history of severe headache and vomiting for 2 weeks. Since CT disclosed a left frontal ICH of >4 cm in diameter, the presenting symptoms were interpreted as signs of intracranial hypertension and surgery was performed urgently. Preoperative MRIs were compatible with the diagnosis of a CCM with repetitive extralesional mass hemorrhage, a diagnosis later confirmed histologically. The patient made an uneventful postoperative neurologic recovery

CCM presentation with ICH or FND were independently associated with the occurrence of ICH after diagnosis of CCMs, whereas age, gender, and CCM multiplicity did not provide any further prognostic information. In detail, the 5 year estimated risk of ICH during untreated follow up was 3.8% for 718 patients with non-brainstem CCMs presenting without ICH or NH-FND, 8.0% for 80 patients with brainstem CCMs presenting without ICH or NH-FND, 18.4% for 327 patients with non-brainstem CCMs presenting with ICH or NH-FND, and 30.8% for 495 people with brainstem CCMs presenting with ICH or NH-FND. The stratification into these 4 groups to predict the 5 year risk of ICH is given in Fig. 4.3.

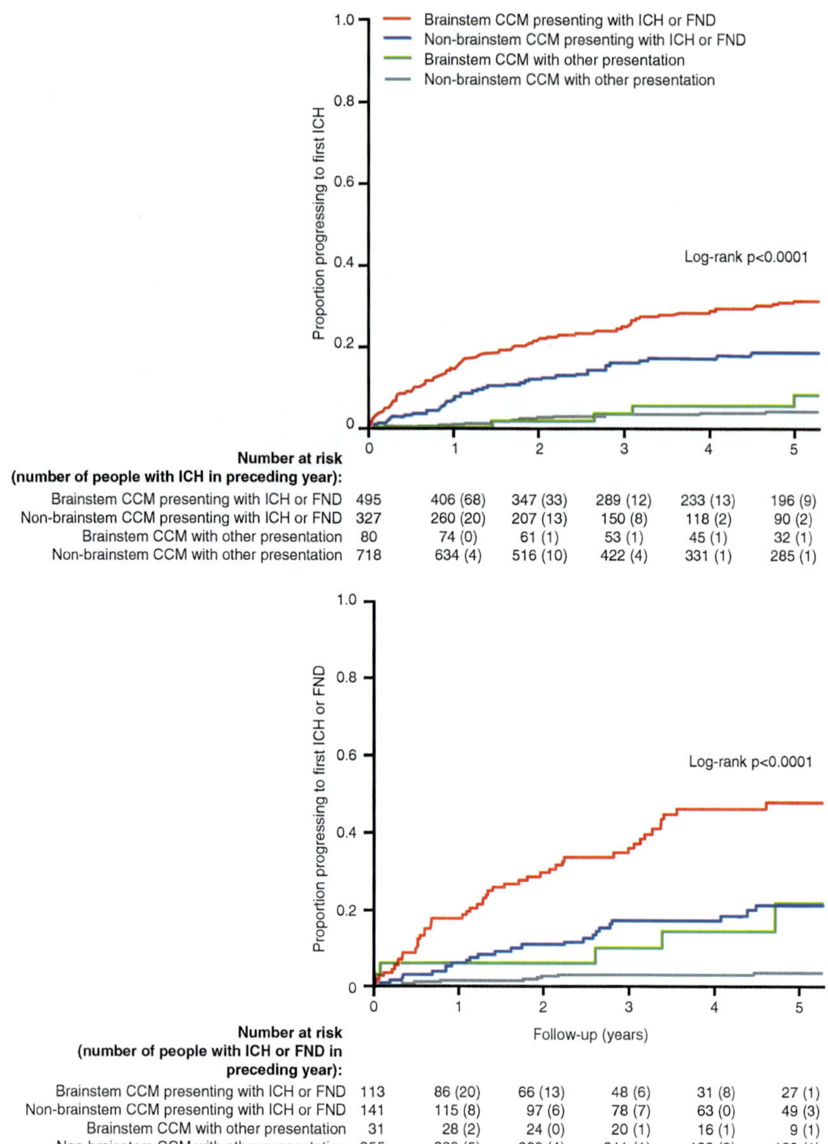


**Fig. 4.3** Stratification into four groups [non-ICH non-brainstem CCM, non-ICH brainstem CCM, ICH non-brainstem CCM, ICH brainstem CCM] to predict the 5 year risk of CCM related ICH. Kaplan-Meier plots of progression to intracranial haemorrhage or to intracranial haemorrhage or focal neurological deficit. Plots show the proportion of people progressing to ICH [left] or ICH or NH-FND [right] during follow-up, stratified by ICH or NH-FND presentation from brainstem CCMs, ICH or NH-FND presentation from non-brainstem CCMs, other presentation from brainstem CCMs, and other presentation from non-brainstem CCMs. *CCM* cerebral cavernous malformation; *FND* focal neurological deficit; *HR* hazard ratio; *ICH* intracranial haemorrhage. Reprint with permission from Horne MA, Flemming KD, Su I, Stapf C, Jeon JP, Li D, Maxwell SS, White P, Christianson TJ, Agid R, Cho WS, Oh CW, Zhang JT, Kim JE, ter Brugge K, Willinsky R, Brown RD Jr, Murray GD, Al Shahi SR, and the Cerebral Cavernous Malformations Individual Patient Data Meta-analysis Collaborators. Clinical course of untreated cerebral cavernous malformations: a meta-analysis of individual patient data. Lancet Neurol 2016, 15.166–173 [26]

Earlier studies are difficult to compare because of the aforementioned methodologic differences. The influence of study design [prospective vs. retrospective] is of relevance, since bleeding rates were either calculated from prospective follow up data or from retrospective natural history registries based on the assumption that the CCMs had been present since birth. Such retrospective calculations assuming a constant ICH risk since birth are inaccurate and underestimate the actual ICH risk of CCMs once they are discovered. Del Curling O Jr. et al. [30] found an annual ICH rate of only 0.25% per patient year and 0.1% per lesion year in a group of 32 patients harboring 76 CCMs discovered in a review of 8131 MRI images performed between 1986 and 1989. Presenting symptoms in these patients included hemorrhage [9%], seizure [50%], headache [34%], and NH-FNDs [22%]. CCMs were incidental findings in 19% and in supratentorial location in 86% of the cases. Robinson JR et al. [21] retrospectively calculated the annual bleeding rate in 66 CCM patients detected on over 14,000 consecutive MRI images performed at the Cleveland Clinic between 1984 and 1989 as 0.7% per lesion year. Presenting symptoms in these patients included seizure [52%], NH-FNDs [46%], and headache [30%]. CCMs were incidental findings in 13.6% and in supratentorial location in 84% of the cases. Zabramski JM et al. [3] calculated a prospective symptomatic bleeding rate of 6.5% per patient year and 1.1% per lesion per year in 31 patients with 128 familial CCMs followed for a period of 2.2 years. Presenting symptoms in these patients included seizure [39%], NH-FNDs [26%], and headache [52%]. CCMs were incidental findings in 39% and in supratentorial location in 91% of the cases. Moriarity JL et al. [24] prospectively reported an annual ICH rate of 3.1% per patient year in a series of 68 CCM patients. Presenting symptoms in these patients included hemorrhage [13%], seizure [49%], NH-FNDs [46%], and headache [65%]. CCMs were incidental findings in only 1.5% and in supratentorial location in 73% of the cases. Porter PJ et al. [31] retrospectively calculated the annual bleeding rate in a series of 173 patients as 1.6% per patient year. Presenting symptoms in these patients included hemorrhage [25%], seizure [36%], NH-FNDs [20%], and headache [6%]. CCMs were incidental findings in 12% and in supratentorial location in 63% of the cases.

The two risk factors for future CCM hemorrhage identified in many individual studies were (1) Initial CCM presentation with hemorrhage [hazard ratio 5.6, 95% confidence interval 3.2–9.7] and (2) CCM location in the brainstem [hazard ratio 4.4, 95% confidence interval 2.3–8.6] [32].

Aiba T et al. [33] retrospectively reviewed 110 CCM patients and found a significantly higher ICH risk among those with previous CCM hemorrhage [CCM presentation as incidental finding or with seizures: 0.39% hemorrhage risk per patient year; CCM presentation with ICH: 22.9% hemorrhage risk per patient year]. In the series of Kondziolka D et al. [22], the retrospective annual bleeding rate—under the assumption that the lesion had been present since birth—was 1.3% among 122 CCM patients [61 CCM hemorrhages in 122 CCM patients during 4550.6 patient years]. In the 61 patients without a prior bleed, the prospective annual hemorrhage rate was 0.6% during a 34 months follow up period, whereas among the 61 patients with a prior bleed, 8 hemorrhages were observed in 7 patients during the follow up period [annual hemorrhage rate of 4.5%, $p = 0.028$]. The prospective annual bleeding rate for the entire series was therefore 2.6% [9 hemorrhages in 341 patient years of prospective observation]. In the meta-analysis by Horne MA et al. [26], the 5 year estimated risk of ICH during untreated follow up was 3.8% for 718 patients with non-brainstem CCMs presenting without ICH or NH-FND, 8.0% for 80 patients with brainstem CCMs presenting without ICH or NH-FND, 18.4% for 327 patients with non-brainstem CCMs presenting with ICH or NH-FND, and 30.8% for 495 people with brainstem CCMs presenting with ICH or NH-FND.

A clustering of CCM rebleeding within the first 2 years after the initial ICH and a decrease of the annual incidence of rebleeding over time has been reported. In the Mayo Clinic cohort assessing the natural history of untreated CCMs [Flemming KD, 4th Bellaria Neurovascular Conference, Bologna 2018], the re-bleeding rates during an 8 year observation period were 18.3% at 0–1 year, 9.2% at 1–2 years, 0.9% at 2–5 years, and 3.1% later than 5 years after the initial ICH, equalling an overall rebleeding rate of 6.2%. In a prospective, population based cohort study including 139 CCM patients, Al-Shahi R et al. [18] identified a 2.4% 5 year risk of first ICH and a 29.5% 5 year risk of recurrent ICH during a 1177 person years follow up period. The 5 year risk of first ICH or NH-FND was 9.3% and the 5 year risk of recurrent ICH or NH-FND was 42.4%. The annual risk of recurrent ICH or NH-FND declined from 19.8% after 1 year to 5.0% after 5 years.

Patients with brainstem CCMs have the highest bleeding rates in the untreated course [hazard ratio 4.4, 95% confidence interval 2.3–8.6] [33]. In the meta-analysis of Taslimi S et al. [34], the annual bleeding rate was 0.3% per person year for non-brainstem CCMs and 2.8% for brainstem CCMs. The annual rebleeding rates were 6.3% for non-brainstem CCMs and 32.3% for brainstem CCMs. These findings are line with the results of previous studies. Fritschi JA et al. [35] reported a symptomatic ICH rate of 2.7% per patient year and a symptomatic rebleeding rate of 21% per patient year in brainstem CCMs. Wang CC et al. [36] described ICH as presenting symptom in 67% of the 137 braistem CCM patients included in their series and reported a 6% hemorrhage rate per patient year and a 60% rebleeding rate per person year. Porter PJ et al. [37] found ICH as presenting symptom in 97% of the 100 brainstem CCM patients and described a 5% hemorrhage rate per person year and a 30% rebleeding rate per person year. Porter PJ et al. further reported a higher symptomatic rebleeding rate in infratentorial than in supratentorial CCMs [3.8% per patient year vs. 0.4% per patient year] as well as in deep [including brainstem, thalamus, and basal ganglia] than in superficial CCMs [4.1% per patient year vs. 0% per patient years]. Li D et al. [38] assessed hemorrhage risks of untreated brainstem CCMs in a population of 331 patients followed for 6.5 years [range 1.0 to 28.6 years, 2151.3 total patient years] and found 185 prospective symptomatic hemorrhages [161 definite and 24 probable] in 131 patients [39.6%]. Thirty-five patients [10.6%] experienced multiple prospective hemorrhages [22 patients experienced 2 episodes, 7 patients experienced 3 episodes, and 6 patients experienced 4 episodes]. There was a trend towards multiple prospective hemorrhages in patients presenting initially with ICH [12.1%] when compared to those patients initially presenting without ICH [7.3%]. The median intervals from diagnosis to the first prospective hemorrhage and from the first to the second prospective hemorrhage were 25.5 and 24.9 months, respectively. The prospective hemorrhage-free survival rate was 92.9% at 6 months, 87.2% at 1 year, 53.0% at 5 years, 23.9% at 10 years, and 10.1%

at 15 years. The significant correlation between the percentage of brainstem CCMs included in a study and the overall incidence of ICH within the study population reported is demonstrated in Fig. 4.4 [34]. Active treatment should be considered after brainstem CCM hemorrhage in lesions surgically accessible, carefully

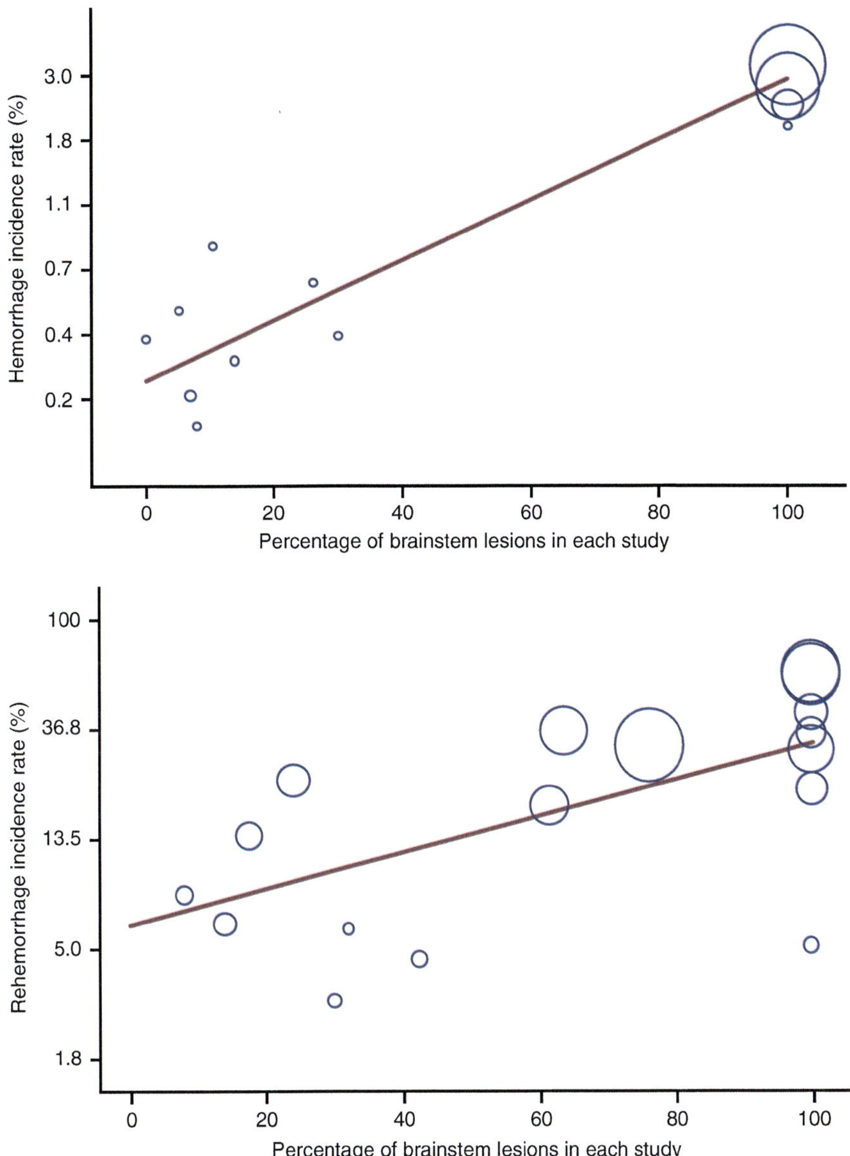

**Fig. 4.4** Correlation between the percentage of brainstem CCMs included and the overall incidence of ICH [top] and recurrent ICH [bottom] reported within a study population. Reprint with permission from Taslimi S, Modabbernia A, Amin-Hanjani S, Barker FG, MacDonald RL. Natural history of cavernous malformation. Systematic review and meta-analysis of 25 studies. Neurology 2016;86:1984–1991 [34]

weighing the aforementioned risks of CCM rebleeding against the expected permanent morbidity of microsurgical resection (Illustrative case 2, Fig. 4.5).

The outcome of CCM hemorrhage depends on the size and location of the ICH. In the meta-analysis of Taslimi S et al. [34], post-hemorrhage full recovery was 38.8% per person year [28.7%–48.8%]. Post-hemorrhage full recovery or

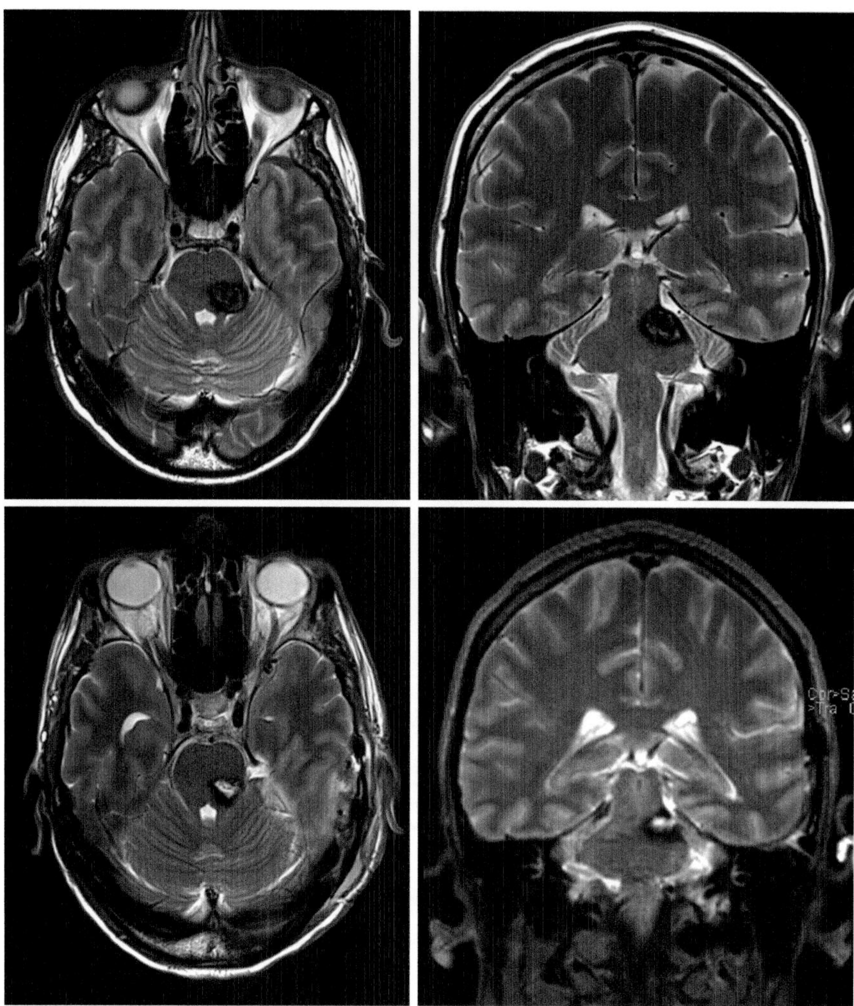

**Fig. 4.5** Illustrative case 2. Brainstem CCM. A 54 year old man developed a rigidity in his right shoulder and right hip during physical training for a running competition. Neurologic examination disclosed a hypesthesia of his left forehead and cheek as well as a right hemihypesthesia in absence of motoric deficits. Since these symptoms persisted for days, a cranial MRI was performed and demonstrated a CCM at the pontomesencephalic junctions with signs of recent intralesional hemorrhage. The patient was referred for further investigation and consultation to our department 8 months later and was operated 3 months thereafter in a modified park bench position via a subtemporal transtentorial approach. The CCM reached the surface of the brainstem and was completely resected as demonstrated on postoperative MRIs. Following a 3 month period of transient symptom aggravation, the patient recovered and finally started running again

minimal disability was 79.5% per person year [74.3%–84.8%]. In the study of Li D et al. [38] describing hemorrhage risks in a population of 331 brainstem CCM patients, the complete recovery rates in patients experiencing none, 1, or more than 1 prospective hemorrhage were 37% [74/200], 17.7% [17/96], and 11.4% [4/35], respectively. The overall cumulative survival rate with complete recovery was 17.1% at 3 months, 24.1% at 6 months, 29.1% at 1 year, and 30.3% at 2 years and thereafter. In a multivariate analysis, the following factors were predictive of favourable outcome: absence of rebleeding [hazard ratio 1.958, 95% confidence interval 1.326–2.892, P = 0.001], younger age [hazard ratio 1.268, 95% confidence interval 1.099–1.463, p = 0.001], and smaller lesion size [hazard ratio 1.578, 95% confidence interval 1.156–2.154, p = 0.004]. Although CCM hemorrhages tend to be intracerebral and of low volume, the case fatalities described in the literature range from 0% [37] to 17% for recurrent ICH in brainstem CCMs [35].

### 4.3.2  *Non-hemorrhagic Focal Neurologic Deficits [NH-FNDs]*

Small CCM hemorrhages into non-eloquent supratentorial parenchyma may be clinically silent and thus a large number of supratentorial CCMs may go undiagnosed unless discovered as incidental findings on MRI or diagnosed in patient presenting with epileptic seizures. With supratentorial lesions, the most common presenting symptom is new onset seizure [23%–79%], whereas NH-FNDs were less frequently encountered [8.2%–46%] [3, 20–22, 24, 30, 31, 33]. Since the cited studies included 9%–32.2% infratentorial CCMs, the NH-FND incidence of supratentorial CCMs may be even lower. With supratentorial lesions, CCM location obviously influences the clinical manifestation and form of CCM related NH-FND.

Reflecting the sensitivity of eloquent surrounding tissue, patients with thalamic and basal ganglia CCMs as well as those with infratentorial CCMs are more likely to present with NH-FNDs. The clinical manifestations of thalamic and basal ganglia CCMs include ICH, slowly progressing NH-FNDs, and hydrocephalus. In the majority of clinical reports, symptomatic ICH is the presenting symptom in >60% of thalamic and basal ganglia CCMs with annual rebleeding rates of 6.1%–15.4% [39]. The most common non-hemorrhagic clinical manifestations of thalamic and basal ganglia CCMs are contralateral motor and sensory deficits [40–43]. Large thalamic and basal ganglia CCMs can further produce signs of hydrocephalus in 15%–25% of the cases due to CSF pathway obstruction or as a result of hemorrhage [39, 40, 43]. Extrapyramidal movement disorders have also been described in cases of basal ganglia CCMs [39–43]. In detail, Akbostanci MC et al. [44] reported the case of a 34 year old female with right hemidystonia who had a CCM at the left thalamo-mesencephalic junction and who was managed conservatively. Lorenzana L et al. [45] described the case of a 17 years of female with dystonia of her right hand who had a 3 cm large CCM in the anterior third of the lentiform nucleus who was cured by surgery. Carpay HA et al. [46] reported the case of an 11 year old male with right hemichorea who had a CCM in the head of the left caudate nucleus and who was cured by surgery. Donmez B et al. [47] described the case of a 63 year old male with right hemichorea who had a left putaminal CCM and who was managed conservatively. Further cases of hemichorea due to CCMs in the contralateral caudate nucleus have been reported by Carella F et al. [48], Lopez-Valdes E et al. [49], and Yakinci C et al. [50]. Hidaka M et al. [51] reported a case of hemiballism due to a contralateral putaminal CCM. Pozzati E et al. [39] described two cases of posterothalamic CCMs which caused involuntary and athetoid movements of the contralateral hand and fingers. Mizutani T et al. [52] reported the case of a patient harboring a hypothalamic CCM observed from 1974 to 1978, presenting with headache, bitemporal hemianopsia, slowly progressive memory loss, and intellectual impairment.

With infratentorial CCMs, most patients not presenting with hemorrhage have NH-FNDs as clinical manifestation, e.g. cranial nerve palsies, hemiparesis, and gait ataxia. Wang CC et al. [36] reported on 137 patients with brainstem CCMs and found as presenting symptoms cranial nerve deficits in 77% and mono- or hemiparesis in 53% of the cases. Among the 29 patients with mesencephalic CCMs in that series, the most common symptoms were diplopia [20/29; 69%], hemiparesis [14/29; 48%], hydrocephalus [11/29; 38%], and ataxia [11/29; 38%]. Infrequent clinical manifestations were with rubral tremor [3/29; 1%], involuntary laughing [1/29; 3.4%], paroxysmal coma [1/29; 3.4%], and Parinaud's syndrome [1/29; 3.4%]. Among the 90 patients with pontine CCMs in that series, the majority presented with deficits of cranial nerves V–VIII [68/90; 76%]. Other common presenting symptoms included hemiparesis [51/90; 57%], hemianesthesia [44/90; 49%], vertigo [40/90; 44%], ataxia [30/90; 33%], diplopia [30/90; 33%], dysphagia [21/90; 23%], and unilateral gaze paralysis [15/90; 16.7%]. All 18 medullary CCMs in that series were associated with dysphagia. Hemiparesis, hemianesthesia, and ataxia were seen in 44% [8/18] of the patients. Of note, intractable hiccups and respiratory depression were seen in 28% [5/18] and 17% [3/18] of the patients with medullary CCMs, respectively. Li D et al. [38] described the functional outcome of untreated brainstem CCMs. The complete improvement rate in that series of 331 patients was highest for diplopia [50/58; 86.2%], followed by dysphagia [33/42; 78.6%], facial numbness [87/112; 77.7%], diplopia [90/118; 76.3%], and facial nerve palsy [55/73; 75.3%]. The complete improvement rate of dysarthria was 71.9% [46/64], of paresthesia 64.4% [121/188], and of motor weakness 61.4% [86/140]. The improvement rate of ataxia was comparably worse [25/53; 43.3%, $p = 0.024$].

### 4.3.3  Cavernoma Related Epilepsy

Approximately half of the patients with intracerebral CCMs present with epilepsy. Definitions for the relationship of epilepsy to CCMs have been proposed [53].

*Definite cavernoma related epilepsy [CRE]* has been defined as epilepsy in patients with at least one CCM and with evidence of a seizure onset zone in the immediate vicinity of the CCM, e.g. a patient with left hand tonic-clonic seizures and a right M1 hand area CCM [32, 53].

*Probable cavernoma related epilepsy [CRE]* has been defined as epilepsy in a patient with at least one CCM and with evidence that epilepsy is focal and arises from the same hemisphere as the CCM but not necessarily in its vicinity. At the same time there is no other cause for the epilepsy, e.g. a patient with a left occipital lobe CCM and a history of a right versive seizure indicating a left hemisphere seizure onset [32, 53].

*Cavernoma unrelated epilepsy* has been defined as epilepsy in a patient with at least one CCM with evidence that the CCM and the epilepsy are not causally related, e.g. a patient with a juvenile myoclonic epilepsy and a right temporal lobe CCM [32, 53].

CCMs appear to be more epileptogenic than other mass lesions [54], although there is no evidence that the space-occupying effect itself leads to epilepsy [53]. Epilepsy in relation to CCMs is thought to be induced by recurrent microhemorrhages, resulting in blood degradation products [hemosiderin] within the perilesional area through leaky endothelial junctions, perilesional gliosis, and inflammation [25, 55–60]. Repeated microhemorrhages in brain tissue surrounding the CCM have been proposed to cause chronic irritation of the underlying cerebral cortex due to iron ions generating free radicals and lipid peroxides. As long as there is sufficient residual perilesional parenchyma, the damaged but still functional cortex may reintegrate and reorganize itself into an epileptogenic network.

Established risk factors for CRE are supratentorial CCM location, cortical CCM involvement, and archicortical/mesiotemporal CCM location. Controversial risk factors are lobar CCM location, CCM multiplicity, and lesion size. A number of studies revealed that 0%–18% of patients with infratentorial CCMs as compared to 50% to 63% of patients with supratentorial CCMs present with seizures [20, 21, 24, 61]. Strong evidence supports cortical CCM involvement as a main risk factor for epilepsy: 57% to 70% of "superficial" supratentorial CCMs as compared to 14%–20% of "deep" supratentorial CCMs were associated with epilepsy [20, 21, 24]. Exclusively subcortial CCMs were highly unlikely to cause CRE in the series of Menzler K et al. [61]. The same group established archicortical CCM localisation as a risk factor for CRE by showing that 8 of 9 patients with a mesiotemporal/archicortical CCM as compared to 41 of 72 patients with a neocortical CCM suffered CRE. Several recent studies have failed to demonstrate a clear cut correlation between lobar CCM localisation and CRE, especially when excluding mesiotemporal CCMs. Conflicting evidence exists about the correlation of CRE to CCM multiplicity and CCM size. Whereas Josephson CB et al. [62] studying a population of 139 CCM patients found that patients with CRE were significantly more likely to have multiple CCMs [43% vs. 6%], Menzler K et al. [61] described a nearly identical rate of CRE among patients with single and multiple CCMs. Whereas Josephson CB et al. [62] found no difference in the occurrence of epilepsy as a function of CCM size, Menzler K et al. [61] reported a significant correlation between CCM diameter including the perilesional hemosiderin rim and the prevalence of CRE.

The estimated risk of a CCM patient to develop CRE varies between 1.5% and 2.4% per patient year. Josephson CB et al. [62] prospectively studying 139 CCM patients found that the 5 year risk of a first ever seizure was 4% in 57 CCM patients presenting incidentally and 6% in 38 CCM patients presenting with ICH or NH-FNDs. For CCMs that have never caused a symptomatic ICH, the risk of a first seizure does not appear to justifiy a prophylactic antiepileptic drug medication. The occurrence of a CCM related ICH or NH-FND does not increase the risk of a first seizure [62]. For adult CCM patients with a first unprovoced seizure, i.e. those who were unaffected by prior ICH or NH-FND, the risk of recurrent seizures was 94% [62] (Fig. 4.6). For the same patient population, the chance of achieving 2 year seizure freedom was 47% [62] (Fig. 4.6). Patients with a first-ever CCM related seizure can be considered to have epilepsy according to the international League Against Epilepsy criteria [63–65].

Most authors favor an initial conservative approach using antiepileptic drugs in CCM patients with a single seizure, since 47%–60% of thesse patients can be well controlled with antiepileptic drugs [62, 66]. In CCM patients it is, however, not necessary to wait until the rigorous criteria of medically refractory epilepsy proposed by the International Liga Against Epilepsy are fulfilled [67] and failure of a single drug trial with an adequate antiepileptic should be considered sufficient to recommend presurgical evaluation and subsequent surgery when indicated. Surgery should not be delayed unnecessarily, since increasing evidence indicates that the time from the first seizure to resection of epileptogenic CCMs and the number of seizures occurring before CCM resection may negatively correlate with the likelihood of a seizure-free outcome [66, 68–73] (Illustrative case 3, Fig. 4.7).

## 4.4 Keypoints

- The most common clinical manifestations of cerebral cavernous malformations [CCMs] include epileptic seizures [50%], symptomatic intracerebral hemorrhage [ICH, 25%], and non-hemorrhagic focal neurologic deficits [NH-FNDs, 25%].
- The estimated 5 year risk of ICH during untreated follow up is around 3.8% for patients with non-brainstem CCMs presenting without ICH or NH-FND, around 8.0% forpatients with brainstem CCMs presenting without ICH or NH-FND, around 18.4% for patients with non-brainstem CCMs presenting with ICH or NH-FND, and around 30.8% for patients with brainstem CCMs presenting with ICH or NH-FND.
- The major predictors for future CCM hemorrhage are previous CCM bleeding and CCM location in the brainstem. CCM location influences the form of CCM related NH-FNDs.
- With supratentorial lesions, CCM location obviously influences the clinical manifestation of CCM related NH-FNDs. Reflecting the sensitivity of eloquent surrounding tissue, patients with thalamic and basal ganglia CCMs as well as those with infratentorial CCMs are more likely to present with NH-FNDs.

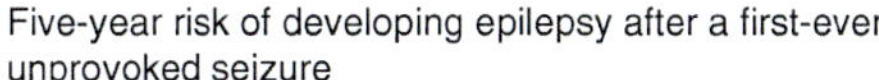


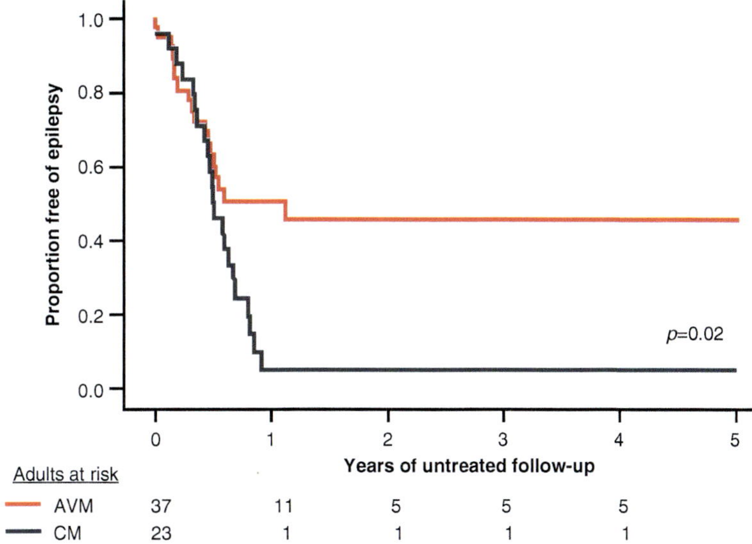


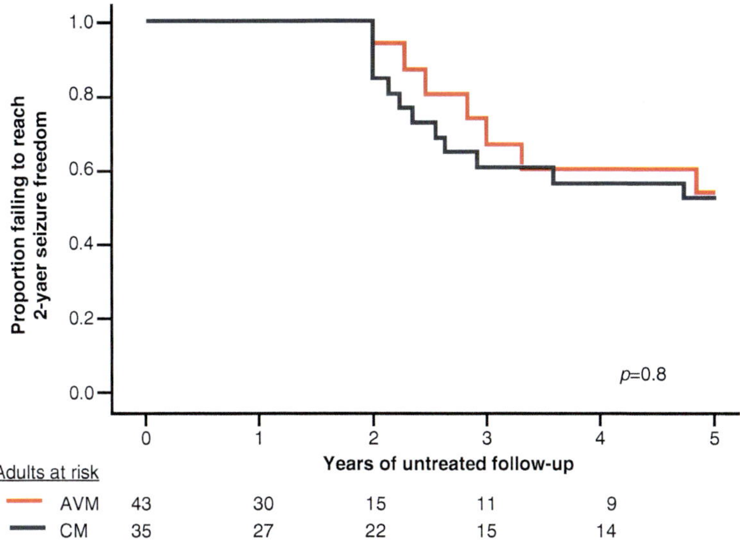


**Fig. 4.6** Chance of epilepsy after first unprovoked CCM related seizure 94%. Chance of seizure free 2 year survival after first unprovoked CCM related seizure 45%. Response to antiepileptic drug medication after first unprovoked CCM related seizure 45%–60%. Reprint with permission from: Josephson CB, Leach JP, Duncan R. Seizure risk from cavernous or arteriovenous malformations. Neurology 2011;76:1548–1554 [62]

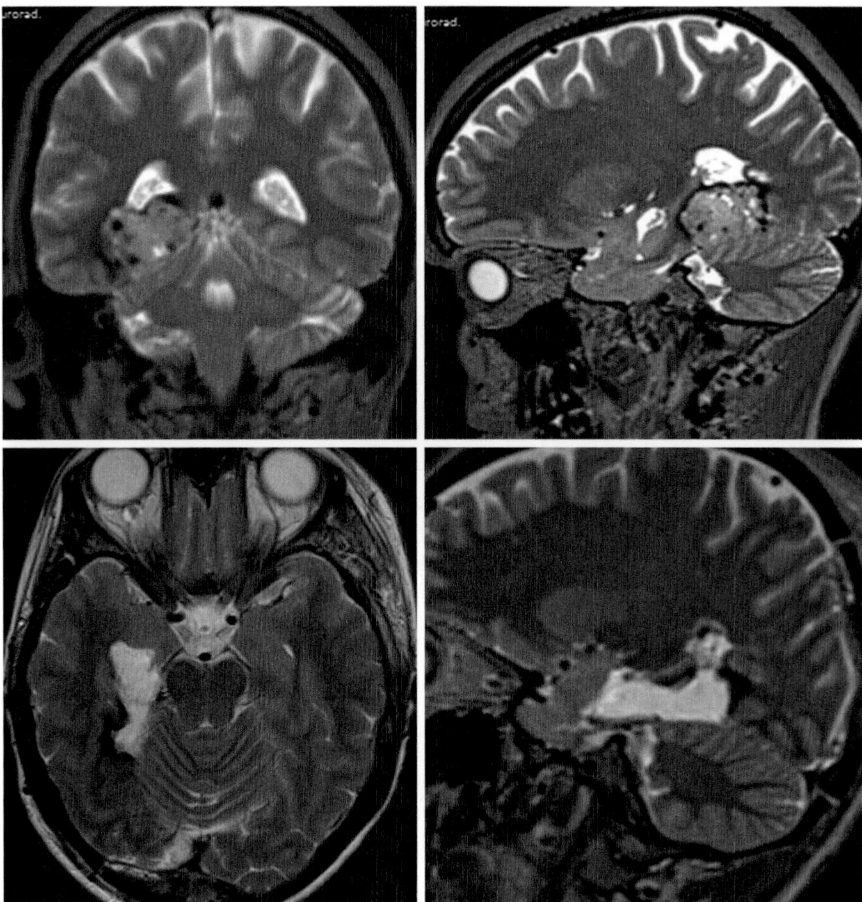

**Fig. 4.7** Illustrative case 3. Cavernoma related epilepsy. A 38 year old mother of two children was referred with an 11 years clinical history of temporal lobe seizures that began at the age of 27. Seizures usually started with an ascending epigastric aura followed by oroalimentary automatisms lasting for less than 5 min. During seizure activity she was disoriented with inadequately reduced responsiveness. During her second pregnancy, the seizure rate increased to one seizure per week. Antiepileptic mediation resulted in a reduced seizure frequency but did not result in seizure control. Neuropsychological testing disclosed both a decline in figural memory as well as an above-average verbal memory. Presurgical epilepsy monitoring localized an epileptic focus in the right temporal lobe and cranial MRI demonstrated an almost 4 cm large CCM in the right parahippocampal gyrus with signs of parenchymal hemosiderin staining in the surrounding temporomesial structures. Surgery was performed with the patient in a modified right sided park bench position with the head turned 45° towards the floor. A right occipital paramedian craniotomy allowed for a retractorless microsurgical CCM resection followed by disconnection of the right hippocampus. Postoperative MRIs demonstrated complete resection of the CCM. Two years later the patient was seizure free without antiepileptic medication. Neuropsychologic testing disclosed further improvements in figural memory

- Established risk factors for cavernoma related epilepsy [CRE] are supratentorial CCM location, cortical CCM involvement, and archicortical/mesiotemporal CCM location.
- The risk to develop CRE varies between 1.5% and 2.4% per patient year. The risk of recurrent seizures is around 94%. The chance of achieving 2 year seizure freedom is around 47%.

# References


1. Jellinger K. Vascular malformations of the central nervous system: a morphological overview. Neurosurg Rev. 1986;9:177–216.
2. Russel DS, Rubinstein IJ. Pathology of tumours of the nervous system. 4th ed. Baltimore: Williams & Wilkins; 1977. p. 116–45.
3. Zabramski JM, Wascher TM, Spetzler RF, et al. The natural history of familial cavernous malformations: results of an ongoing study. J Neurosurg. 1994;80:422–32.
4. Batra S, Lin D, Recinos PF, et al. Cavernous malformations: natural history, diagnosis and treatment. Nat Rev Neurol. 2009;5:659–70.
5. Little JR, Awad IA, Jones SC. Vascular pressures and cortical blood flow in cavernous angioma of the brain. J Neurosurg. 1990;73:555–9.
6. Morris Z, Whiteley WN, Longstreth WT Jr, et al. Incidental findings on brain magnetic resonance imaging: systematic review and meta-analysis. BMJ. 2000;339:b3016.
7. Otten P, Pizzolato GP, Rilliet B, et al. 131 cases of cavernous angioma (cavernomas) of the CNS, discovered by retrospective analysis of 24,535 autopsies. Neurochirurgie. 1989;35:82–3.
8. Al-Holou WN, O'Lynnger TM, Pandey AS, et al. Natural history and imaging prevalence of cavernous malformations in children and young adults. J Neurosurg Pediatr. 2012;9:198–205.
9. Bertalanffy H, Benes L, Miyazawa T, et al. Cerebral cavernomas in the adult. Review of the literature and analysis of 72 surgically treated patients. Neurosurg Rev. 2002;25:1–53.
10. Gross BA, Lin N, Du R, et al. The natural history of intracranial cavernous malformations. Neurosurg Focus. 2011;30(6):E24.
11. Brown RD Jr, Wiebers DO, Torner JC, et al. Incidence and prevalence of intracranial vascular malformations in Olmsted County, Minnesota, 1965 to 1992. Neurology. 1996;46:949–52.
12. Al-Shahi R, Bhattacharya JJ, Currie DG. Prospective, population-based detection of intracranial vascular malformations in adults: the Scottish Intracranial Vascular Malformation Study (SIVMS). Stroke. 2003;34:1163–9.
13. Choquet H, Pawlikowska L, Lawton MT, et al. Genetics of cerebral cavernous malformations: current status and future perspectives. J Neurosurg Sci. 2015;59:211–20.
14. Pagenstecher A, Stahl S, Sure U, et al. A two-hit mechanism causes cerebral cavernous malformations: complete inactivation of CCM1, CCM2, or CCM 3 in affected endothelial cells. Hum Mol Genet. 2009;18:911–8.
15. Flemming KD, Bovis GK, Meyer FB. Aggressive course of multiple de novo cavernous malformations. J Neurosurg. 2011;115:1175–8.
16. Flemming KD, Link MJ, Christianson TJ, et al. Prospective haemorrhage risk of intracerebral cavernous malformations. Neurology. 2012;78:632–6.
17. Gastelum E, Sear K, Hills N, et al. Rates and characteristics of radiographically detected intracerebral cavernous malformations after cranial radiation therapy in pediatric cancer patients. J Child Neurol. 2015;30:842–9.
18. Al-Shahi R, Hall JM, Horne MA. Untreated clinical course of cerebral cavernous malformations: a prospective, population-based cohort study. Lancet Neurol. 2012;11:217–24.

19. Moore SA, Brown RD, Christianson T, et al. Long-term natural history of incidentally discovered cavernous malformation in a single-center cohort. J Neurosurg. 2014;120:1188–92.
20. Kim DS, Park YG, Choi JU. An analysis of the natural history of cavernous malformations. Surg Neurol. 1997;48:9–17.
21. Robinson JR, Awad IA, Little JR. Natural history of the cavernous angioma. J Neurosurg. 1991;75:709–14.
22. Kondziolka D, Lunsford LD, Kestle JRW. The natural history of cerebral cavernous malformations. J Neurosurg. 1995;83:820–4.
23. Labauge P, Brunerau L, Lévy C, et al. The natural history of familial cerebral cavernomas: a retrospective MRI study of 40 patients. Neuroradiology. 2000;42:327–32.
24. Moriarity JL, Wetzel M, Clatterbuck RE, et al. The natural history of cavernous malformations: a prospective study of 68 patients. Neurosurgery. 1999;44:1166–73.
25. Washington CW, McCoy KE, Zipfel GJ. Update on the natural history of cavernous malformations and factors predicting aggressive clinical presentation. Neurosurg Focus. 2010;29(3):E7.
26. Horne MA, Flemming KD, Su I, et al. Clinical course of untreated cerebral cavernous malformations: a meta-analysis of individual patient data. Lancet Neurol. 2016;15:166–73.
27. Al-Shahi R, Berg MJ, Morrison L, et al. Hemorrhage from cavernous malformations of the brain. Definition und reporting standards. Stroke. 2008;39:3222–30.
28. Leigh R, Wityk RJ. Special problems in cavernous malformations: migraine, pregnancy, hormonal replacement, anticoagulation, NSAIDs. In: Rigamonti D, editor. Cavernous malformations of the central nervous system. Cambridge: Cambridge University Press; 2011. p. 185–91.
29. Gross BA, Du R. Cerebral cavernous malformations: natural history and clinical management. Expert Rev Neurother. 2015;15:1–7.
30. Del Curling O Jr, Kelly DL Jr, Elster AD. An analysis of the natural history of cavernous angiomas. J Neurosurg. 1991;75:702–8.
31. Porter PJ, Willinsky RA, Harper W, et al. Cerebral cavernous malformations: natural history and prognosis after clinical deterioration with or without haemorrhage. J Neurosurg. 1997;87:190–7.
32. Akers A, Al Shahi SR, Awad IA, et al. Synopsis of guidelines for the clinical management of cerebral cavernous malformations: consensus recommendations based on systematic literature review by the angioma alliance scientific advisory board clinical experts panel. Neurosurgery. 2017;80:665–76.
33. Aiba T, Tanaka R, Koike T, et al. Natural history of intracranial cavernous malformations. J Neurosurg. 1995;83:56–9.
34. Taslimi S, Modabbernia A, Amin-Hanjani S, et al. Natural history of cavernous malformation. Systematic review and meta-analysis of 25 studies. Neurology. 2016;86:1984–91.
35. Fritschi JA, Reulen HJ, Spetzler RF, et al. Cavernous malformations of the brain stem: a review of 139 cases. Acta Neurochir. 1994;130:35–46.
36. Wang CC, Liu A, Zhang JT, et al. Surgical management of brain-stem cavernous malformations: report of 137 cases. Surg Neurol. 2003;59:444–54.
37. Porter RW, Detwiler PW, Spetzler RF, et al. Cavernous malformations of the brainstem: experience with 100 patients. J Neurosurg. 1999;90:50–8.
38. Li D, Hao SY, Jia GJ, et al. Hemorrhage risks and functional outcomes of untreated brainstem cavernous malformations. J Neurosurg. 2014;121:32–41.
39. Pozzati E. Thalamic cavernous malformations. Surg Neurol. 2000;53:30–9.
40. Gross BA, Batjer HH, Awad IA, et al. Cavernous malformations of the basal ganglia and thalamus. Neurosurgery. 2009;65:7–18.
41. Gross BA, Smith ER, Scott RM, et al. Cavernous malformations of the basal ganglia in children. J Neurosurg Pediatr. 2013;12:171–4.
42. Steinberg GK, Chang SD, Gewirtz RJ, et al. Microsurgical resection of brainstem, thalamic and basal ganglia angiographically occult vascular malformations. Neurosurgery. 2000;46:260–70.
43. Mathiesen T, Edner G, Kihlström L, et al. Deep and brainstem cavernomas: a consecutive 8-year series. J Neurosurg. 2003;99:31–7.

44. Akbostanci MC, Ygĭt A, Ulkatan S, et al. Cavernous angioma presenting with hemidystonia. Clin Neurol Neurosurg. 1998;100:234–7.
45. Lorenzana L, Cabezudo JM, Porras LF, et al. Focal dystonia secondary to cavernous angioma of the basal ganglia: case report and review of the literature. Neurosurgery. 1992;31:1108–11.
46. Carpay HA, Arts WF, Kloet A. Hemichorea reversible after operation in a boy with cavernous angioma in the head of caudate nucleus. J Neurol Neurosurg Psychiatry. 1994;57:1547–8.
47. Donmez B, Cakmur R, Uysal U, et al. Putaminal cavernous angioma presenting with hemichorea. Mov Disord. 2004;19:1379–80.
48. Carella F, Caraceni T, Girotti F. Hemichorea due to a cavernous angioma of the caudate. Case report of an aged patient. Ital J Neurol Sci. 1992;13:783–5.
49. López-Valdés E, Posada IJ, Muñoz A, et al. Acute hemichorea caused by a cavernous angioma in the caudate. Neurologia. 1998;13:205–6.
50. Yakinci C, Durmaz Y, Korkut M, et al. Cavernous hemangioma in a child presenting with hemichorea: response to pimozide. J Child Neurol. 2001;16:685–8.
51. Hidaka M, Shimoda M, Sato O, et al. Case report: hemiballism due to a putaminal cavernous hemangioma. No To Shinkei. 1989;41:1135–9.
52. Mizutani T, Goldberg HI, Kerson LA, et al. Cavernous hemangioma in the diencephalon. Arch Neurol. 1981;38:379–82.
53. Rosenow F, Alonso-Vanegas MA, Baumgartner C, et al. Surgical task force, commission on therapeutic strategies of the ILAE. Cavernoma-related epilepsy: review and recommendations for management-report of the surgical task force of the ILAE commission on therapeutic strategies. Epilepsia. 2013;54:2025–35.
54. Leone MA, Ivashynka AV, Tonini MC, ARES (Alcohol Related Seizures) study group, et al. Risk factors for a first epileptic seizure symptomatic of brain tumour or brain vascular malformation. A case control study. Swiss Med Wkly. 2011;141:w13155.
55. Awad I, Jabbour P. Cerebral cavernous malformations and epilepsy. Neurosurg Focus. 2006;21(1):e7.
56. Reid SA, Sypert GW, Boggs WM. Histopathology of the ferric-induced chronic epileptic focus in cat: a Golgi study. Exp Neurol. 1979;66:205–19.
57. Willmore LJ, Sypert GW, Munson JB. Recurrent seizures induced by cortical iron injection: a model of posttraumatic epilepsy. Ann Neurol. 1978;4:329–36.
58. Clatterbuck RE, Eberhart CG, Crain BJ, et al. Ultrastructural and immunocytochemical evidence that an incompetent blood-brain barrier is related to the pathophysiology of cavernous malformations. J Neurol Neurosurg Psychiatry. 2001;71:188–92.
59. von Essen C, Rydenhag B, Nystrom B, et al. High levels of glycine and serine as a cause of the seizure symptoms of cavernous angiomas? J Neurochem. 1996;67:260–4.
60. Lange SC, Neafsey EJ, Wyler AR. Neuronal activity in chronic ferric chloride epileptic foci in cats and monkey. Epilepsia. 1980;21:251–4.
61. Menzler K, Chen X, Thiel P, et al. Epileptogenicity of cavernomas depends on (archi-) cortical localization. Neurosurgery. 2010;67:918–24.
62. Josephson CB, Leach JP, Duncan R. Seizure risk from cavernous or arteriovenous malformations. Neurology. 2011;76:1548–54.
63. Al-Shahi R. The outlook for adults with epileptic seizure(s) associated with cerebral cavernous malformations or arteriovenous malformations. Epilepsia. 2012;53(Suppl.4):34–42.
64. Josephson CB, Rosenow F, Al-Shahi SR, et al. Intracranial vascular malformations and epilepsy. Semin Neurol. 2015;35:224–34.
65. Fisher RS, van Emde BW, Blume W, et al. Epileptic seizures and epilepsy: definitions proposed by the International League Against Epilepsy (ILAE) and the International Bureau for Epilepsy (IBE). Epilepsia. 2005;46:470–2.
66. Stavrou I, Baumgartner C, Frischer JM, et al. Long-term seizure control after resection of supratentorial cavernomas: a retrospective single-center study in 53 patients. Neurosurgery. 2008;63:888–96.

67. Kwan P, Arzimanoglou A, Berg AT, et al. Definition of drug resistant epilepsy: consensus proposal by the ad hoc task force of the ILAE commission on therapeutic strategies. Epilepsia. 2010;51:1069–77.
68. Casazza M, Broggi G, Franzini A, et al. Supratentorial cavernous angiomas and epileptic seizures: preoperative course and postoperative outcome. Neurosurgery. 1996;39:26–32.
69. Chang EF, Gabriel RA, Potts MB, et al. Seizure characteristics and control after microsurgical resection of supratentorial cerebral cavernous malformations. Neurosurgery. 2009;65:31–7.
70. Stefan H, Walter J, Kerling F, et al. Supratentorial cavernoma and epileptic seizures. Are there predictors for postoperative seizure control? Nervenarzt. 2004;75:755–62.
71. Cappabianca P, Alfieri A, Maiuri F, et al. Supratentorial cavernous malformations and epilepsy: seizure outcome after lesionectomy on a series of 35 patients. Clin Neurol Neurosurg. 1997;99:179–83.
72. Schroeder HW, Gaab MR, Runge U. Supratentorial cavernous angiomas and epileptic seizures: preoperative course and postoperative outcome. Neurosurgery. 1997;40:885.
73. Yeon JY, Kim JS, Choi SJ, et al. Supratentorial cavernous angiomas presenting with seizures: surgical outcomes in 60 consecutive patients. Seizure. 2009;18:14–20.

# Chapter 5
# Neuroimaging of Cerebral Cavernous Malformations

Ioannidis Ioannis, Nasis Nikolaos, and Andreou Alexandros

## 5.1 Introduction

Cerebral cavernous malformations (CCMs), also known as cavernous angiomas, cavernomas, «occult» or cryptic vascular malformations is a distinct vascular disorder that occur mainly in the brain and less often in the spinal cord [1, 2]. They are one of the four major types of vascular malformations, together with developmental venous anomalies, arteriovenous malformations and capillary telangiectasias [3].

CCMs occur in 0.4–0.8% of the general population according to series of autopsies, and they account for 5–15% of all cerebral vascular malformations. They are also the second most common type of vascular malformations after developmental venous anomalies (DVAs) which are often found in association with cavernous malformations [1, 4]. There is no male or female preponderance and usually appear between the second and fifth decade of life [5].

CCMs occur in two forms: (a) a sporadic, and (b) a familial form. Multiple lesions are more often occur in familial cases (90%), and in around 12–20% of sporadic cases [6].

The typical size of CCMs range from 0.01 to 1.7 cm [4]. In rare instances CCMs grow to very large sizes without any major associated symptoms, eventually becoming giant CCMs. Dimensional threshold although not well defined, is widely accepted to be 6 cm. However, only 10% of lesions remain stable overtime: 35% increase and 55% decrease during a mean follow-up of 2 years. The dynamic behavior exhibited by these lesions is likely the result of both hemorrhage and hemorrhage resolution, as well as the disordered growth of their cells of origin [6].

I. Ioannis (✉) · N. Nikolaos · A. Alexandros
Department of Neurosurgery & Interventional Neuroradiology, Hygeia Hospital,
Marousi, Athens, Greece
e-mail: iioannidis@hygeia.gr

© Springer Nature Switzerland AG 2020
O. Bradáč, V. Beneš (eds.), *Cavernomas of the CNS*,
https://doi.org/10.1007/978-3-030-49406-3_5

CMs are more often supratentorial (65–80%) than infratentorial [4]. Frontal and temporal lobes are the most common supratentorial locations, while pons and cerebellum are the most common infratentorial locations. Cavernomas have been reported in many different locations. Intraventricular CCMs are rare, accounting for 2–10% of patients with cerebral cavernomas. Subarachnoid, subdural and even extradural lesions as well as lesions in the cavernous sinus have been reported [7].

CMs may be found in association with other vascular malformations like developmental venous anomaly (DVA) in 8%–36% of lesions, or capillary telangiectasia [4]. When associated with DVAs, CMs are more likely to bleed. This has been attributed to a higher intraluminal pressure within the lesion associated with DVA [8].

Histologically, cavernomas are composed of dilated, blood-filled vascular channels, variable in size (30–50 μm) lined by a thin and weak endothelium. They typically lack mural elements of mature vascular structures, predisposing to hemorrhage [9]. The main histological feature of cavernomas is the absence of intervening parenchymal tissue, which distinguishes these lesions from capillary telangiectasias [2]. They are not encapsulated, but well separable from brain parenchyma. However, the surrounding brain is gliotic, and it is usually stained with hemosiderin from prior hemorrhages. Blood flow across CCMs is slow and as a result, intraluminal thrombosis of varying stages is usually identified. Calcifications are common both within vessel walls and within the adjacent parenchyma [10].

Very rarely, CCMs present as cystic lesions. Recurrent minor, local hemorrhage within the sinusoids is considered as possible cause. Various features of cystic degeneration may be seen (multiple cysts within the solid component of the CCM, or large cyst in combination with small nodules) [11].

Many patients with CCMs are asymptomatic and incidentally discovered during radiological investigation. The incidence of asymptomatic cavernomas is not precisely known, but according to several reports it seems to be as high as 40% [4, 5]. Seizures are reported as the most common symptom (38–55%), followed by focal neurological deficits in 12–45%, acute haemorrhage in 4–32%, and chronic headaches in 5–52% [12]. Clinically evident hemorrhage is the most concerning presentation of CCMs. The estimated annual risk of symptomatic hemorrhage from CCMs is in the range 0.5%–1.1% per year for each lesion [5, 13].

## 5.2   Neuroimaging

Neuroimaging plays a crucial role in diagnosis and follow-up of CCMs. Prior to the advent of computed tomography (CT), and MRI the diagnosis of CCMs was challenging. These lesions are not generally detected on angiograms because of very slow blood flow or spontaneous thrombosis. CT has a low sensitivity, especially in small lesions. On the other hand, MRI is now considered as the imaging modality of choice for detection and characterization of CCMs [14] (Fig. 5.1).

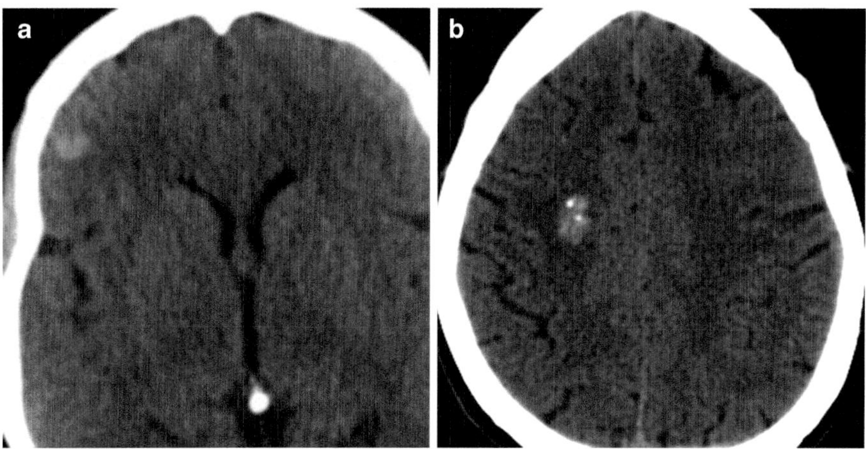

Fig. 5.1 Computed tomography (CT) appearance of cerebral cavernous malformations (CCMs). (a) Head non-contrast CT shows a mildly hyperdense lesion in the right frontal lobe. (b) CT shows a hyperdense right frontal white matter lesion with focal calcification. None of these lesions is associated with adjacent edema or mass effect

## 5.3 Cerebral Angiography

CCMs are typically not seen during conventional digital subtraction angiography (DSA) and are therefore classically referred to as occult or cryptic lesions. This is the result of small feeding arteries or draining veins, slow-flow, and thrombi within vascular spaces [14].

An avascular mass with displacement of adjacent vessels, more prominent if the lesion has hemorrhaged, can sometimes be identified. In less than 10% an abnormal capillary blush into the late venous phase can be demonstrated [15]. Increased sensitivity for a blush has been reported with prolonged injection. Despite advances in angiographic techniques, studies report approximately 20–85% of cases failed to exhibit abnormal angiographic findings or findings are not specific, and therefore DSA plays little if any role in the diagnosis of CCMs [1].

Angiography is indicated mainly for the evaluation of cerebral hematoma when the diagnosis of CCMs is uncertain by MRI or CT, but it is not recommended as part of the standard evaluation of CCMs [16].

## 5.4 Computed Tomography (CT)

CT scans with or without contrast administration are often normal and detects only 30–50% of CCMs, especially in the absence of recent hemorrhage or calcification, and if the lesion is small (<1 cm) [17].

CT findings are often nonspecific and depend on the amount of internal thrombosis, hemorrhage and calcification. If the lesion is large enough it appears as a hyperdense, well-circumscribed lesion, sometimes with internal calcifications. Because the density of blood on CT depends on clot formation, the attenuation of a cavernoma changes with time [14]. There is usually no mass effect, or perilesional edema (Fig. 5.1). In patients with recent hemorrhage the cavernoma may be visible as a lesion with a distinct density, located eccentrically in the hematoma.

Minimal or no enhancement is evident following intravenous contrast administration.

Differential diagnosis from calcified brain tumors, mainly oligodendrogliomas is often challenging [1, 14].

## 5.5  Magnetic Resonance Imaging (MRI)

MR imaging is both sensitive and specific for the detection, characterization and follow-up of CCMs [1, 18].

The appearance of cavernomas varies depending on the stage of the hemorrhage and the sequence utilized. Additionally, high-field MR imaging at 3.0 Tesla provides better resolution of CCMs than that on 1.5-Tesla images [16, 19].

Conventional MR imaging sequences (T2 weighted fast spin echo and T1-weighted fast spin echo) can accurately identify CCMs and provide useful information about the morphology and the age of the blood products associated with these lesions [20, 21]. A typical cavernoma have a popcorn-like appearance with a well delineated reticulated nucleus of mixed signal intensities on T2WI, representing blood products in different stages of evolution within variable sized caverns, and different velocities of blood flow [14]. The heterogeneous core is surrounded by hemosiderin deposition in the adjacent brain parenchyma due to repeated microhemorrhages, and manifests as a peripheral ring of hypo-intensity on T2WI and to a lesser extent on T1WI (Figs. 5.2, 5.3, 5.4, and 5.5). Overall, the combination of the mixed signal core with a rim of decreased signal intensity is highly suggestive of cavernomas [1]. CCMs with subacute hemorrhage are hyperintense on T1-WI. Perilesional edema or significant mass effect are usually not present, unless acute hemorrhage has occurred [21].

The most sensitive sequence to detect CCMS is gradient echo T2*-weighted studies [22, 23]. CCMs demonstrate greater signal loss on T2* weighted GRE (Fig. 5.4), compared to spin-echo sequences [23]. This is due to the greater sensitivity of gradient-echo technique to paramagnetic susceptibility effect associated with blood breakdown products including hemosiderin. Thus, gradient-echo imaging is

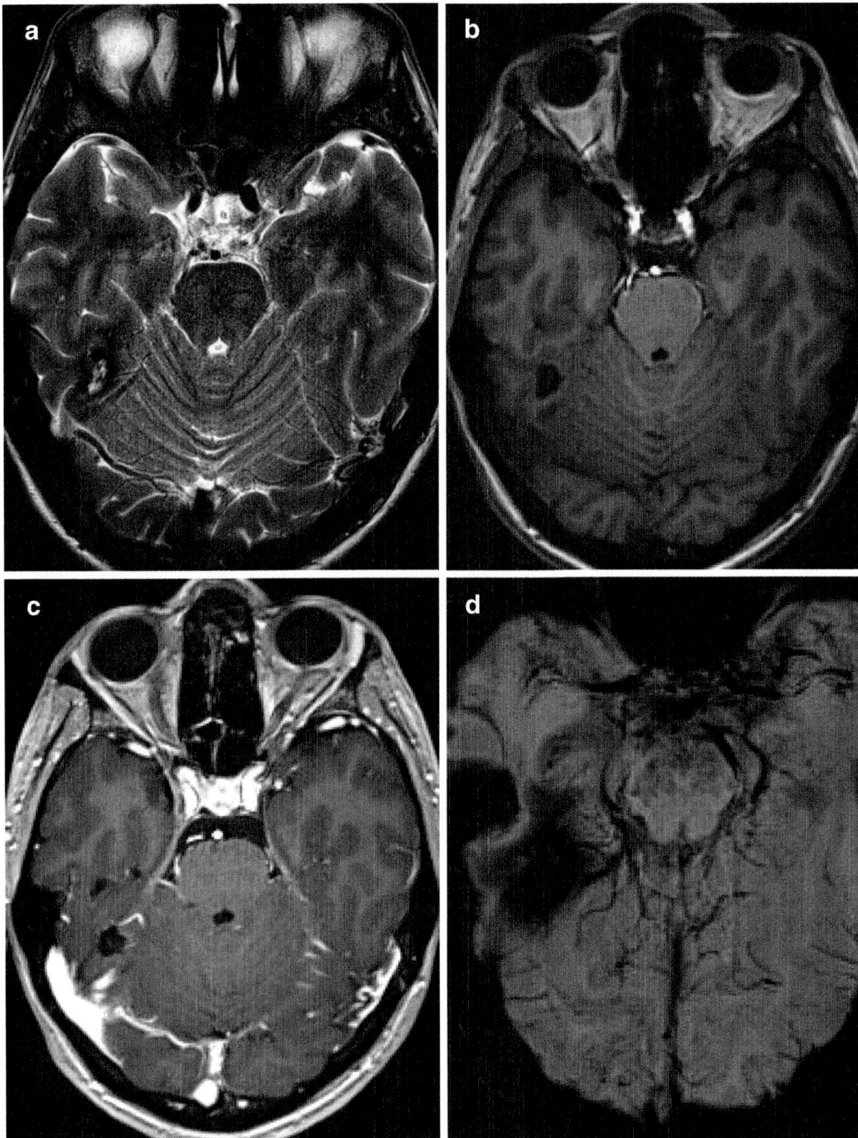

**Fig. 5.2** MRI appearance of a classic right temporal lobe cavernoma on various pulse sequences. Axial T2—weighted (**a**) and T1-weighted (**b**) images show the typical mixed popcorn pattern of a cavernoma. The heterogeneous core and peripheral dark rim of hemosiderin is much more visible on T2-weighted image. Post-gadolinium T1-weighted image (**c**) does not show any significant enhancement. The susceptibility-weighted image (**d**) shows a blooming artifact, which is denoted by the large area of dark signal

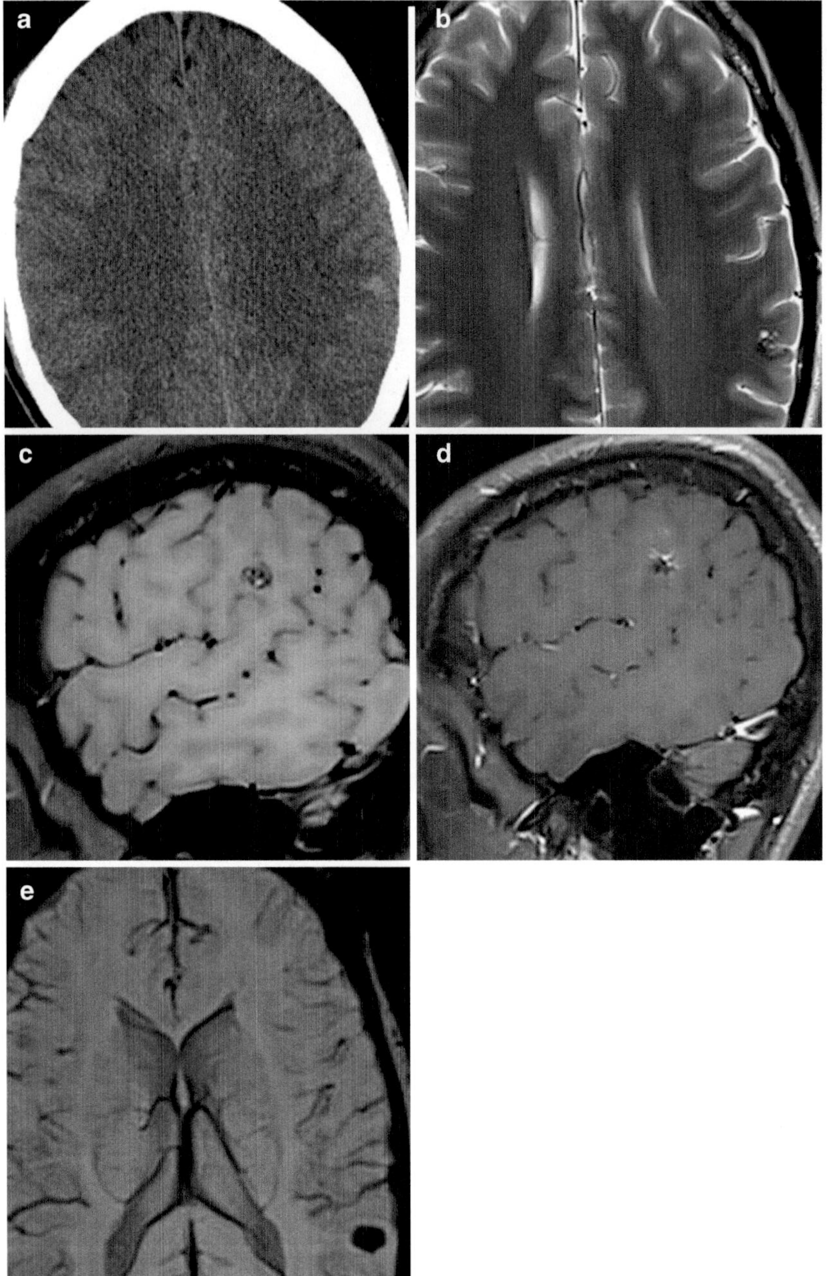

**Fig. 5.3** Cavernous malformations as depicted on CT and MRI. CT (**a**) shows a small mildly hyperdense lesion without surrounding edema and mass effect in the left parietal lobe. T2-weighted (**b**) and T1-weighted (**c**) MR images show the characteristic appearance of a cavernoma. On the post-gadolinium T1-weighted image (**d**) branching venous structures representing developmental venous anomaly adjacent to the cavernous malformation. More exaggerated dark signal is seen on susceptibility-weighted imaging (**e**)

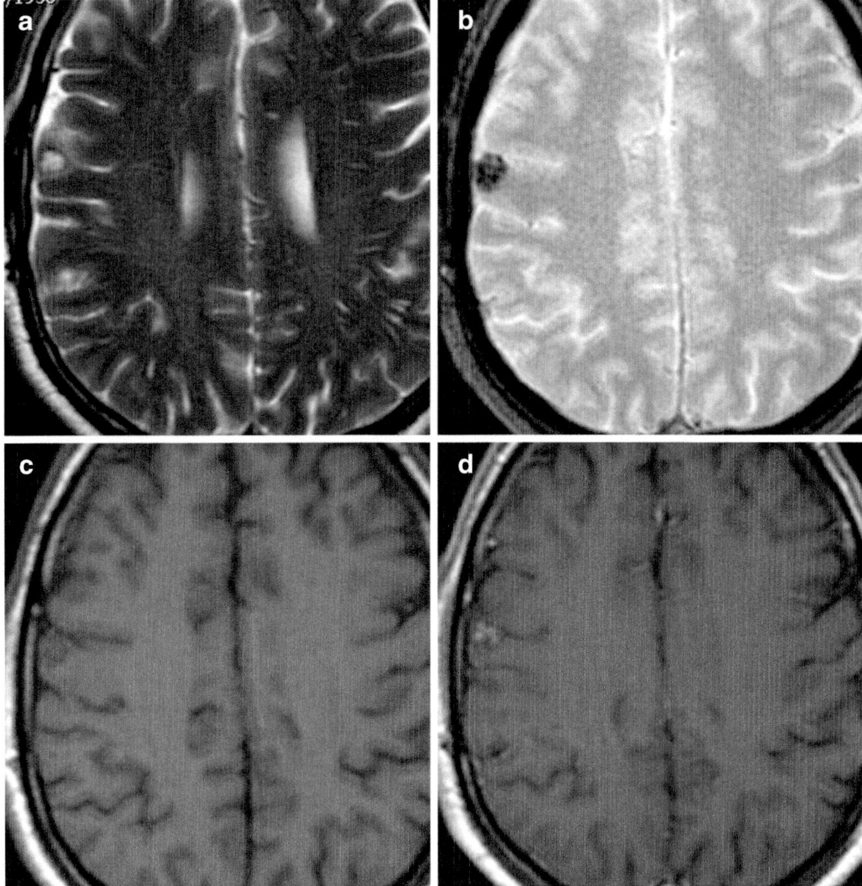

**Fig. 5.4** Cavernoma in various MR pulse sequences. (**a**) T2W images show the typical appearance with a hyperintense core and a peripheral dark rim due to hemosiderin. (**b**) T2* GRE sequence shows a larger area of dark signal due to. susceptibility artifact. (**c**) T1 W image and image show an iso- to slightly hypointense relative to the adjacent brain parenchyma lesion. Small cavernomas can easily be missed. (**d**) Post-gadolinium T1 W image shows inhomogeneous central enhancement

the sequence of choice for demonstrating multiple small lesions which are characteristic of the familial type of CCMs and they are not detected with standard spin-echo protocols [23]. Susceptibility-weighted imaging (SWI) is assembled from both magnitude and phase images from a high-resolution, 3D velocity-compensated GRE sequence. The SWI sequence is more sensitive than the GRE T2* sequence in detecting CCMs [24] (Figs. 5.2 and 5.3). A threefold increase in the number of CCMs detected on SWI images compared to T2*-weighted GRE images has been reported. Moreover, SWI can delineate the margins of lesions better than a conventional T2* gradient-echo sequence and detects the peripherally located CCMs better.

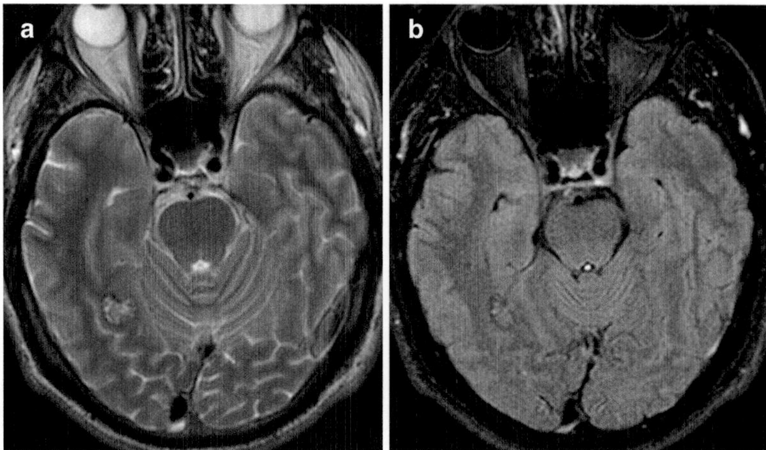

**Fig. 5.5** Right temporal lobe cavernoma. (**a**) T2-weighted image shows the hyperintense core and the peripheral dark rim. (**b**) T2-weighted FLAIR image shows the hyperintense central area. The hemosiderin hypointense rim is usually not clearly depicted

CCMs demonstrate variable contrast enhancement on MRI, ranging from none to moderate [21] (Fig. 5.4). It has been reported that delayed contrast enhancement is evident in most of the lesions, and it is therefore necessary to delay the interval between contrast injection and the start of the scanning procedure [14, 25]. Contrast-enhanced MR however might be useful in revealing concomitant DVAs or capillary telangiectasias [21] (Figs. 5.3 and 5.7).

Cystic degeneration of CCMS is very unusual and the radiographic appearance vary widely from a cystic lesion accompanied by a characteristic nodule to a heterogeneous mass composed of both components.

CCMs have been classified into four types based on MRI findings and pathological features [26]. **Type I** lesions are characterized by subacute hemorrhage and demonstrate a hyperintense core on T1WI and mixed hyper-/hypointense on T2WI (Figs. 5.6 and 5.8). In **Type II** lesions, loculated areas of hemorrhage of varying age are surrounded by gliotic parenchyma and hemosiderin. Type II lesions on both T1 and T2 WI demonstrate a reticulated core with mixed-signal intensity, with a well-circumscribed hypointense ring, mainly on T2 WI, reflecting hemosiderin stain. The **Type III** lesions are iso- or hypointense on T1WI and hypointense on T2WI in and around the lesions compatible with chronic hemorrhage or hemosiderin. **Type IV** lesions are poorly visualized on T1 and T2 and are best seen as punctate hypointense foci on gradient echo sequences. The clinical significance of the MR classification is unclear, although it has been reported a correlation between clinical severity and the appearance on MRI. Patients with type I or II had a significantly

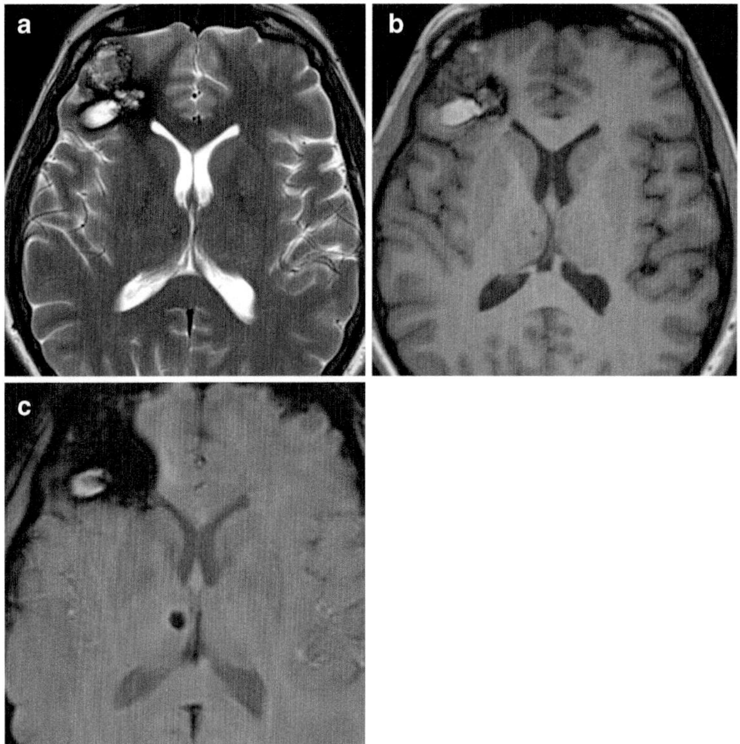

**Fig. 5.6** Right frontal cavernoma. (**a**) T2-weighted image, (**b**) T1-weighted image demonstrate the characteristic features of the lesion, and (**c**) SWI shows a 'blooming artifact'. An area of hyperintensity on both T2 and T1—weighted images suggestive of subacute (extracellular methemoglobin) blood products are also present. SWI shows an additional right thalamic dark lesion, less apparent in the T2 and T1 weighted images

higher hemorrhage rate than type III and IV [26, 27] (Figs. 5.2, 5.3, 5.4, 5.5, 5.6, 5.7, and 5.8).

MRI is the modality of choice and a typical CCM can easily be recognized [20]. The diagnosis with certainty may be problematic when an acute hematoma is present, because the appearance may be distorted. In an acute intracerebral hematoma MRI should be performed as early as possible. Evidence of former, repeated episodes of hemorrhage, the presence of a characteristic hemosiderin ring, and encapsulation are indicative of an underlying CCM. In patients with intracerebral hematoma but with imaging non-pathognomonic of a cavernoma, follow-up MRI is suggested, if immediate surgical intervention is not warranted.

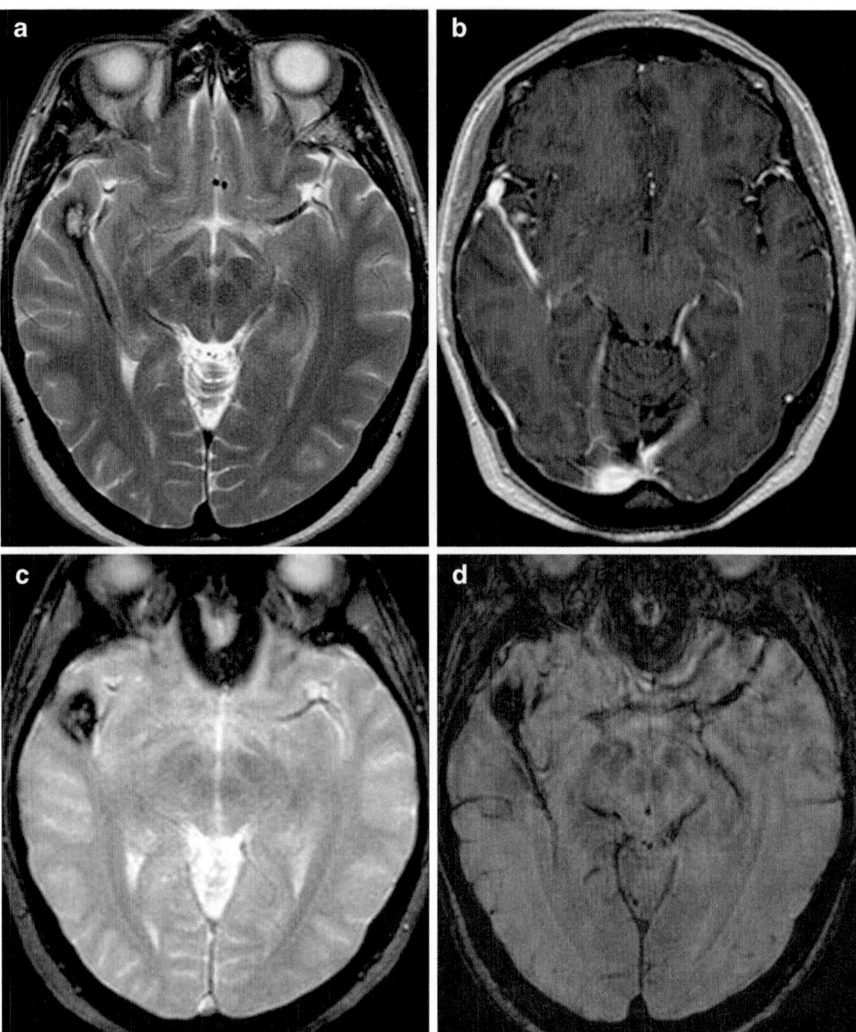

**Fig. 5.7** Magnetic resonance imaging appearance of a right temporal lobe cavernous malformation with a coexisting developmental venous anomaly (DVA) on various pulse sequences. (**a**) T2-weighted image shows the typical the popcorn appearance of a cavernoma with a peripheral hypointense rim. A curvilinear flow void is depicted adjacent to the cavernoma. (**b**) On contrast enhanced T1-weighted image the cavernoma shows a punctate area of enhancement centrally. There is, however, linear enhancement of the adjacent venous structure. The latter feature is consistent with a coexisting DVA. Cavernoma is better depicted on SWI (**d**) than on T2* GRE scan (**c**). Additionally, SWI shows the DVA

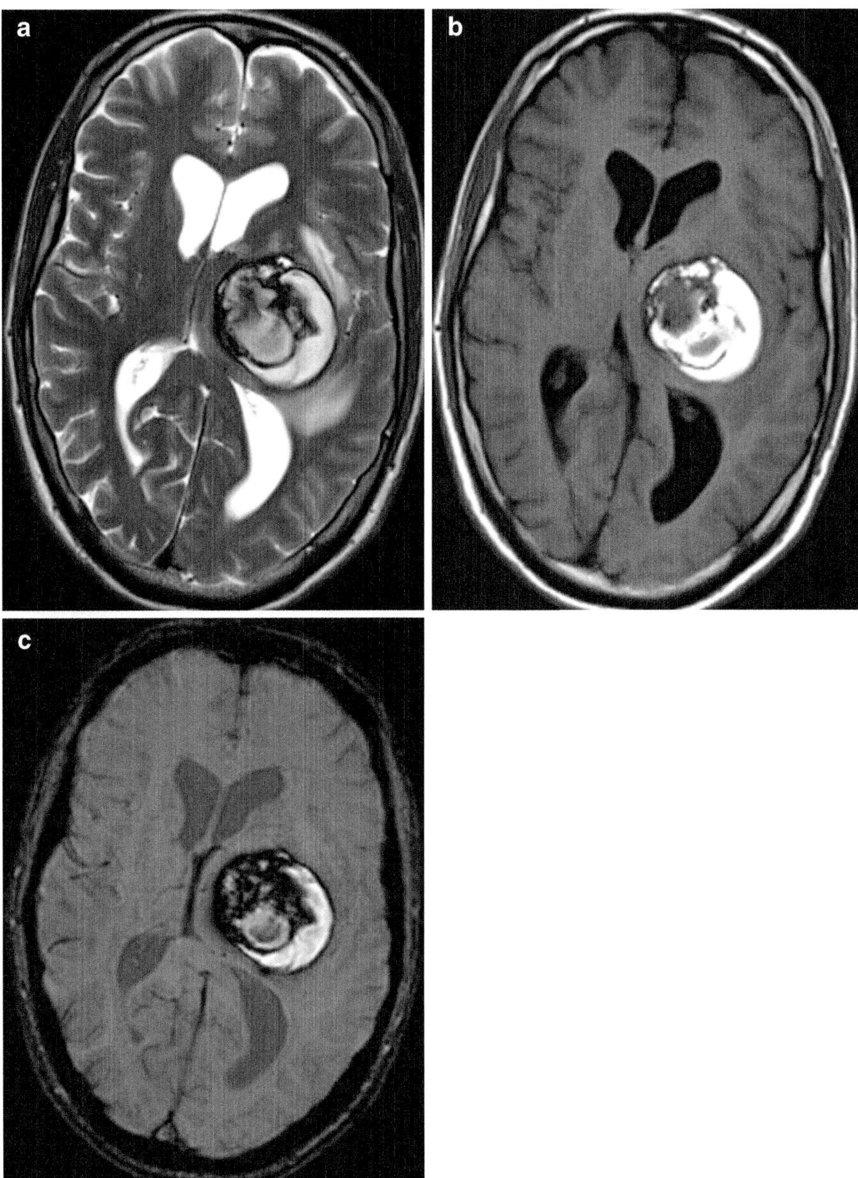

**Fig. 5.8** Symptomatic hemorrhage due to left thalamic cavernoma. (**a**) T2-weighted MR imaging, (**b**) T1-weighted MR imaging and (**c**) susceptibility weighted image show a multilobulated intra-parenchymal hematoma with mild mass effect and perifocal edema. Blood products at various stages can be observed which is indicative of a cavernous malformation than of other types of vascular malformations. Surgical pathology confirmed that the lesion was a cavernous malformation

# References


1. Wang KY, Idowu OR, Lin DDM. Radiology and imaging for cavernous malformations. Handb Clin Neurol. 2017;143:249–66.
2. Dillon WP. Cryptic vascular malformations: controversies in terminology, diagnosis, pathophysiology, and treatment. Am J Neuroradiol. 1997;18:1839–46.
3. McCormick WF. The pathology of vascular ("arteriovenous") malformations. J Neurosurg. 1966;24:807–16.
4. Maraire JN, Awad IA. Intracranial cavernous malformations: lesion behavior and management strategies. Neurosurgery. 1995;37:591–605.
5. del Curling O, Kelly DL, Elster A. An analysis of the natural history of cavernous angiomas. J Neurosurg. 1991;75:702–8.
6. Clatterbuck RE, Moriarity JL, Elmaci I, Lee RR, Breiter SN, Rigamonti D. Dynamic nature of cavernous malformations: a prospective magnetic resonance imaging study with volumetric analysis. J Neurosurg. 2000;93(6):981–6.
7. Engelmann R, Batra S, Li A, Camara-Quintana J, Rigamonti D. Epidemiology and natural history of cavernous malformations. In: Rigamonti D, editor. Cavernous malformations of the nervous system. Cambridge: Cambridge University; 2011. p. 9–14.
8. Abdulrauf S, Kaynar M, Awad I. A comparison of the clinical profile of cavernous malformations with and without associated venous malformations. Neurosurgery. 1999;44:41–46; discussion 46–47.
9. McCormick WF, Hardman JM, Boulter TR. Vascular malformations ("angiomas") of the brain, with special reference to those occurring in the posterior fossa. J Neurosurg. 1968;28:241–51.
10. Batra S, Crain B, Engelmann R, Camara-Quintana J, Rigamonti D. Pathology of cavernous malformations. In: Rigamonti D, editor. Cavernous malformations of the nervous system. Cambridge: Cambridge University; 2011. p. 1–7.
11. Kim IC, Kwon KY, Rhee JJ, Lee JW, Hur JW, Lee HK. Giant cystic cerebral cavernous malformation with multiple calcification - case report. J Cerebrovasc Endovasc Neurosurg. 2013;15(3):255–9.
12. Batra S, Lin D, Recinos PF, Zhang J, Rigamonti D. Cavernous malformations: natural history, diagnosis and treatment nature reviews. Neurology. 2009;5:659–70.
13. Robinson JR, Awad IA, Little JR. Natural history of the cavernous angioma. J Neurosurg. 1991;75:709–14.
14. Küker W, Forsting M. Cavernomas and capillary telangiectasias. In: Forsting M, Wanke I, editors. Intracranial vascular malformations and aneurysms. From diagnostic work-up to endovascular therapy. 2nd ed. Berlin: Springer. p. 19–50.
15. Savoiardo M, Strada L, Passerini A. Intracranial cavernous hemangioma: neuroradiologic review of 36 operated cases. Am J Neuroradiol AJNR. 1983;4:945–50.
16. Cortés Vela JJ, Concepción Aramendía L, Ballenilla Marco F, Gallego León JI, González-Spínola San Gil J. Cerebral cavernous malformations: spectrum of neuroradiological findings. Radiologia. 2012;54(5):401–9.
17. Vaquero J, Salazar J, Martínez R, Martínez P, Bravo G. Cavernomas of the central nervous system: clinical syndromes, CT scan diagnosis and prognosis after surgical treatment. Acta Neurochir. 1987;85:29–33.
18. Rigamonti D, Drayer BP, Johnson PC, et al. The MRI appearance of cavernous malformations (angiomas). J Neurosurg. 1987;67:518–24.
19. Novak V, Chowdhary A, Abduljalil A, Novak P, Chakeres D. Venous cavernoma at 8 Tesla MRI. Magn Reason Imaging. 2003;21(9):1087–9.
20. Lin DDM, Abdalla W. Neuroimaging of cavernous malformations. In: Rigamonti D, editor. Cavernous malformations of the nervous system. Cambridge: Cambridge University; 2011. p. 49–63.
21. Batra S, Lin D, Recinos PF, et al. Cavernous malformations: natural history, diagnosis and treatment. Nat Rev Neurol. 2009;5:659–70.

22. Labauge P, Laberge S, Brunereau L, et al. Hereditary cerebral cavernous angiomas: clinical and genetic features in 57 French families. Societe Francaise de Neurochirurgie. Lancet. 1998;352:1892–7.
23. Brunereau L, Leveque C, Bertrand P, et al. Familial form of cerebral cavernous malformations: evaluation of gradient-spin-echo (GRASE) imaging in lesion detection and characterization at 1.5T. Neuroradiology. 2001;43:973–9.
24. Lee BC, Vo KD, Kido DK, et al. MR high-resolution blood oxygenation level-dependent venography of occult (low-flow) vascular lesions. Am J Neuroradiol. 1999;20:1239–42.
25. Thiex R, et al. Giant cavernoma of the brain stem: value of delayed MR imaging after contrast injection. Eur Radiol. 2003;13(Suppl 6):L219–25.
26. Zabramski JM, Wascher TM, Spetzler RF, et al. The natural history of familial cavernous malformations: results of an ongoing study. J Neurosurg. 1994;80:422–32.
27. Nikoubashman O, Di Rocco F, Davagnanam I, Mankad K, Zerah M, Wiesmann M. Prospective hemorrhage rates of cerebral cavernous malformations in children and adolescents based on MRI appearance. Am J Neuroradiol. 2015;36(11):2177–83.

# Chapter 6
# Natural History of Cavernous Malformations

**Juri Kivelev and Mika Niemelä**

## 6.1 Epidemiology

Among the vascular malformations of the brain and spine, cavernomas constitute 10–15% [1]. Their incidence in the general population is estimated to range between 0.16% and 0.8% [2–8]. Prior to modern imaging, the diagnosis of cavernoma was rare and usually confirmed only at operative exploration or autopsy. Several classic autopsy studies have reported the incidence of cavernomas in the general population. In 1984, McCormick found 19 cavernomas in 5.734 autopsies reporting an incidence of 0.34% [4]. Just a few years later, in a consecutive series of 24.535 autopsies, Otten et al. reported 131 cavernoma cases, yielding an incidence of 0.53% [9]. With the advent of MRI in clinical practice reliable imaging of the cavernoma in living persons became possible, and a fairly similar incidence was noted. In 1991, Del Curling et al. analyzed 8131 MRIs and found 32 cavernomas, the incidence thus being 0.39% [2]. In the same year, Robinson et al. published their work, where 14.035 MRIs were reviewed and 66 patients with cavernoma were uncovered, yielding an incidence of 0.47% [10]. More recent systematic review and meta-analysis of incidental findings on brain MRI showed 23 cavernomas out of 15,599 participants yielding an incidence of 0.16% [8].

Cavernomas have been reported to occur in all age groups including young children and have been even detected in utero [11–14]. According to Lanzino et al. up to 25% of cavernomas are diagnosed in pediatric age [15]. In the study of 14,936 consecutive patients 25 years of age or younger, Al-Holou et al. showed that imaging prevalence of CM may increase with advancing age during childhood [7].

J. Kivelev (✉)
Department of Neurosurgery, Neurocenter, Turku University Hospital, Turku, Finland

M. Niemelä
Department of Neurosurgery, Helsinki University Hospital, Helsinki, Finland
e-mail: mika.niemela@hus.fi

© Springer Nature Switzerland AG 2020
O. Bradáč, V. Beneš (eds.), *Cavernomas of the CNS*,
https://doi.org/10.1007/978-3-030-49406-3_6

According to their results imaging prevalence of cavernomas in children younger than 1 year was 3.4 times lower when compared to the patients aged 18–25 years. These findings correspond with previously published surgical series of pediatric cavernomas, since most of cavernomas in these studies were diagnosed in the second decade of life [11, 14, 16–19]. Population-based annual detection rate of cavernomas has been estimated at 0.56 per 100,000 per year for adults older than 16 years of age [20]. So far, no population-based studies on the incidence of cavernomas in Finland have been performed. In the neurosurgical department of Helsinki University Central Hospital (serving 1.8 million inhabitants), 383 consecutive patients with cavernoma were treated over the 30 years. This represents a cumulative incidence of 0.62% in this given district during 30 years. Taking into account, that the Finnish population is epidemiologically quite homogeneous the same incidence probably exists in other parts of the country.

## 6.2   The Role of Pathologic Features in Understanding Natural History

According to the pathological classification of neurovascular malformations suggested by McCormick in 1966, lesions are divided to five major groups: (1) teleangiectasias; (2) varices; (3) cavernous malformations; (4) arteriovenous malformations (AVMs); and (5) venous angiomas [21]. This classification has thereafter been modified: varices (varicose veins) have been combined with venous malformations/venous angiomas, and such lesions have been renamed to developmental venous anomaly (DVA). Although pathological criteria have been suggested for every type of malformation their structural criteria and nomenclature are somewhat ambiguous and variable. Furthermore, reports of transitional or mixed forms exist in the literature and all of the above-mentioned malformations can coexist with each other.

From a macroscopic viewpoint, cavernomas are well-defined lesions and because of their lobulated appearance often resemble a mulberry (Fig. 6.1). They do not invade the neural tissue. In contrast to AVMs, large feeding arteries or draining veins are not common; therefore, blood flow inside the lesion is low. Their mean size is usually 1–2 cm, with a range from punctate to gigantic examples. The biggest lesion in our practice was 5 cm in diameter. There are anecdotal cases of huge lesions, with the cavernoma occupying an entire lobe or even several lobes of the brain [22, 23].

In fact, in 2008, Kan et al. published an overview of 36 collected cases of giant cavernomas emphasizing the extreme rarity of such lesions [24]. Although no agreement exists regarding terminology, the authors applied the term "giant cavernoma" to lesions exceeding 4 cm in diameter, which seems to be rational. Despite of generally accepted opinion of more aggressive clinical course in large and giant lesions, the natural history of these type of cavernomas remain uncovered.

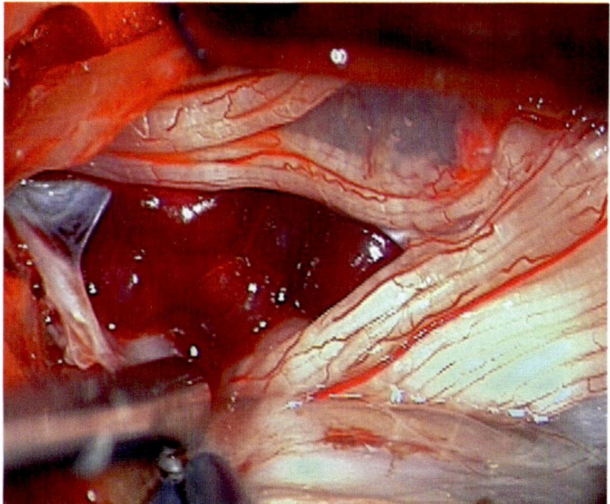

**Fig. 6.1** Intraoperative view of the spinal cavernoma surrounded by nerve roots

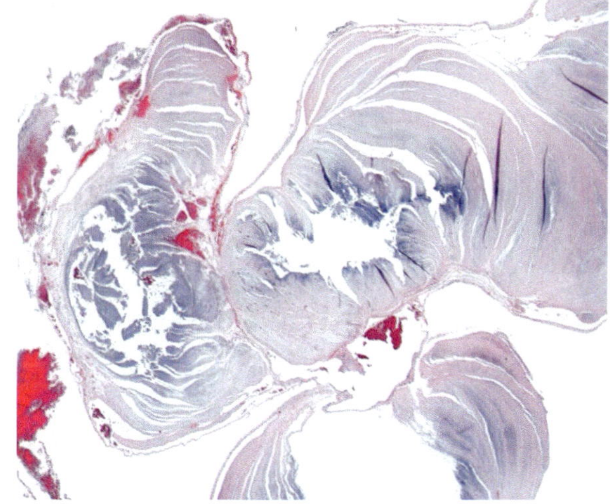

**Fig. 6.2** Microscopic view of a cavernoma. The dilated vessels without intervening neural parenchyma are lined by thin endothelium and surrounded by collagenous fibrotic tissue with blue deposits of iron (hemosiderin) after hemorrhages

In a typical case, the lesion's core consists of unequal sinusoids or caverns filled with blood that are separated by fine fibrous strands. Intraluminal thrombosis with subsequent organization is typical and this area appears more solid. Calcifications and even bone formation may also exist [23]. Adjacent neural tissue is very typically discolored due to accumulation of blood breakdown products after repetitive microhemorrhages.

Microscopically, cavernomas are sinusoid structures with thin walls, which are composed of collagen lined by a single layer of endothelium [23]. Outside the lumen there are often macrophages containing iron pigment, hemosiderin, phagocytosed after microbleeds (Fig. 6.2). Electron microscopy has shown that endothelia may be fenestrated or there are gaps at intercellular junction, all these alterations indicating defective blood-brain barrier [25, 26]. The basal lamina outside the endothelium may be lacking or is abnormal, and astrocytic endfeet are often absent.

Vascular permeability and iron leakage seems to play central role in pathogenesis of cavernomas when considering natural history of the disease [27]. Recent advances in MR-imaging with utilization of dynamic contrast-enhanced quantitative permeability (DCEQP) and quantitative susceptibility mapping (QSM) allowed investigation of permeability dynamics in longitudinal clinical studies [27–34]. These studies have shown reliable interobserver and cross-platform agreement and close correlation of QSM with actual iron concentration in resected cavernoma specimens and in phantoms [33]. Furthermore, some studies confirmed higher background brain permeability most notably in white matter away from lesions in familial cases as compared with sporadic cavernomas and non-cavernoma controls, consistent with germline heterozygosity in the former cases [32]. According to Girard et al., significant lesional permeability increases at follow-up correlated with interval hemorrhage or growth [27]. This corresponds with hypothesis that enhanced vascular permeability is associated with and may drive cavernomas hemorrhagic proliferation. Using a high MRI sensitivity technique, authors showed higher regional brain permeability than contralateral homologous regions in anatomical locations initially lacking cavernomas which later developed de novo lesions.

Some histological subtypes of cavernomas have been identified and a certain degree of variability in their natural history has been reported in the literature: (1) *Cystic form*, which is predisposed to bleeding and growth and occurs commonly in the posterior fossa [35, 36]. This form is very rare, and only 25 cases of cystic cavernoma have been reviewed to date [37]. The mechanisms of formation of large cysts are not understood; presumably, osmotic transport of the fluid into the cyst combined with microhemorrhages induces progressive enlargement of the lesion (Fig. 6.3). This type is more frequent in females and elderly patients; (2) *Dural-based form*, which is usually encountered in the middle fossa close to the cavernous sinus or within it, in the cerebellopontine angle, or on the tentorium and convexities,

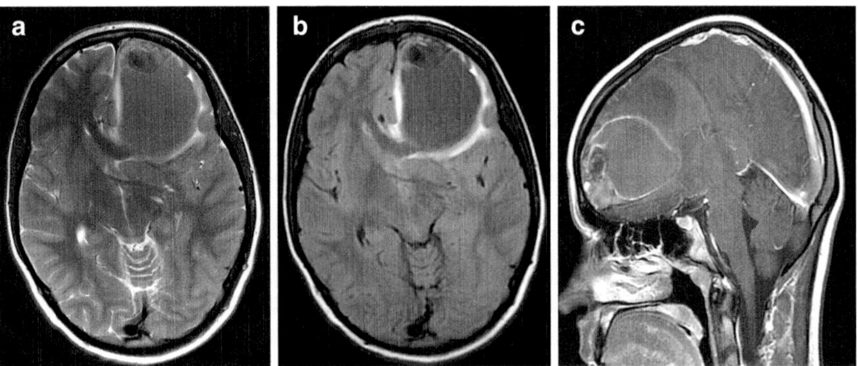

**Fig. 6.3** MRI of the frontal cavernoma with large cystic component. (**a**) T2-weighted image, axial view; (**b**) T1-weighted image, axial view; (**c**) T1-weighted image with Gadolinium contrast, sagittal view

is prone to an aggressive clinical course [38–41]. Middle fossa lesions may have abundant vascular supply and tend to bleed profusely when excised [41]; (3) *Hemangioma calcificans* is typically found in the temporal lobe and, as reflected by its name, is strongly calcified with a low risk of hemorrhage, while still being highly epileptogenic [42].

## *6.2.1   Associated Vascular Abnormalities*

Natural history of cavernomas may be affected by associated vascular abnormalities. The most frequent entity associated with cavernomas appears to be DVA [43–45]. It may be found in up to 25% of cavernoma patients [46, 47]. Previous studies have shown conjunction of cavernoma development with venous architecture or pathophysiology related to DVA [46, 48–50]. Brinjikji et al. in their study performed in Mayo clinic hypothesized that the prevalence of DVA-associated cavernomas increases with age [51]. This trial included 1689 individuals with 116 being affected by DVA-associated cavernomas. Authors could identify strong statistically significant association between age and the prevalence of DVA-associated cavernomas. Indeed, in the group of 0–10 year-old patients the prevalence of DVA-associated cavernomas was 0.8% but in the group of patient older than 70 years respective jumped to 11.6% [51]. Based on these findings authors concluded that (1) DVA-associated cavernomas are not congenital lesions, (2) de novo cavernomas' formation associated with DVA is likely the rule rather than exception, (3) various age-related changes in the cerebral venous system could trigger the formation of cavernomas associated with DVA [51]. These conclusions are consonant with previous reports where the trigger for microhemorrhages is generally thought to be local venous hypertension resulting from local thrombosis, stenosis or changes in DVA architecture [43] Moreover, severe medullary venous tortuosity, medullary venous stenosis or sharp angles between radicular vein and the dominant medullary venous drainage are associated with a higher prevalence of cavernomas associated with DVA [52, 53] Dammann et al. utilized 7-Tesla MRI in their study of DVA-associated cavernomas showing a strong correlation of a typical DVA with the cavernomas at the same draining territory with negative genetic screening thus indicating sporadic disease [54]. Based on repetitive patterns of distribution over the brain and association/nonassociation with DVA authors suggested naming the patterns cluster type (sporadic form) and scattered-type (familial form). Study results indicated that in patients with cluster-type distribution the existence of an underlying familial form of the disease is extremely unlikely but a scattered-type distribution is suggestive for familial disease [54].

Another common cavernoma-associated vascular abnormality is a capillary teleangiectasia. Some similarities between these malformations (multiplicity, pontine involvement, familial variety) give reason to consider teleangiectasias as a precursor of cavernomas [23, 55].

## 6.3 Genetics and Molecular Biology in Natural History of Cavernomas

Primary evidence of hereditary mechanisms underlying cavernoma formation was elucidated in the early 1980s, when investigators detected several families of Hispanic origin who suffered from cavernomas [56–58]. These studies convincingly showed that cavernomas can present as a familial form with an autosomal dominant pattern of inheritance. Extensive laboratory research has been initiated to address the genetic substrate of this phenomenon, and genes predisposing patients for cavernomas (*CCM1, CCM2 and CCM3*) have been identified (Table 6.1). Already in 1995, Günel et al. discovered *CCM1* confirming genetic mechanism of the disease [60]. All three genes are likely involved in the same molecular pathway providing interplay between the neural and glial elements (neurons and astrocytes) and the endothelium of the CNS [61]. Biallelic somatic mutations of the same genes in cavernoma endothelial cells likely contribute to lesion genesis in both familial and sporadic forms of the disease [62, 63]. Functions of each gene were studied and certain changes in protein interactions and consequent pathologic appearances in cytoarchitecture within the cavernoma were addressed.

**Table 6.1** Genetic background of cavernomas

| [59] Genes, clinical penetrance | Affected chromosome loci | Alternative name | Ultrastructural profile |
|---|---|---|---|
| *CCM1*, 60–88% | 7q21 | KRIT1 (Krev-1 interaction trapped 1) | KRIT1 protein localizes specifically to the vascular endothelium. Expresses in foots processes of astrocytes, forming BBB. Involved in integrin signaling. Encodes a microtubule-associated protein, binds ß-catenin, integrin cytoplasmic domain associated protein-$1\alpha$ (ICAP-$1\alpha$), stabilizes interendothelial junctions associated with actin stress fibers. Involved in angiogenesis. |
| *CCM2*, 100% | 7p13-15 | MGC4607 Malcavernin; OSM (osmosensing scaffold for mitogen-activated protein kinase kinase kinase 3, or MEKK3) | Expressed in arterial and microvascular endothelium, in brain pyramid cells and in astrocytes. Mimics CCM1. Provides cellular responses to osmotic stress, binds CCM1 and MEKK3 acting like scaffolding protein signaling through p38 after extracellular stimulation. p38 pathway involved in cell proliferation and differentiation to apoptosis. Modulates mitogen-activated protein (MAP) kinase and Ras homolog gene family, member A (RhoA) GTPase signaling. Involved in angiogenesis. |
| *CCM3*, 63% | 3q25-27 | PDCD10 (programmed cell death 10) | Provides cell proliferation and transformation, involved in apoptotic signaling, modulates extracellular signal-related kinase (ERK). Involved in angiogenesis. |

The *CCM1* gene (alternative name KRIT 1) is located at chromosome locus 7q and stabilizes the interendothelial junctions associated with actin stress fibers [64]. Through integrin signaling, *CCM1* possibly mediates bidirectional signaling between the extracellular matrix and the cellular cytoskeleton [61]. It is expressed in arterial and microvascular endothelium of the CNS and more than 90 mutations of *CCM1* have been reported [65, 66]. The natural history of cavernomas originated due to *CCM1* seems to be the least severe when compared with *CCM2 and CCM3* gene's mutations [6].The *CCM2* gene (or malcavernin) located at 7p, probably determines cellular responses to osmotic stress [64]. In a study by Plummer et al., *CCM2* expression in the brain was found to be primarily neuronal, but not endothelial [67]. This finding suggests that cavernomas may arise from abnormalities in surrounding neuronal and glial cells rather than in vascular endothelium [68].

The *CCM3* gene is located at the chromosome locus 3q (called programmed cell death 10 or PDCD10) and is encountered in up to 15% of familial cavernomas [69, 70]. It determines cell proliferation and transformation (cancer cell lines), together with modulating extracellular signal-regulated kinase [64]. *CCM3* mutation carries have a greater chance of spontaneous mutation, an increased cavernoma burden and a younger mean age of presentation, which is often associated with clinical hemorrhage. There is also a significant association with other manifestations including skin cavernomas, scoliosis, spinal cord cavernomas, cognitive disability, and benign brain tumor including meningioma, vestibular schwannoma, and astrocytoma. The impact of *CCM3* on the natural history of the disease may be devastating as was shown by Shenkar et al. who found an exceptionally high aggressiveness of the disease in this cohort of patients [70]. According to their study, lesion burden on susceptibility weighted imaging (SWI) MRI was extraordinarily high, with 33% of *CCM3* mutation carriers harboring more than 100 lesions and 78% harboring more than 20 lesions. Mean number of lesions on T2-MRI was 31, whereas the mean lesion count in individuals with *CCM1* and *CCM2* mutations was only 5.1. Moreover, the annual rate of de novo lesions in *CCM3* cohort was eight times as high as in *CCM1* and *CCM2* group (2.36 vs 0.3, respectively) [70].

Carriers of the mutated genes have cavernomas on MRI in up to 69% of cases [59]. Thus, the presence of mutations in the above-mentioned genes is necessary but not sufficient for the development of the cavernoma [71]. Knudson's "two-hit" mechanism, proposed to explain this phenomenon, suggests an external trigger ("second hit") that exacerbates the disease in a given region [64, 71, 72]. Loss of one of the alleles ("first hit") is the result of a germline mutation, and loss of the second allele ("second hit") will occur somatically within the brain [66]. Several factors have been assumed to have "second-hit" abilities. For example, a somatic mutation in the second copy of the gene or a mutation in another gene acting in the same cellular pathway is considered to be the most probable trigger of the disease [64, 73]. Clinical observations of de novo cavernomas after radiotherapy confirm that environmental factors also play a role in "second hits". Angiogenic factors, inflammatory agents and breakdown of the blood-brain barrier may also be responsible for the development of cavernomas [22, 64, 74–77].

## 6.4   Natural History of Irradiation-Induced Cavernomas

Cavernomas are cerebral irradiation-related late complication. Already in 1994, Ciricillo et al. first suggested that cavernomas could be induced by radiotherapy [78, 79]. Later on, Nimjee et al. conducted a literature review on de novo formation of cavernomas after radiation therapy and found 76 patients—most of them children—with different pathologies of the CNS who developed de novo cavernomas [80]. The mean latency period was 8.9 years and the mean radiation dose 60.45 Gy. In recent study of Di Giannatale et al., authors analyzed a cohort of 108 *CCM* gene mutation negative pediatric patients who received brain radiotherapy due to primary tumor and 31.5% of patients developed cavernoma during follow-up [79]. In this study, mean latency period between radiation therapy and the development of the cavernomas was 4.8 years. Interestingly, irradiation in the first decade of life caused cavernomas after a mean follow-up of 5 years and when performed in second decade of life—after a mean of only 3 years follow-up. In 17% of radiation-induced cavernomas, authors found enlargement of the size over time and 7% had bled. There was strong predominance of these cavernomas to occur in hemispheres unlike in basal ganglia or cerebellum. According to authors results, cavernomas occur most frequently after irradiation of medulloblastoma. The vast majority of radiation-induced lesions remain clinically silent and seem to have lower incidence of seizures than sporadic cavernomas. Based on these data, authors recommend close observation for asymptomatic lesions in children.

## 6.5   Radiological Features in View of Natural History Research

In 1956, Crawford and Russel proposed the term "cryptic cerebrovascular malformations", in which cavernomas were traditionally grouped [81]. This subset of neurovascular lesions included cavernomas, thrombosed arteriovenous malformations, venous malformations, capillary teleangiectasias, and other mixed forms. The main reason why these "cryptic" or "occult" lesions got this name was based on their scarce appearance or, more commonly, invisibility in the angiographic view. Although some authors were able to find some prominent draining veins [81] or small homogeneous finely stippled areas of contrast medium, no pathognomonic angiographic features could be shown [82]. Due to the low blood flow inside the nidus, lesions are negative on the CT angiography (CTA), except for large ones that may even displace major vessels causing a mass-effect.Routine use of CT scanning in patients with acute neurological events contributed considerably to preliminary diagnosis of cavernomas. However, the sensitivity of CT in cavernoma diagnostics is low, and specificity ranges from only 30%–50% [81]. A true breakthrough in cavernoma diagnostics began with the widespread use of MR imaging, which appeared to be the most sensitive tool for revealing a cavernoma throughout the cerebrospinal axis. MRI allows cavernomas to be reliably diagnosed not only after acute neurological decline but also in asymptomatic incidental cases. Thus, the number of detected cavernoma patients has increased dramatically and extensive MRI-based epidemiological studies have been performed [2, 10]. The MR appearance of a cavernoma can be quite variable depending commonly on the amount of hemorrhage.

Lesions commonly present in the T1- and T2-weighted sequences with a reticulated "popcorn ball" appearance of mixed hyper- and hypointense blood-containing locules [81]. The hemorrhage-resolving stage significantly affects the MR appearance of the cavernoma, as stated by Zabramski et al. [83]. The authors proposed a practical classification of MR features of cavernomas, corresponding to pathological features of the lesion and including four major types (Table 6.2). Type I lesions represent subacute hemorrhage, which makes them identifiable on CT as well. On T1- and T2-weighted MR images, they are hyperintense at the initial stage, while with hematoma aging and methemoglobin is converted to ferritin and hemosiderin (Fig. 6.4). Changing of paramagnetic features starts from the margin of the

**Table 6.2**  Grading of cavernomas according to MRI appearance as proposed by Zabramski et al.

| Type | MRI features | Pathology features |
|---|---|---|
| I | T1: hyperintense core<br>T2: hyper- or hypointense core | Subacute hemorrhage |
| II | T1: reticulated mixed signal core<br>T2: reticulated mixed signal core with surrounding hypointense rim | Lesions with thrombosis of varying ages |
| III | T1: iso- or hypointense<br>T2: hypointense lesion with hypointense Rim magnifying size of lesion | Chronic hemorrhage with hemosiderin staining within and around lesion |
| IV | T1: not seen<br>T2: not seen<br>GRE: punctate hypointense lesion | Tiny cavernoma or teleangiectasia |

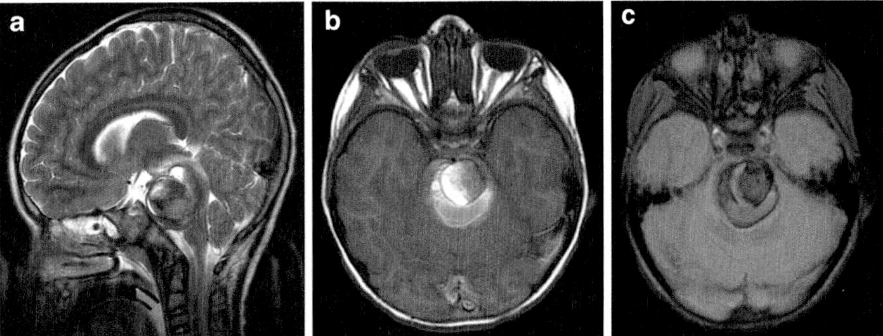

**Fig. 6.4**  MRI of a 4 year-old patient with acute somnolence and hemiparesis. (**a**) T2-weighted image, sagittal view; (**b**) T1 –weighted image, axial view; (**c**) T2*-GRE image showing a pontine cavernoma with a hemorrhage

hematoma, which leads to a decrease in the size of the hyperintense core and the appearance of a hypointense halo around the lesion, known as the hemosiderotic rim. In cases of major extralesional bleeding, a definitive description of the cavernoma apart from the hematoma is seldom possible, usually indicating follow-up imaging and re-evaluation of the lesion. Type II cavernomas constitute the most recognizable group, with a classical reticulated core of mixed signal that is surrounded by a hypointense ring seen in T1- and T2-weighted images (Fig. 6.5). This appearance is considered as a pathognomonic sign of a cavernoma and reflects the existence of partial thrombosis and organization of intralesional blood within the sinusoids sometimes combined with calcification.

Meanwhile, on CT images type II lesions are visualized quite poorly. Type III lesions look hypointense on either T1- or T2-weighted images, representing chronic hemorrhage (Fig. 6.6). They are not identifiable on CT, except for large lesions containing calcifications. Type IV lesions are best visualized on hemosiderin-sensitive sequences, like T2*-gradient echo, and look like punctate hyperintense lesions (Fig. 6.7). Still no consensus exists regarding the pathological substrate of these lesions. Earlier considered as capillary teleangiectasias [55, 83], some recent evidence shows these lesions to be true cavernomas, which can even convert into other radiological types [74]. Type IV lesions more often exist in multiple forms, especially with family history [84]. It was generally accepted that Type IV cavernomas are totally benign lesions which are asymptomatic and do not require any clinical or radiological follow-up. However, in 2013 Nikoubashman et al. published their study confirming that these "black spot" Type IV cavernomas are anything but benign compared to other cavernoma types and should not be underestimated, especially in *CCM* gene mutation carries [85]. Authors analyzed a group of 70 pediatric

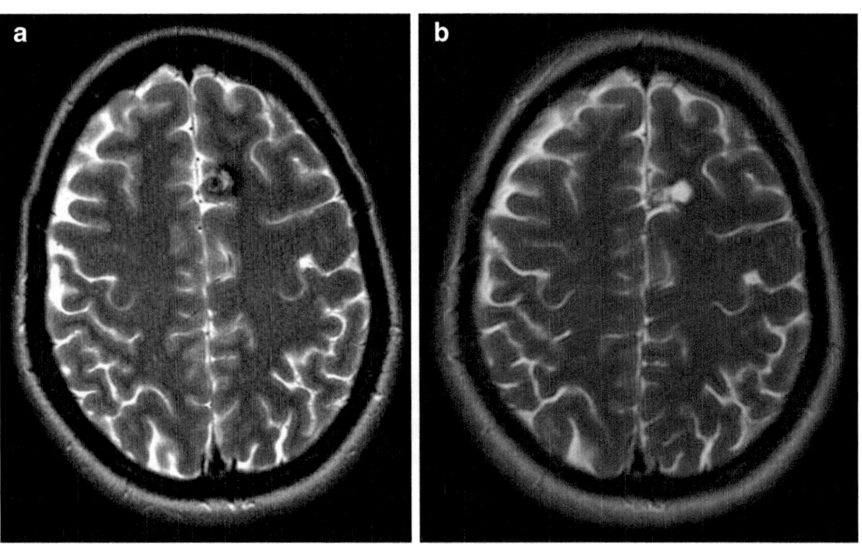

**Fig. 6.5** A type II frontal cavernoma with typical. (**a**) Preoperative view. (**b**) Postoperative view

**Fig. 6.6** Sagittal view of type III frontal "pop-corn" appearance cavernoma. T1-weighted image

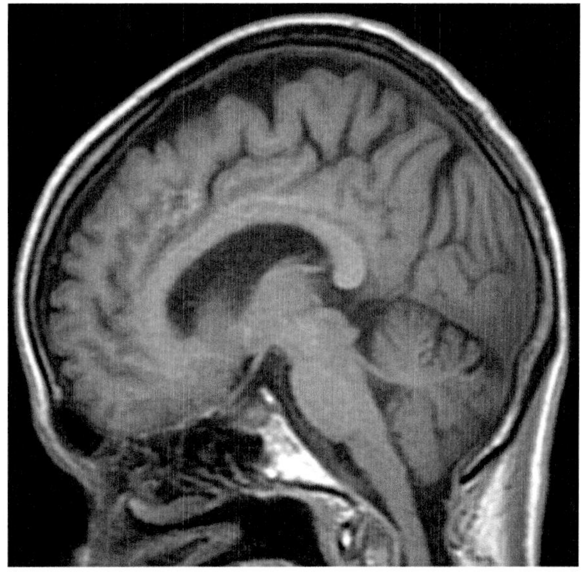

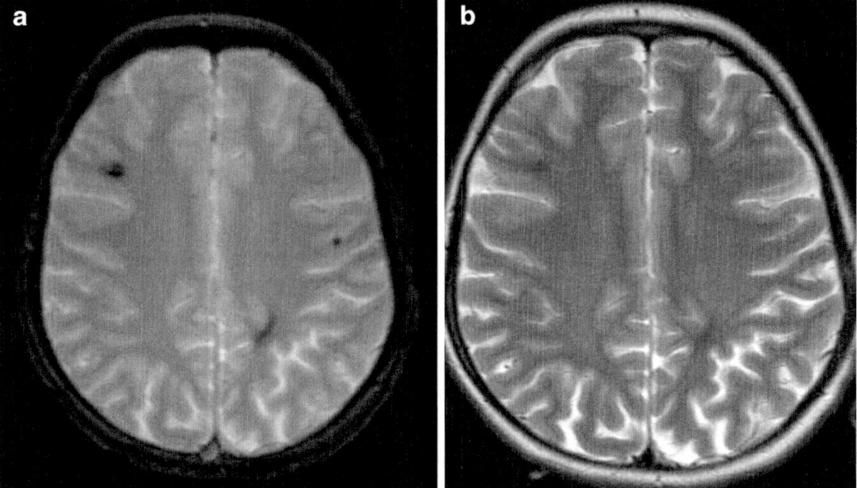

**Fig. 6.7** Left frontal cavernoma of type IV. (**a**) T2*-GRE image, (**b**) T2-weighted image (a lesion is not visible)

patients with 18 individuals having totally 187 Type IV cavernomas. After mean follow-up of 5.5 years authors found 70 de novo lesions and 10 radiological events of hemorrhage thus yielding a hemorrhage rate from Type IV cavernomas of 0.7% per lesion-year. Despite of the fact that authors could not elucidate any evidences of Type IV cavernomas clinical manifestation, their hemorrhage and de novo burden potential obviously should be taken into account when planning treatment strategy.

Based on these finding authors recommend annual MRI-examinations for pediatric patients with black spot cavernomas in strategically important areas, such as, the brainstem, in order to anticipate possible future clinical symptoms [85].

## 6.6 Symptomatology

Cavernomas can be diagnosed at any age, but are most common in individuals aged 20–50 years [3, 82, 86] with a peak at 30 years [66]. They occur in both genders with equal frequency [87] . Most patients present with a sporadic single lesion. Supratentorial lesions comprise 70–90% of all locations [3, 9]. Meanwhile, in 10–40% of cases cavernomas are familial, and thus, often multiple [5, 58]. The natural course of cavernomas seems to be relatively benign. Fatal outcome of the disease is very uncommon, occurring mostly in cases of huge lesions affecting critical brain structures that disrupt after profuse bleeding. Usually, cavernomas are characterized by three major clinical patterns – epileptic disorders, focal neurological deficits, and hemorrhage, which can present separately or in different combinations.

### 6.6.1 *Epileptic Disorders*

Seizures are the most frequent clinical presentation of supratentorial cavernomas, occurring in 41–80% of patients [6, 88, 89]. It is not uncommon that seizures occur after a cavernoma hemorrhage. Interestingly, seizure incidence in patients suffering from AVM is 20–40%, and from gliomas 10–30% which are only half of that in cavernoma patients [90, 91]. Cavernomas do not invade parenchyma and are not intrinsically epileptogenic; thus, epileptogenicity is probably due to perifocal changes in the adjacent brain parenchyma. Typical for cavernoma perifocal collection of blood breakdown products combined with inflammatory alterations and gliotic changes seems to be an organic substrate of epileptogenicity in these patients [88]. Iron ions have a role in producing free radicals and lipid peroxides, which affect functioning of certain cell receptors [92, 93]. The subsequent cascade of changes includes a marked increase in excitatory neurotransmitter amino acids [94]. Such activation has also been discovered in electrophysiological studies, which have shown more than two times higher evoked activity values in cavernoma-neighboring neurons than in cells around glial tumors.

Patients with cavernomas can present with any type of seizures. For unknown reasons, cavernoma-associated seizures are more likely intractable than those related to other vascular malformations [90, 91]. The variability of the seizure disorder may be related to the location of the lesion, its size, history of hemorrhage, and patients' age. For example, temporal lobe lesions tend to cause seizures more frequently and have an obvious propensity to intractable epilepsy [88]. Less favorable seizure outcome was noted in younger persons and women [89]. Long-lasting epileptic disorders with high frequency of seizures in certain cases can lead to development of secondary epileptogenic foci located in remote brain regions [88]. Notably, the risk of recurrent seizures appears to be as high as 5.5% per patient-year [95].

The appearance of the epileptic syndrome in cavernoma patients is not included in the framework of the "all-or-nothing" concept, as patients with supratentorial lesions can be asymptomatic until hemorrhage or some environmental provocative factor triggers epileptic activity. Furthermore, patients with a similar location, size, or radiological appearance of the lesion may have completely different patterns of epilepsy. This variability is sharply emphasized in multiple cavernoma patients, as any of the supratentorial lesions carries a potential risk of epileptogenicity.

To date, there has been only one study examining seizures as an endpoint in cavernoma natural history [6]. Namely, in 2011 Josephson et al. published a prospective population-based study on 139 adults diagnosed with cavernomas and found a 5-year risk of first-ever seizure to be 6% in patients presenting with cavernoma-related intracerebral hemorrhage (ICH) or focal neurological deficit (FND) and 4% in incidentally diagnosed cavernomas [96]. Among the adults who never experienced ICH/FND and presented with or developed epilepsy, the proportion achieving 2-year seizure-free state over 5 years was 47%. Consequently, adult individuals with cavernomas may have a high risk of epilepsy after first-ever seizure and roughly half achieve 2-year seizure freedom over 5 years after epilepsy diagnosis.

### 6.6.2  Focal Neurological Deficits

Appearance of focal neurological deficits in cavernoma patients is not uncommon when lesions affect the motor cortex, speech areas, basal ganglia, brain stem and spinal cord. Due to their relatively small size and slow growth, cavernomas themselves rarely cause fast deterioration, even though patients complain of fluctuating appearance of symptoms with frequent spontaneous relief and subsequent deterioration. Acute decline usually occurs after a cavernoma hemorrhage into surrounding parenchyma, compressing or destroying it.

### 6.6.3  Hemorrhage

Cavernomas have a well-known tendency to bleed. In some very rare cases, hemorrhage can be fatal. Usually it is well tolerated depending on the volume, nearness to critical structures, patients' age, and comorbidities. The term "cavernoma hemorrhage" in the literature is quite confusing and depends on the interpretation of the radiological signs of the lesion on CT and MRI when acute onset of the symptoms occurs. The presence of a thrombus may give a false impression of acute bleeding in projection of the cavernoma. Hemorrhagic events occurring in cavernoma patients are divided into two groups: intra- and extralesional bleeding. An intralesional (or encapsulated) hemorrhage is limited to the border of the lesion and causes enlargement of the cavernoma. Probably, the surrounding hemosiderotic parenchyma, which is strengthened by gliosis, takes a role in preventing the hemorrhage from spreading outside into healthy parenchyma. This can lead to formation of a capsule, which behaves like a membrane of a chronic subdural hematoma, osmotically attracting fluid and leading to enlargement of the cavernoma. A weakened capsule compatible with hemodynamic stress is a possible factor predisposing to more prominent bleeding that invades nearby brain areas [97, 98]. An extralesional (or overt, gross) hemorrhage extends beyond the hemosiderin ring and on MRI shows signs of acute or subacute bleeding (Fig. 6.4). This "true" intracerebral bleeding can cause marked disruption of surrounding tissue and lead to permanent deficits depending on the location. Both intra- and extralesional hemorrhages usually manifest with acute onset of headaches accompanied by focal deficit or seizures.

In the pre-MRI era, within the framework of cryptic vascular malformations, cavernomas were considered lesions with very high hemorrhage potential. Early series showed hemorrhage incidence in cavernoma patients to be up to 65% [99, 100]. However, most of the studies were influenced by significant patient selection bias and mixing of different pathological entities; as a rule, patients were studied after acute symptoms and hemorrhage and could have even had an AVM, which carries a higher risk of profuse hemorrhage than a cavernoma. In more recent studies based on MRI findings with recruited asymptomatic patients, the extralesional hemorrhage rate appears to be quite low, on average 1% per patient-year in lesions with supratentorial location (range 0.25%–2.5%) [2, 10, 20, 83, 101–105] (Table 6.3). In familial cases, bleeding rates may vary depending on the cavernoma

**Table 6.3** Reported symptomatic hemorrhage rates of cerebral cavernomas

| First author, year | Annual hemorrhage rate (%) | Study design |
|---|---|---|
| Del Curling, 1991 | 0.1 | Retrospective |
| Robinson, 1991 | 0.7 | Prospective |
| Zabramski, 1994 | 1.2 | Prospective |
| Kondziolka, 1995 | 1.3 | Retrospective |
| | 2.6 | Prospective |
| | 0.6 | For incidental lesion |
| Aiba, 1995 | 0–0.4 | Prospective |
| Porter, 1999 | 5 | Retrospective |
| | | Brain stem lesion |
| Labauge, 2000 | 2.5 | Retrospective, familial forms |
| Kupersmith, 2001 | 2.46 | Brain stem lesions |
| Labauge, 2001 | 4.3 | Prospective, familial forms |
| Cantu, 2005 | 1.7 | Retrospective, Hispanic population |
| Al-Shahi Salman, 2012 | 0.5 | Prospective |
| Jeon, 2014 | 4.5 | Prospective |

genotype. Notably, Denier et al. in 2006, found that *CCM3* carriers are more prone than *CCM2* and *CCM1* patients to develop cerebral hemorrhages, especially at a younger age [106]. Furthermore, the authors showed that in patients with multiple cavernomas *CCM1* was associated with a higher number of lesions than *CCM2* and *CCM3*. Thus, the overall risk of hemorrhage in these patients is increased due to cumulative risks from each lesion.

Lesions of the infratentorial compartment and particularly the brain stem are characterized by higher bleeding rates than their supratentorial counterparts, ranging from 2.5% to 13.6% per patient-year [107]. Interestingly, larger lesion size (>1 cm), early age at presentation (<35 years), and coexistence of DVA were found to be associated with higher hemorrhage rates [108]. Nevertheless, the mechanisms of higher bleeding risk of cavernomas in infratentorial compartment remain obscure.

After initial decline, caused by extralesional bleeding, many patients recover well, but some can experience re-bleedings. Lesions of the brain stem seem to be more prone to re-bleed. The risk of having recurrent extralesional hemorrhage in this selected group varies from 5.1% to 60% per patient-year [107]. Aiba et al. found that younger women exhibited a higher incidence of re-bleeding, possibly caused by hormonal factors [109]. Of note, Kalani et al. in 2013 showed no increased hemorrhage risk during pregnancy thus concluding that a history of cavernoma is not a contraindication to pregnancy or vaginal delivery [110].

In contrast to previous studies, Barker et al. proposed the concept of temporal clustering of the hemorrhages after the initial event [111]. Using sophisticated statistical analysis in 141 patients, the authors discovered quantitative evidence of a spontaneous decline in the hazard of cavernoma re-hemorrhage approximately 2 years after the first hemorrhage.

According to some case reports, anticoagulant therapy may affect natural history of cavernomas increasing hemorrhage rates [112]. Opposite to that, Schneble et al. in prospective study of 87 cavernoma patients did not explore any additional hemorrhage risk related to anticoagulant therapy [113]. With a general trend towards population aging, the amount of cavernoma patients who need to be treated by anticoagulants will most likely be significantly higher than earlier. In view of modern data, such cavernoma patients do not possess additional risks of clinical deterioration due to hemorrhage and, thus should be managed accordingly. Xie et al. in 2018 summarized published data on hemorrhage risk factors subdividing them into three groups [107]:

1. Hemorrhage risk factors. Include history of previous ictus and location in brainstem.
2. Possible risk factors. Include female sex, younger age, perilesional edema on MRI, large lesion size, co-existence of DVA, hemodynamic change or high blood pressure
3. No risk factors. Include pregnancy, multiplicity, antiplatelet or antithrombotic use.

This simple classification reflects modern understanding of factors which may affect cavernoma natural history. According to these data, only a history of previous hemorrhage and brainstem location constitutes "true" increased risk of re-hemorrhage whereas other variables are not enough strong to change natural history of the disease. Obviously further larger international multicenter prospective studies are needed to have unbiased data on disease course.

## 6.7 Challenges in Natural History Research

Large series of untreated asymptomatic cavernoma patients with long-term follow-up are missing. However, due to advances in neuroradiology, the number of such patients coming to be evaluated in neurosurgical practice is increasing. This is supplemented by the growing amount of cases earlier considered to be rare, and, thus not thoroughly investigated. The comprehensive investigation of disease natural history is obviously of superior interest making cavernoma management safe and effective in each individual case. Modern data suggest cavernomas to be fairly benign lesions which however, may carry risks of epilepsy, hemorrhage, or focal neurological deficits.

Significant drawback of the current research on cavernoma natural history lies in self-limitation of retrospective studies when significant biases are established at primary stage of collecting data. Indeed, even considered incidental, such cavernoma cases represent only a limited subset of disease carrier population. Accumulating literature data shows enormous heterogeneity of genetic, ultrastructural, clinical and radiological features of cavernomas. This may be related not only to intrinsic complexity of the disease but also to biased data collection and over/underestimating of the risks or safety of the pathology. Moreover, data collection may be altered by socio-economic factors and local healthcare system organization issues such as unequal access to MR-imaging in general population. This may obviously disfigure understanding of disease incidence and can cause misinterpretation of factors affecting natural history.

Great variability of factors determining cavernoma natural course justifies a healthy level of skepticism when assessing conclusions of older studies. Alterations in genetic background (e.g. relatively "calm" *CCM1* gene mutations vs. "angry" *CCM3* gene mutations), in MRI features (e.g. Zabramski typing), or differences related to location along neuroaxis (e.g. supratentorial vs. brainstem and spinal cord) constitute enormously ramified summation of different variables of the disease, as we realize nowadays. The exploration and comprehensive analysis of all factors' combinations and interactions was probably the most difficult and hence hardly achievable task in earlier research. Fortunately, modern IT-technologies like "artificial intelligence"-based systems are getting more and more closer to clinical studies. Automatized collection of population-based medical data and thorough analysis of all possible factors in large series of cavernoma patients (Big Data analysis) will allow the results to become obviously more reliable and applicable to each individual patient.

**Key Points**

- Natural history of cavernomas is predetermined by genetics, ultrastructural features, location along the neural axis and hemodynamic alteration in the lesion and surrounding brain. In most cases, cavernomas have benign clinical course.
- Seizures are the most frequent clinical presentation of supratentorial cavernomas, occurring in 41%–80% of patients. Adult individuals may have a high risk of epilepsy after first-ever seizure and roughly half achieve 2-year seizure freedom over 5 years after epilepsy diagnosis.
- Overt cavernoma hemorrhage rate appears to be quite low, on average 1% per patient-year in lesions with supratentorial location (range 0.25%–2.5%). Lesions of the infratentorial compartment and particularly the brain stem are characterized by higher bleeding rates ranging from 2.5% to 13.6% per patient-year.
- A history of hemorrhage and brainstem location increases the risk of hemorrhage. Female sex, younger age, perilesional edema on MRI, large lesion size, co-existence of DVA, hemodynamic change or high blood pressure are possible risk factors for bleeding.

# References


1. Washington CW, McCoy KE, Zipfel GJ. Update on the natural history of cavernous malformations and factors predicting aggressive clinical presentation. Neurosurg Focus. 2010 Sep;29(3):E7.
2. Del Curling O Jr, Kelly DL Jr, Elster AD, Craven TE. An analysis of the natural history of cavernous angiomas. J Neurosurg. 1991 Nov;75(5):702–8.
3. Giombini S, Morello G. Cavernous angiomas of the brain. Account of fourteen personal cases and review of the literature. Acta Neurochir. 1978;40(1–2):61–82.
4. McCormick WF. Pathology of vascular malformations of the brain. In: Wilson CB, Steihn BM, editors. Intracranial arteriovenous malformations. Baltimore: Williams & Wilkins; 1984.
5. Pozzati E, Acciarri N, Tognetti F, Marliani F, Giangaspero F. Growth, subsequent bleeding, and de novo appearance of cerebral cavernous angiomas. Neurosurgery 1996;38(4):662–9; discussion 669-70.
6. Akers A, Al-Shahi Salman R, Awad IA, Dahlem K, Flemming K, Hart B, et al. Synopsis of guidelines for the clinical management of cerebral cavernous malformations: consensus recommendations based on systematic literature review by the Angioma Alliance Scientific Advisory Board Clinical Experts Panel. Neurosurgery. 2017;80(5):665–80.
7. Al-Holou WN, O'Lynnger TM, Pandey AS, Gemmete JJ, Thompson BG, Muraszko KM, et al. Natural history and imaging prevalence of cavernous malformations in children and young adults. J Neurosurg Pediatr. 2012;9(2):198–205.
8. Morris Z, Whiteley WN, Longstreth WT Jr, Weber F, Lee YC, Tsushima Y, et al. Incidental findings on brain magnetic resonance imaging: systematic review and meta-analysis. BMJ. 2009 Aug 17;339:b3016.
9. Otten P, Pizzolato GP, Rilliet B, Berney J. 131 cases of cavernous angioma (cavernomas) of the CNS, discovered by retrospective analysis of 24,535 autopsies. Neurochirurgie. 1989;35(2):82–3. 128–31.
10. Robinson JR, Awad IA, Little JR. Natural history of the cavernous angioma. J Neurosurg. 1991 Nov;75(5):709–14.

11. Bhardwaj RD, Auguste KI, Kulkarni AV, Dirks PB, Drake JM, Rutka JT. Management of pediatric brainstem cavernous malformations: experience over 20 years at the hospital for sick children. J Neurosurg Pediatr. 2009 Nov;4(5):458–64.
12. Kon T, Mori H, Hasegawa K, Nishiyama K, Tanaka R, Takahashi H. Neonatal cavernous angioma located in the basal ganglia with profuse intraoperative bleeding. Childs Nerv Syst. 2007 Apr;23(4):449–53.
13. Gangemi M, Longatti P, Maiuri F, Cinalli G, Carteri A. Cerebral cavernous angiomas in the first year of life. Neurosurgery 1989;25(3):465–8; discussion 468-9.
14. Scott RM, Barnes P, Kupsky W, Adelman LS. Cavernous angiomas of the central nervous system in children. J Neurosurg. 1992 Jan;76(1):38–46.
15. Lanzino G, Spetzler RF, editors. Cavernous malformations of brain and spinal cord. New York: Thieme; 2008.
16. Abla AA, Lekovic GP, Turner J, de Oliveira JG, Porter R, Spetzler RF. Advances in the treatment and outcome of brain stem cavernous malformation surgery: a case series of 300 surgically treated patients. Neurosurgery. 2011 Feb;68:403–14.
17. Herter T, Brandt M, Szuwart U. Cavernous hemangiomas in children. Childs Nerv Syst. 1988 June;4(3):123–7.
18. Lee JW, Kim DS, Shim KW, Chang JH, Huh SK, Park YG, et al. Management of intracranial cavernous malformation in pediatric patients. Childs Nerv Syst. 2008 Mar;24(3):321–7.
19. Xia C, Zhang R, Mao Y, Zhou L. Pediatric cavernous malformation in the central nervous system: report of 66 cases. Pediatr Neurosurg. 2009;45(2):105–13.
20. Al-Shahi Salman R, Hall JM, Horne MA, Moultrie F, Josephson CB, Bhattacharya JJ, et al. Untreated clinical course of cerebral cavernous malformations: a prospective, population-based cohort study. Lancet Neurol. 2012 Mar;11(3):217–24.
21. McCormick WF, Nofzinger JD. "Cryptic" vascular malformations of the central nervous system. J Neurosurg. 1966 May;24(5):865–75.
22. Gault J, Awad IA, Recksiek P, Shenkar R, Breeze R, Handler M, et al. Cerebral cavernous malformations: somatic mutations in vascular endothelial cells. Neurosurgery 2009;65(1):138–44; discussion 144-5.
23. Russel DS, Rubenstein LJ, editors. Pathology of tumors of the nervous system. 5th ed. Baltimore: Williams & Wilkins; 1989.
24. Kan P, Tubay M, Osborn A, Blaser S, Couldwell WT. Radiographic features of tumefactive giant cavernous angiomas. Acta Neurochir 2008;150(1):49–55; discussion 55.
25. Tu J, Stoodley MA, Morgan MK, Storer KP. Ultrastructural characteristics of hemorrhagic, nonhemorrhagic, and recurrent cavernous malformations. J Neurosurg. 2005 Nov;103(5):903–9.
26. Clatterbuck RE, Moriarity JL, Elmaci I, Lee RR, Breiter SN, Rigamonti D. Dynamic nature of cavernous malformations: a prospective magnetic resonance imaging study with volumetric analysis. J Neurosurg. 2000 Dec;93(6):981–6.
27. Girard R, Fam MD, Zeineddine HA, Tan H, Mikati AG, Shi C, et al. Vascular permeability and iron deposition biomarkers in longitudinal follow-up of cerebral cavernous malformations. J Neurosurg. 2017 July;127(1):102–10.
28. de Rochefort L, Liu T, Kressler B, Liu J, Spincemaille P, Lebon V, et al. Quantitative susceptibility map reconstruction from MR phase data using bayesian regularization: validation and application to brain imaging. Magn Reson Med. 2010 Jan;63(1):194–206.
29. Hart BL, Taheri S, Rosenberg GA, Morrison LA. Dynamic contrast-enhanced MRI evaluation of cerebral cavernous malformations. Transl Stroke Res. 2013 Oct;4(5):500–6.
30. Larsson HB, Courivaud F, Rostrup E, Hansen AE. Measurement of brain perfusion, blood volume, and blood-brain barrier permeability, using dynamic contrast-enhanced $T(1)$-weighted MRI at 3 tesla. Magn Reson Med. 2009 Nov;62(5):1270–81.
31. Mikati AG, Tan H, Shenkar R, Li L, Zhang L, Guo X, et al. Dynamic permeability and quantitative susceptibility: related imaging biomarkers in cerebral cavernous malformations. Stroke. 2014 Feb;45(2):598–601.

32. Mikati AG, Khanna O, Zhang L, Girard R, Shenkar R, Guo X, et al. Vascular permeability in cerebral cavernous malformations. J Cereb Blood Flow Metab. 2015 Oct;35(10):1632–9.

33. Tan H, Liu T, Wu Y, Thacker J, Shenkar R, Mikati AG, et al. Evaluation of iron content in human cerebral cavernous malformation using quantitative susceptibility mapping. Investig Radiol. 2014 July;49(7):498–504.

34. Tan H, Zhang L, Mikati AG, Girard R, Khanna O, Fam MD, et al. Quantitative susceptibility mapping in cerebral cavernous malformations: clinical correlations. AJNR Am J Neuroradiol. 2016 July;37(7):1209–15.

35. Bellotti C, Medina M, Oliveri G, Barrale S, Ettorre F. Cystic cavernous angiomas of the posterior fossa. Report of three cases. J Neurosurg. 1985 Nov;63(5):797–9.

36. Pozzati E, Gaist G, Poppi M, Morrone B, Padovani R. Microsurgical removal of paraventricular cavernous angiomas. Report of two cases. J Neurosurg. 1981 Aug;55(2):308–11.

37. Ohba S, Shimizu K, Shibao S, Nakagawa T, Murakami H. Cystic cavernous angiomas. Neurosurg Rev 2010 Oct. 33(4):395-400

38. Kudo T, Ueki S, Kobayashi H, Torigoe H, Tadokoro M. Experience with the ultrasonic surgical aspirator in a cavernous hemangioma of the cavernous sinus. Neurosurgery. 1989 Apr;24(4):628–31.

39. Meyer FB, Lombardi D, Scheithauer B, Nichols DA. Extra-axial cavernous hemangiomas involving the dural sinuses. J Neurosurg. 1990 Aug;73(2):187–92.

40. Rigamonti D, Pappas CT, Spetzler RF, Johnson PC. Extracerebral cavernous angiomas of the middle fossa. Neurosurgery. 1990 Aug;27(2):306–10.

41. Vives KP, Gunel M, Awad I. Surgical management of supratentorial cavernous malformation. In: Winn RH, editor. Youmans neurological surgery. 5th ed. Philadelphia: Saunders; 2004. p. 2305–20.

42. Johnson PC, Wascher TM, Golfinos J, Spetzler RF. Definition and pathologic features. In: Awad I, Barrow DL, editors. Cavernous malformations. Park Ridge, IL: American Association of Neurological Surgeons; 1993. p. 1–9.

43. Perrini P, Lanzino G. The association of venous developmental anomalies and cavernous malformations: pathophysiological, diagnostic, and surgical considerations. Neurosurg Focus. 2006 July 15;21(1):e5.

44. Porter RW, Detwiler PW, Spetzler RF, Lawton MT, Baskin JJ, Derksen PT, et al. Cavernous malformations of the brainstem: experience with 100 patients. J Neurosurg. 1999 Jan;90(1):50–8.

45. Topper R, Jurgens E, Reul J, Thron A. Clinical significance of intracranial developmental venous anomalies. J Neurol Neurosurg Psychiatry. 1999 Aug;67(2):234–8.

46. Wurm G, Schnizer M, Fellner FA. Cerebral cavernous malformations associated with venous anomalies: surgical considerations. Neurosurgery. 2005;57(1 Suppl):42–58. discussion 42–58.

47. Abdulrauf SI, Kaynar MY, Awad IA. A comparison of the clinical profile of cavernous malformations with and without associated venous malformations. Neurosurgery 1999;44(1):41–6; discussion 46–7.

48. Cakirer S. De novo formation of a cavernous malformation of the brain in the presence of a developmental venous anomaly. Clin Radiol. 2003 Mar;58(3):251–6.

49. Campeau NG, Lane JI. De novo development of a lesion with the appearance of a cavernous malformation adjacent to an existing developmental venous anomaly. AJNR Am J Neuroradiol. 2005 Jan;26(1):156–9.

50. Desal HA, Lee SK, Kim BS, Raoul S, Tymianski M, TerBrugge KG. Multiple de novo vascular malformations in relation to diffuse venous occlusive disease: a case report. Neuroradiology. 2005 Jan;47(1):38–42.

51. Brinjikji W, El-Masri AE, Wald JT, Flemming KD, Lanzino G. Prevalence of cerebral cavernous malformations associated with developmental venous anomalies increases with age. Childs Nerv Syst. 2017 Sep;33(9):1539–43.

52. Hong YJ, Chung TS, Suh SH, Park CH, Tomar G, Seo KD, et al. The angioarchitectural factors of the cerebral developmental venous anomaly; can they be the causes of concurrent sporadic cavernous malformation? Neuroradiology. 2010 Oct;52(10):883–91.
53. Yu T, Liu X, Lin X, Bai C, Zhao J, Zhang J, et al. The relation between angioarchitectural factors of developmental venous anomaly and concomitant sporadic cavernous malformation. BMC Neurol. 2016 Sep 22;16(1):183.
54. Dammann P, Jabbarli R, Wittek P, Oppong MD, Kneist A, Zhu Y, et al. Solitary sporadic cerebral cavernous malformations: risk factors of first or recurrent symptomatic hemorrhage and associated functional impairment. World Neurosurg. 2016 July;91:73–80.
55. Rigamonti D, Johnson PC, Spetzler RF, Hadley MN, Drayer BP. Cavernous malformations and capillary telangiectasia: a spectrum within a single pathological entity. Neurosurgery. 1991 Jan;28(1):60–4.
56. Hayman LA, Evans RA, Ferrell RE, Fahr LM, Ostrow P, Riccardi VM. Familial cavernous angiomas: natural history and genetic study over a 5-year period. Am J Med Genet. 1982 Feb;11(2):147–60.
57. Mason I, Aase JM, Orrison WW, Wicks JD, Seigel RS, Bicknell JM. Familial cavernous angiomas of the brain in an Hispanic family. Neurology. 1988 Feb;38(2):324–6.
58. Rigamonti D, Hadley MN, Drayer BP, Johnson PC, Hoenig-Rigamonti K, Knight JT, et al. Cerebral cavernous malformations. Incidence and familial occurrence. N Engl J Med. 1988 Aug 11;319(6):343–7.
59. Denier C, Labauge P, Brunereau L, Cave-Riant F, Marchelli F, Arnoult M, et al. Clinical features of cerebral cavernous malformations patients with KRIT1 mutations. Ann Neurol. 2004 Feb;55(2):213–20.
60. Gunel M, Awad IA, Finberg K, Anson JA, Steinberg GK, Batjer HH, et al. A founder mutation as a cause of cerebral cavernous malformation in Hispanic Americans. N Engl J Med. 1996 Apr 11;334(15):946–51.
61. Seker A, Pricola KL, Guclu B, Ozturk AK, Louvi A, Gunel M. CCM2 expression parallels that of CCM1. Stroke. 2006 Feb;37(2):518–23.
62. McDonald DA, Shi C, Shenkar R, Gallione CJ, Akers AL, Li S, et al. Lesions from patients with sporadic cerebral cavernous malformations harbor somatic mutations in the CCM genes: evidence for a common biochemical pathway for CCM pathogenesis. Hum Mol Genet. 2014 Aug 15;23(16):4357–70.
63. Akers AL, Johnson E, Steinberg GK, Zabramski JM, Marchuk DA. Biallelic somatic and germline mutations in cerebral cavernous malformations (CCMs): evidence for a two-hit mechanism of CCM pathogenesis. Hum Mol Genet. 2009 Mar 1;18(5):919–30.
64. Leblanc GG, Golanov E, Awad IA, Young WL. Biology of vascular malformations of the brain NINDS workshop collaborators. Biology of vascular malformations of the brain. Stroke. 2009 Dec;40(12):e694–702.
65. Guzeloglu-Kayisli O, Amankulor NM, Voorhees J, Luleci G, Lifton RP, Gunel M. KRIT1/ cerebral cavernous malformation 1 protein localizes to vascular endothelium, astrocytes, and pyramidal cells of the adult human cerebral cortex. Neurosurgery 2004;54(4):943–9; discussion 949.
66. Labauge P, Denier C, Bergametti F, Tournier-Lasserve E. Genetics of cavernous angiomas. Lancet Neurol. 2007 Mar;6(3):237–44.
67. Plummer NW, Squire TL, Srinivasan S, Huang E, Zawistowski JS, Matsunami H, et al. Neuronal expression of the Ccm2 gene in a new mouse model of cerebral cavernous malformations. Mamm Genome. 2006 Feb;17(2):119–28.
68. Mindea SA, Yang BP, Shenkar R, Bendok B, Batjer HH, Awad IA. Cerebral cavernous malformations: clinical insights from genetic studies. Neurosurg Focus. 2006 July 15;21(1):e1.
69. Craig HD, Gunel M, Cepeda O, Johnson EW, Ptacek L, Steinberg GK, et al. Multilocus linkage identifies two new loci for a mendelian form of stroke, cerebral cavernous malformation, at 7p15-13 and 3q25.2-27. Hum Mol Genet. 1998 Nov;7(12):1851–8.

70. Shenkar R, Shi C, Rebeiz T, Stockton RA, McDonald DA, Mikati AG, et al. Exceptional aggressiveness of cerebral cavernous malformation disease associated with PDCD10 mutations. Genet Med. 2015 Mar;17(3):188–96.
71. Guclu B, Ozturk AK, Pricola KL, Seker A, Ozek M, Gunel M. Cerebral venous malformations have distinct genetic origin from cerebral cavernous malformations. Stroke. 2005 Nov;36(11):2479–80.
72. Pagenstecher A, Stahl S, Sure U, Felbor U. A two-hit mechanism causes cerebral cavernous malformations: complete inactivation of CCM1, CCM2 or CCM3 in affected endothelial cells. Hum Mol Genet. 2009 Mar 1;18(5):911–8.
73. Gunel M, Awad IA, Anson J, Lifton RP. Mapping a gene causing cerebral cavernous malformation to 7q11.2-q21. Proc Natl Acad Sci USA. 1995 July 3;92(14):6620–4.
74. Clatterbuck RE, Eberhart CG, Crain BJ, Rigamonti D. Ultrastructural and immunocytochemical evidence that an incompetent blood-brain barrier is related to the pathophysiology of cavernous malformations. J Neurol Neurosurg Psychiatry. 2001 Aug;71(2):188–92.
75. Shi C, Shenkar R, Batjer HH, Check IJ, Awad IA. Oligoclonal immune response in cerebral cavernous malformations. Laboratory investigation. J Neurosurg. 2007 Nov;107(5):1023–6.
76. Sure U, Butz N, Schlegel J, Siegel AM, Wakat JP, Mennel HD, et al. Endothelial proliferation, neoangiogenesis, and potential de novo generation of cerebrovascular malformations. J Neurosurg. 2001 June;94(6):972–7.
77. Tu YK, Liu HM, Chen SJ, Lin SM. Intramedullary cavernous haemangiomas: clinical features, imaging diagnosis, surgical resection and outcome. J Clin Neurosci. 1999 May;6(3):212–6.
78. Ciricillo SF, Cogen PH, Edwards MS. Pediatric cryptic vascular malformations: presentation, diagnosis and treatment. Pediatr Neurosurg. 1994;20(2):137–47.
79. Di Giannatale A, Morana G, Rossi A, Cama A, Bertoluzzo L, Barra S, et al. Natural history of cavernous malformations in children with brain tumors treated with radiotherapy and chemotherapy. J Neuro-Oncol. 2014 Apr;117(2):311–20.
80. Nimjee SM, Powers CJ, Bulsara KR. Review of the literature on de novo formation of cavernous malformations of the central nervous system after radiation therapy. Neurosurg Focus. 2006 July 15;21(1):e4.
81. Osborne AG. Cavernous malformations. In: Osborne AG, editor. Diagnostiv imaging. Brain. 1st ed. Amirsys Inc: Salt Lake City, UT; 2004.
82. Voigt K, Yasargil MG. Cerebral cavernous haemangiomas or cavernomas. Incidence, pathology, localization, diagnosis, clinical features and treatment. Review of the literature and report of an unusual case. Neurochirurgia (Stuttg). 1976 Mar;19(2):59–68.
83. Zabramski JM, Wascher TM, Spetzler RF, Johnson B, Golfinos J, Drayer BP, et al. The natural history of familial cavernous malformations: results of an ongoing study. J Neurosurg. 1994 Mar;80(3):422–32.
84. Brunereau L, Labauge P, Tournier-Lasserve E, Laberge S, Levy C, Houtteville JP. Familial form of intracranial cavernous angioma: MR imaging findings in 51 families. French Society of Neurosurgery. Radiology. 2000 Jan;214(1):209–16.
85. Nikoubashman O, Wiesmann M, Tournier-Lasserve E, Mankad K, Bourgeois M, Brunelle F, et al. Natural history of cerebral dot-like cavernomas. Clin Radiol. 2013 Aug;68(8):e453–9.
86. Taslimi S, Modabbernia A, Amin-Hanjani S, Barker FG, Macdonald RL. Natural history of cavernous malformation: systematic review and meta-analysis of 25 studies. Neurology. 2016 May 24;86(21):1984–91.
87. Hsu FP, Rigamonti D, Huhn SL. Epidemiology of cavernous malformations. In: Awad I, Barrow DL, editors. Cavernous malformations. Park Ridge, IL: American Association of Neurological Surgeons; 1993. p. 18.
88. Awad I, Jabbour P. Cerebral cavernous malformations and epilepsy. Neurosurg Focus. 2006 July 15;21(1):e7.
89. Cohen DS, Zubay GP, Goodman RR. Seizure outcome after lesionectomy for cavernous malformations. J Neurosurg. 1995 Aug;83(2):237–42.

90. Awad IA, Robinson JR. Cavernous malformations and epilepsy. In: Awad IA, Barrow DL, editors. Cavernous malformation. Park Ridge, IL: American Association of Neurological Surgeons; 1993.

91. Awad IA, Rosenfeld J, Ahl J, Hahn JF, Luders H. Intractable epilepsy and structural lesions of the brain: mapping, resection strategies, and seizure outcome. Epilepsia. 1991 Mar–Apr;32(2):179–86.

92. Singh R, Pathak DN. Lipid peroxidation and glutathione peroxidase, glutathione reductase, superoxide dismutase, catalase, and glucose-6-phosphate dehydrogenase activities in $FeCl_3$-induced epileptogenic foci in the rat brain. Epilepsia. 1990 Jan–Feb;31(1):15–26.

93. Willmore LJ, Sypert GW, Munson JV, Hurd RW. Chronic focal epileptiform discharges induced by injection of iron into rat and cat cortex. Science. 1978 June 30;200(4349):1501–3.

94. von Essen C, Rydenhag B, Nystrom B, Mozzi R, van Gelder N, Hamberger A. High levels of glycine and serine as a cause of the seizure symptoms of cavernous angiomas? J Neurochem. 1996 July;67(1):260–4.

95. Moriarity JL, Wetzel M, Clatterbuck RE, Javedan S, Sheppard JM, Hoenig-Rigamonti K, et al. The natural history of cavernous malformations: a prospective study of 68 patients. Neurosurgery 1999;44(6):1166–71; discussion 1172-3.

96. Josephson CB, Leach JP, Duncan R, Roberts RC, Counsell CE, Al-Shahi Salman R, et al. Seizure risk from cavernous or arteriovenous malformations: prospective population-based study. Neurology. 2011 May 3;76(18):1548–54.

97. Barrow DL, Krisht A. Cavernous malformation and hemorrhage. In: Awad IA, Barrow DL, editors. Cavernous malformations. Park Ridge, IL: American Association of Neurological Surgeons; 1993. p. 65–85.

98. Steiger HJ, Markwalder TM, Reulen HJ. Clinicopathological relations of cerebral cavernous angiomas: observations in eleven cases. Neurosurgery. 1987 Dec;21(6):879–84.

99. Wakai S, Ueda Y, Inoh S, Nagai M. Angiographically occult angiomas: a report of thirteen cases with analysis of the cases documented in the literature. Neurosurgery. 1985 Oct;17(4):549–56.

100. Yamasaki T, Handa H, Yamashita J, Paine JT, Tashiro Y, Uno A, et al. Intracranial and orbital cavernous angiomas. A review of 30 cases. J Neurosurg. 1986 Feb;64(2):197–208.

101. Kondziolka D, Lunsford LD, Kestle JR. The natural history of cerebral cavernous malformations. J Neurosurg. 1995 Nov;83(5):820–4.

102. Labauge P, Brunereau L, Levy C, Laberge S, Houtteville JP. The natural history of familial cerebral cavernomas: a retrospective MRI study of 40 patients. Neuroradiology. 2000 May;42(5):327–32.

103. Porter PJ, Willinsky RA, Harper W, Wallace MC. Cerebral cavernous malformations: natural history and prognosis after clinical deterioration with or without hemorrhage. J Neurosurg. 1997 Aug;87(2):190–7.

104. Jeon JS, Kim JE, Chung YS, Oh S, Ahn JH, Cho WS, et al. A risk factor analysis of prospective symptomatic haemorrhage in adult patients with cerebral cavernous malformation. J Neurol Neurosurg Psychiatry. 2014 Dec;85(12):1366–70.

105. Cantu C, Murillo-Bonilla L, Arauz A, Higuera J, Padilla J, Barinagarrementeria F. Predictive factors for intracerebral hemorrhage in patients with cavernous angiomas. Neurol Res. 2005 Apr;27(3):314–8.

106. Denier C, Labauge P, Bergametti F, Marchelli F, Riant F, Arnoult M, et al. Genotype-phenotype correlations in cerebral cavernous malformations patients. Ann Neurol. 2006 Nov;60(5):550–6.

107. Xie MG, Li D, Guo FZ, Zhang LW, Zhang JT, Wu Z, et al. Brainstem cavernous malformations: surgical indications based on natural history and surgical outcomes. World Neurosurg. 2018 Feb;110:55–63.

108. Kupersmith MJ, Kalish H, Epstein F, Yu G, Berenstein A, Woo H, et al. Natural history of brainstem cavernous malformations. Neurosurgery 2001;48(1):47–53; discussion 53-4.

109. Aiba T, Tanaka R, Koike T, Kameyama S, Takeda N, Komata T. Natural history of intracranial cavernous malformations. J Neurosurg. 1995 July;83(1):56–9.
110. Kalani MY, Zabramski JM. Risk for symptomatic hemorrhage of cerebral cavernous malformations during pregnancy. J Neurosurg. 2013 Jan;118(1):50–5.
111. Barker FG, Amin-Hanjani S, Butler WE, Lyons S, Ojemann RG, Chapman PH, et al. Temporal clustering of hemorrhages from untreated cavernous malformations of the central nervous system. Neurosurgery 2001;49(1):15–24; discussion 24-5.
112. Pozzati E, Zucchelli M, Marliani AF, Riccioli LA. Bleeding of a familial cerebral cavernous malformation after prophylactic anticoagulation therapy. Case report. Neurosurg Focus. 2006 July 15;21(1):e15.
113. Schneble HM, Soumare A, Herve D, Bresson D, Guichard JP, Riant F, et al. Antithrombotic therapy and bleeding risk in a prospective cohort study of patients with cerebral cavernous malformations. Stroke. 2012 Dec;43(12):3196–9.

# Chapter 7
# Hemispherical Cavernomas in Non-Eloquent and Eloquent Areas

**Bill H. Wang, Burkhard S. Kasper, and Ekkehard M. Kasper**

## 7.1  Overview

Cerebral cavernous malformations (CCMs) are vascular malformations that consist of thin hyalinized vascular channels without intervening brain parenchyma [1, 2]. Please see Chap. 2 for more details regarding CCM definition and histological structure. These lesions are surrounded by hemosiderin deposits and a gliotic margin and may be thrombosed [3]. CCMs form one of the major clinicopathologic categories of vascular malformations of the central nervous system [4, 5]. In fact, CCMs are the most common clinically symptomatic vascular anomaly and constitute approximately 10%–15% of all vascular malformations [5–7]. Their incidence is roughly 0.4%–0.8% of the general population based on autopsy and large scale MR studies [6–8]. They occur throughout the entire age spectrum with a mean patient age at presentation in the fourth decade of life [9]. Approximately 25% of CCMs occur in children [10]. While the location of CCMs is quite variable, 70%–80% of CCMs have a supratentorial origin [3].

With the increasing availability of MR imaging, the frequency of diagnosis of CM has risen significantly. In fact, prior to MR imaging, the diagnosis of CMMs was less common, and their evaluation either limited to CT scans or by pathology at the time of surgery [11]. Due to this, most patients were symptomatic at the time of diagnosis with an intracerebral hemorrhage or seizure. However,

B. H. Wang (✉)
Hamilton General Hospital, McMaster University, Hamilton, ON, Canada
e-mail: wangb100@mcmaster.ca

B. S. Kasper
University of Erlangen, Erlangen, Germany

E. M. Kasper
McMaster University, Hamilton, ON, Canada

© Springer Nature Switzerland AG 2020
O. Bradáč, V. Beneš (eds.), *Cavernomas of the CNS*,
https://doi.org/10.1007/978-3-030-49406-3_7

improvements in radiographic imaging have led not only to the increased diagnosis of symptomatic lesions, but also to the incidental discovery of CMs, with as much as 40% of these lesions now being diagnosed incidentally [7]. The specific risk to patients harboring CCMs rests in the occurrence of recurrent microhemorrhages that can lead to headaches, focal neurological deficits, or seizures. Rarely they present with large enough intracerebral hemorrhages to cause coma or death, but deep-seated midline CMM or brain stem lesions can cause profound neurological decline.

The hemosiderin deposits from recurrent microhemorrhages exert an epileptogenic effect on the surrounding brain, causing irritation and gliosis to the parenchyma and leading to epilepsy in some patients (Fig. 7.1) [9]. For more details, please see Chap. 4 for clinical presentation and Chap. 5 for imaging characteristics.

Due to lack of abnormal vasculature seen on formal angiography, CCMs have often been referred to as *cryptic* or *occult vascular malformations*. This is a term typically used to describe any vascular malformation that cannot be seen on diagnostic angiography [2]. These vascular lesions are not visualized with diagnostic cerebral angiography given their low-pressure and low-flow properties [2, 12].

A detailed review of the genetics and natural history of CCMs can be found in Chaps. 3 and 6 respectively. In brief, cavernous malformations occur in two forms: *sporadic* and *familial*. In the sporadic form, the patient usually has only a single lesion and there is no family history of the disorder. In 40%–60% of case the familial form is suggested, characterized by multiple lesions and a frequent family history of seizures [13]. Three distinct gene foci on chromosomes 7q, 7p, and 3 have been linked to familial CCMs encoding for three separate genes: CCM1/KRIT1, CCM2/MGC4607, and CCM3/PDCD10 [13, 14]. Familial CCMs exhibit a Mendelian autosomal dominant inheritance pattern due to a heterozygous loss-of-function mutation, and the identified proteins encoded by CCM genes appear to interact with the cytoskeleton and inter-endothelial cell junction proteins during angiogenesis [1, 13, 14].

Patients diagnosed with CCMs have differing risks for ICH based on the specific location of their CCMs and prior hemorrhage status. Results from observational studies vary greatly on the reported risk of subsequent hemorrhage for CCMs depending on the specific design of each study. Prospective studies have demonstrated a rate of hemorrhage between 0.8% and 3.8% per year for hemispheric lobar lesions [15–18]. This rate increases to as much as 7%–8.9% per year in the patients who are initially presenting with hemorrhage [15–18]. A recent meta-analysis of individual patient data revealed that the 5-year risk of ICH is 3.8% for a non-brainstem CCM *without* prior evidence of ICH or focal neurological deficits (FND); 8.0% for brainstem CCM *without* evidence of ICH or FND; 18.4% for non-brainstem CCM *with* prior evidence of ICH or FND; 30.8% for brainstem CCM *with* prior ICH or FND [19]. Additional factors that influence the risk of ICH include patient sex and hereditary status [20] (Fig. 7.2).

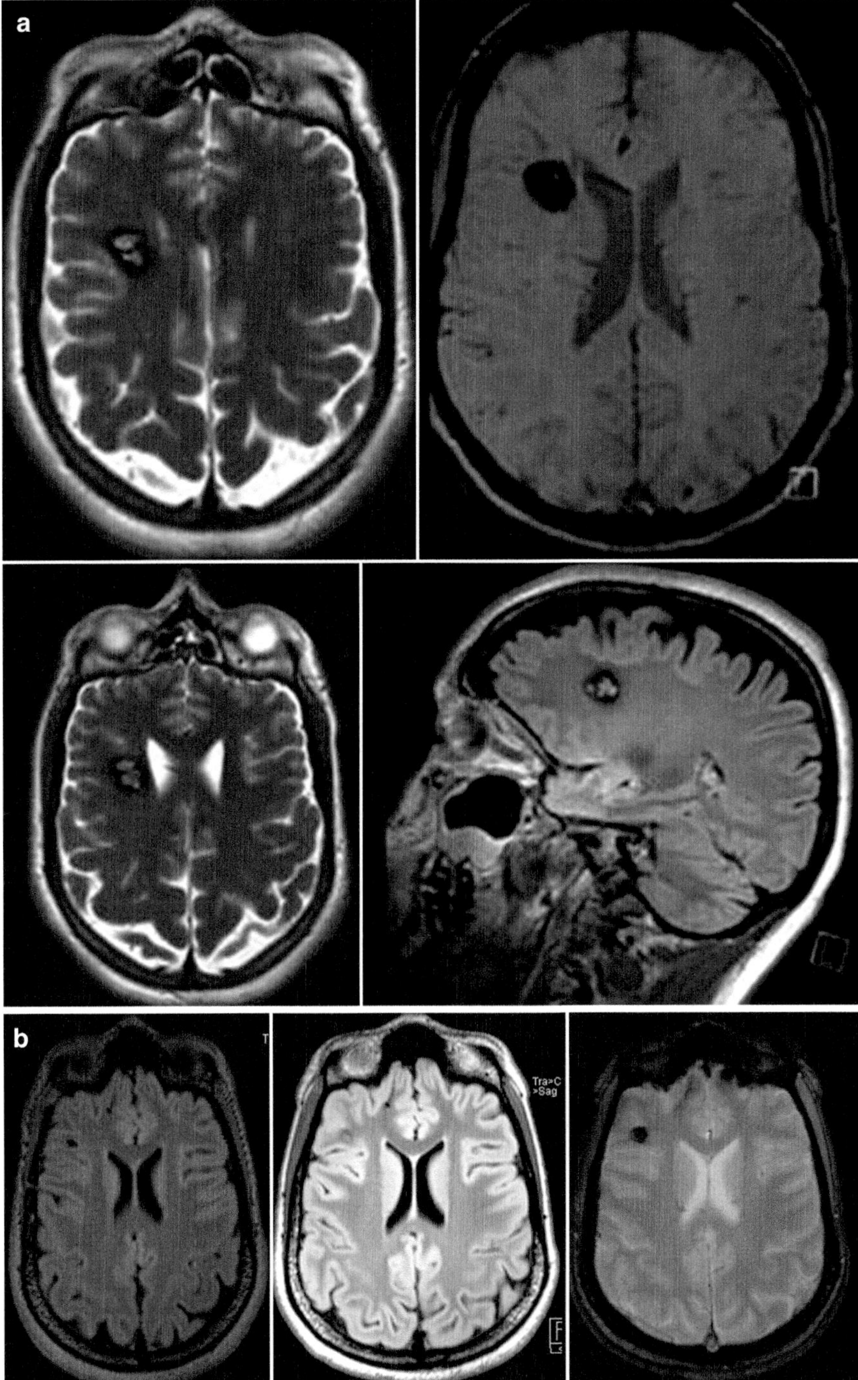

**Fig. 7.1** Supratentorial hemispheric cavernoma. (**a**) PreOP images in axial T2 sequences and axial and sagittal SWI- sequences. (**b**) PostOP PreOP images in axial FLAIR sequences and axial SWI- sequences

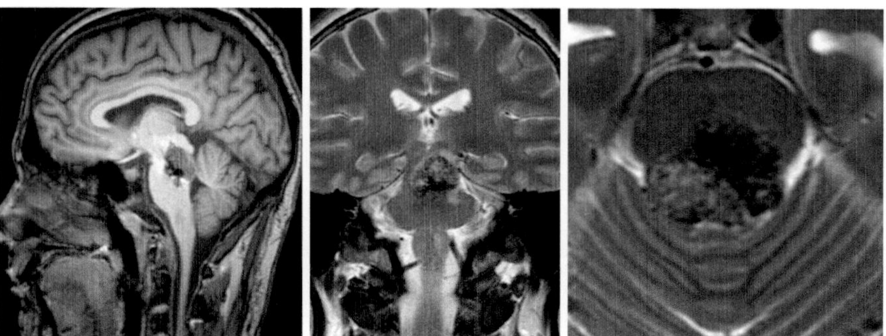

**Fig. 7.2** Infratentorial brain stem cavernoma in Sagitall FLAIR and coronal and axial T2

## 7.2 Treatment Considerations

Treatment options for patients with CCM include observation, microsurgical resection, and at times stereotactic radiosurgery. Because of the differing risk profile for ICH, the risks associated with microsurgical excision [21–23] and stereotactic radiosurgery [24] need to be weighed against that of natural history when considering treatment. This is further confounded by the fact that most ICH from CCM's tend to be focally limited and remain comparatively small (average volume ~1.8 cm$^3$), and patients tend to have good functional outcomes [25]. Furthermore, the annual risk of recurrent ICH appears to subside within 2–5 years after the initial ICH [19, 26, 27]. This phenomenon is sometimes referred to as "temporal clustering" where the risk of a second hemorrhage is proportional to the temporal proximity of the initial hemorrhage. When looking over time periods for CCMs, Barker et al. reported a decline in the observed hemorrhage risk at about 2–3 years after the initial hemorrhagic event [26]. These authors documented a decrease in bleeding rates from 2.1% per month to 0.8% per month after 28 months. Temporal clustering is important especially when analyzing treatment options with delayed efficacy such as radiosurgery, when the risk of hemorrhage may already decline based on natural history alone during the waiting period.

## 7.3 Observation

Some patients with CCMs should be followed conservatively. Almost all asymptomatic lesions are observed because they can remain asymptomatic indefinitely. Asymptomatic lesions are frequently discovered as incidental findings on imaging or in association with another symptomatic lesion. Patients with asymptomatic lesions, or a vague compliant such as headaches, can be reassured that the expected natural history is likely to be relatively benign and do not necessarily require treatment [2]. If a hemorrhage occurs, it is usually small and very rarely results in major neurologic deficit. This is in keeping with the recommendation from the Angioma Alliance 2017 guidelines on treatment of CCMs [28]. The Angioma Alliance is a non-profit patient support organization that has established DNA/tissue bank and patient registry for the use of researchers investigating CCMs [29]. After a thorough review of literature, the expert panel concluded that surgical resection is not recommended for asymptomatic CCM, especially if located in eloquent, deep, or brainstem areas. Surgical resection is also not recommended in cases with multiple asymptomatic CCMs. The overall evidence was given class III, level B.

A closer look at the available body of evidence reveals that - despite decades of neurosurgical experience in resection of cavernomas—results from studies supporting this modality of CCM treatment remain conflicting. When looking at existing studies that comprise at least 20 symptomatic CCM patients, none were identified as high quality evidence to demonstrate dramatic benefit or harm of surgery [28]. Only around a dozen studies were found eligible and most of them did not show clinically or statistically significant differences in death or functional outcome after CCM excision [30]. A few studies showed beneficial effects of surgical resection of CCM in the setting of seizures or epilepsy, bearing in mind the presence of varying degrees of bias in the studies [30, 31]. Moultrie et al. looked at surgical excision compared to conservative management in a nonrandomized population-based study using National Health Services (NHS) data in Scotland [31]. The study revealed poorer outcome over the subsequent 5 years after surgery, and higher risk of symptomatic bleeds and focal neurological deficits in the surgical group compared to the conservative management group [31]. However, the baseline health of the surgical arm was not clearly described and patients often had more severe presentation from their CCM in the surgical group, making the study inherently biased towards poorer outcomes in the surgical group.

Case series reported in the literature generally advocate for conservative management of asymptomatic CCMs [9]. One systematic review documented an overall risk of 6% for death or symptomatic stroke after CCM resection [30, 31]. This exceeds the analogous natural risk (3.8% over 5 years) of a CCM that has never bled. The same postoperative risk becomes more favorable compared to the risk associated with recurrent ICH after a first CCM bleed (18.4% over 5 years) [19]. The risk of resection varies greatly with CCM location, and this plays an important role when contemplating surgical resection. Resection is generally recommended for symptomatic, easily accessible CCMs due to the increased risk of recurrent hemorrhage after the first bleed, and the relatively low morbidity associated with surgery in comparison [19, 32, 33].

Another group that may be observed consists of those patients with symptomatic lesions in eloquent or deep area where the risks of surgery are deemed to be significant. For these patients, observation can be a viable option if the CCMs do not cause recurrent ICH or progressive neurological function. Some patients, who initially presented with seizures or headache with a lesion in eloquent cortex without recurrent hemorrhage have also been observed. A subset of these patients can also be candidates for surgery, as discussed in the following sections. The decision about which treatment is appropriate depends on a detailed evaluation of the clinical presentation and discussion with the patient.

For patients who are observed, some form of regular sequential imaging and clinical follow up is recommended. The time interval of imaging is not well defined, but most authors seem to agree on yearly MRI's to monitor any changes such as de novo CCMs, lesion growth, or new (micro)hemorrhages. A careful neurological history and physical exam should also be performed to determine if the patient had truly been asymptomatic during the follow-up period [9].

## 7.4   Surgical Resection

No clear consensus has been reached regarding the role of surgical treatment for CCMs. Incidental lesions have traditionally been observed due to the morbidity associated with surgical resection. The current guideline recommendations are mostly based on case series, and no Level 1 evidence exists on the management of this disease entity. However, asymptomatic CCMs must be closely monitored for either new clinical symptoms or a change in radiographic appearance. Many originally asymptomatic patients may experience symptomatic hemorrhage or seizures.

Factors that promote surgical resection of CCM of the cerebrum include: [9]

- Medically intractable seizures
- Progressive neurological decline
- Clinically significant hemorrhage in noneloquent cortex
- Second clinically significant hemorrhage in eloquent cortex
- Patient risk adversity with anxiety causing functional impairment
- Young patient age
- Female sex

Factors that serve as relative contraindications to surgical resection include:

- Asymptomatic CCM
- Multiple incidental or familial lesions

Despite the low annual rate of hemorrhage of CCMs, the cumulative life-time risk for patient is not trivial, especially in younger patients. For certain patients, depending on their lifestyle, occupation, or mindset, an incidental lesion often be a source of great anxiety and stress. The intrinsic psychological burden for some patients may outweigh the risk of surgical morbidity once the diagnosis of CCM is made. For a young patient with a solitary lesion in an easily accessible location, surgical resection presents an opportunity for a cure. Surgery would obviate the need for regular imaging and follow-ups as well as prevent even a small chance of serious sequelae from the lesion. It may even simplify pregnancy management in women or any anticoagulation management that may be needed later in life. Because the risk of surgery is low for lesions in many cortical locations, there are groups of patients in whom surgery should be considered.

The currently accepted indications for surgical resection of CCMs in the cerebral hemispheres include recurrent hemorrhage, progressive neurologic deterioration, and intractable epilepsy, unless the location is associated with an unacceptably high surgical risk [9, 28]. For patients with epilepsy, several studies showed that pure CCM resection (lesionectomy) results in postoperative seizure control rate of 70%–90% [34, 35]. The management of patient with CCMs causing epilepsy is covered in greater detail in Chap. 9. For patients presenting with recurrent hemorrhage, the management of intracerebral and intraventricular hemorrhage associated with CCM should follow the most current evidence-based guidelines. This includes early blood pressure control, reversal of coagulopathy, control of intracranial pressure, and the evacuation of hemorrhages causing impending herniation or posterior fossa compression [36]. With respect to the CCMs, it is important to weigh the risk of surgery vs the natural history of the CCM in each specific clinical scenario and CCM location.

Many surgical series on CCMs have demonstrated good results with operative management, with low surgical morbidity or mortality among patients with lesions in the cerebral hemispheres. Amin-Hanjani et al. reported in their series of 94 patients who underwent surgical resection for 94 CCMs no deaths, a 20.6% rate of transient neurological deficits, and a 6.2% rate of permanent morbidity [21]. In the subgroup of patient with CCMs in the cerebral hemispheres, the rate of transient neurological deficits decreases to only 4.8% while the rate of permanent disability decreases to 3.2%. For CCMs in supratentorial noneloquent regions, the risk of new neurological sequelae is equivalent to living with the CCM for 1–2 years after a first bleed [31]. On the other hand, performing surgical resection of CCMs in more eloquent locations is associated with higher risk, equivalent to living with the CCM for upwards of 5–10 years after a first bleed. Patients with a reasonable life expectancy and CCMs in eloquent cortex can still be potentially good candidates from surgical resection, although a detailed discussion needs to take place in order to address the risk, benefits and expectations.

When surgical resection of a CCM is performed in the hemisphere, the lesion can usually be removed entirely with low morbidity. This procedure is facilitated by microsurgical dissection in the gliotic tissue that surrounds the lesion, allowing a distinct plane of cleavage to be developed through microsurgical techniques, bipolar coagulation, and the use of finely regulated suction. Once the lesion is exposed, internally decompression of the cavernoma can be initially performed. This is followed by retraction of the capsule into the area of the decompression, which may help avoid undue pressure on the surrounding normal parenchyma. If the CCM is densely calcified, an ultrasonic surgical aspirator may be helpful for debulking. Bleeding is usually not a significant problem during resection and can be adequately addressed with a combination of bipolar coagulation and tamponade with cottonoid patties.

For lesions that are in a deep sulcus or some distance away from the cortical surface, splitting a cortical fissure may be possible rather than performing a full corticectomy to approach the lesion. Intraoperative image guidance (stereotaxy) should be used for all cases to minimize the size of cortical resection and disruption of normal brain tissue. For lesions that are deeper and harder to localize, intraoperative ultrasound can sometimes serve as a useful adjunct to help locate the lesion.

For CCMs located in eloquent cortex, pre-operative planning will help minimize the risk of neurological deficits post-resection. This includes updated MRI with isovolumetric sequences for image-guidance. The planned surgically corridor should ideally avoid direct cortisectomy over eloquent cortex if possible. The development of gliotic plane should be handled with extra caution with debulking of central portion of the CCMs first to avoid retraction injury of surrounding eloquent cortex. Depending on the location, some hemosiderin stained brain may need to be left behind to preserve function. This can be potentially challenging in cases where the primarily goal of surgery is control of epilepsy where the hemosiderin stained brain can remain as a potential seizure focus. Please see Chap. 9 for more detailed discussion regarding CCM and epilepsy.

## 7.5 Conclusions

Cerebral cavernous malformations (CCMs) are increasingly been diagnosed as incidental lesions on noninvasive imaging studies. Patients with CCMs may also present with seizures or hemorrhage. Truly incidental CCMs should be managed conservatively and followed-up with serial (yearly) MR imaging. The treatment of symptomatic CCMs is generally image-guided resection. Some recommendations regarding the treatment of CCMs include: intractable seizures or progressive neurological deficit, after the first clinically significant hemorrhage in noneloquent areas, and after the second clinically significant hemorrhage in eloquent areas including the brainstem. The current body of evidence is not adequate to make clear decision, the surgeon's clinical judgment and discussion with patient is required for optimal care.

## References


1. Yadla S, Jabbour PM, Shenkar R, et al. Cerebral cavernous malformations as a disease of vascular permeability: from bench to bedside with caution. Neurosurg Focus. 2010;29:E4. https://doi.org/10.3171/2010.5.FOCUS10121.
2. Raychaudhuri R, Batjer HH, Awad IA. Intracranial cavernous angioma: a practical review of clinical and biological aspects. Surg Neurol. 2005;63:319–28. https://doi.org/10.1016/j.surneu.2004.05.032.
3. D'Angelo VA, De Bonis C, Amoroso R, et al. Supratentorial cerebral cavernous malformations: clinical, surgical, and genetic involvement. Neurosurg Focus. 2006;21:e9.
4. Rigamonti D, Drayer BP, Johnson PC, et al. The MRI appearance of cavernous malformations (angiomas). J Neurosurg. 1987;67:518–24. https://doi.org/10.3171/jns.1987.67.4.0518.
5. Vernooij MW, Ikram MA, Tanghe HL, et al. Incidental findings on brain MRI in the general population. N Engl J Med. 2007;357:1821–8. https://doi.org/10.1056/NEJMoa070972.

6. Washington CW, McCoy KE, Zipfel GJ. Update on the natural history of cavernous malformations and factors predicting aggressive clinical presentation. Neurosurg Focus. 2010;29:E7. https://doi.org/10.3171/2010.5.FOCUS10149.
7. Recinos PF, Lin D, Batra S, et al. Cavernous malformations: natural history, diagnosis and treatment. Nat Rev Neurol. 2009;5:659–70. https://doi.org/10.1038/nrneurol.2009.177.
8. Otten P, Pizzolato GP, Rilliet B, et al. 131 cases of cavernous angioma (cavernomas) of the CNS, discovered by retrospective analysis of 24,535 autopsies. Neurochirurgie. 1989;35:82.
9. Dalyai RT, Ghobrial G, Awad I, et al. Management of incidental cavernous malformations: a review. Neurosurg Focus. 2011;31:E5. https://doi.org/10.3171/2011.9.FOCUS11211.
10. Mottolese C, Hermier M, Stan H, et al. Central nervous system cavernomas in the pediatric age group. Neurosurg Rev. 2001;24:55–71. https://doi.org/10.1007/PL00014581.
11. Voigt K, Yaşargil MG. Cerebral cavernous haemangiomas or cavernomas. Incidence, pathology, localization, diagnosis, clinical features and treatment. Review of the literature and report of an unusual case. Neurochirurgia. 1976;19:59.
12. Hentati A, Matar N, Dridi H, et al. Bilateral orbital cavernous hemangioma. Asian J Neurosurg. 2018;13:1222. https://doi.org/10.4103/ajns.AJNS_96_17.
13. Campbell PG, Jabbour P, Yadla S, et al. Emerging clinical imaging techniques for cerebral cavernous malformations: a systematic review. Neurosurg Focus. 2010;29:E6. https://doi.org/10.3171/2010.5.FOCUS10120.
14. Storkebaum E, Quaegebeur A, Vikkula M, et al. Cerebrovascular disorders: molecular insights and therapeutic opportunities. Nat Neurosci. 2011; https://doi.org/10.1038/nn.2947.
15. Steiner L, Karlsson B, Yen C, et al. Radiosurgery in cavernous malformations: anatomy of a controversy. J Neurosurg. 2010;113:16. https://doi.org/10.3171/2009.11.JNS091733.
16. Porter PJ, Willinsky RA, Harper W, et al. Cerebral cavernous malformations: natural history and prognosis after clinical deterioration with or without hemorrhage. J Neurosurg. 1997;87:190–7. https://doi.org/10.3171/jns.1997.87.2.0190.
17. Kondziolka D, Lunsford LD, Kestle JR. The natural history of cerebral cavernous malformations. J Neurosurg. 1995;83:820–4. https://doi.org/10.3171/jns.1995.83.5.0820.
18. Robinson JR, Awad IA, Little JR. Natural history of the cavernous angioma. J Neurosurg. 1991;75:709–14. https://doi.org/10.3171/jns.1991.75.5.0709.
19. Horne MA, Flemming KD, Su I-C, Stapf C, Jeon JO, Li D, Maxwell SS, White P, Christianson TJ, Agid R, Cho W-S, Oh CW, Wu Z, Zhang J-T, Kim JE, ter Brugge K, Willinsky R, Brown RD, Murray GD, Al-Shahi Salman R. Clinical course of untreated cerebral cavernous malformations: a meta-analysis of individual patient data. Lancet Neurol. 2016;15:166–73. https://doi.org/10.1016/S1474-4422(15)00303-8.
20. Cavalcanti DD, Kalani MYS, Martirosyan NL, et al. Cerebral cavernous malformations: from genes to proteins to disease. J Neurosurg. 2012;116:122–32. https://doi.org/10.3171/2011.8.JNS101241.
21. Amin-Hanjani S, Ogilvy CS, Ojemann RG, et al. Risks of surgical management for cavernous malformations of the nervous system. Neurosurgery. 1998;42:1220–7. https://doi.org/10.1097/00006123-199806000-00007.
22. Garrett M, Spetzler RF. Surgical treatment of brainstem cavernous malformations. Surg Neurol. 2009;72:S9. https://doi.org/10.1016/j.surneu.2009.05.031.
23. Ojemann RG, Ogilvy CS. Microsurgical treatment of supratentorial cavernous malformations. Neurosurg Clin N Am. 1999;10:433–40. https://doi.org/10.1016/S1042-3680(18)30177-3.
24. Kondziolka D, Flickinger JC, Lunsford LD. Radiosurgery for cavernous malformations. Prog Neurol Surg. 2007;20:220.
25. Cordonnier C, Al-Shahi Salman R, Bhattacharya JJ, et al. Differences between intracranial vascular malformation types in the characteristics of their presenting haemorrhages: prospective, population-based study. J Neurol Neurosurg Psychiatry. 2008;79:47–51. https://doi.org/10.1136/jnnp.2006.113753.

26. Barker FG, Amin-Hanjani S, Butler WE, et al. Temporal clustering of hemorrhages from untreated cavernous malformations of the central nervous system. Neurosurgery. 2001;49:15–25. https://doi.org/10.1097/00006123-200107000-00002.

27. Flemming KD, Link MJ, Christianson TJH, et al. Prospective hemorrhage risk of intracerebral cavernous malformations. Neurology. 2012;78:632–6. https://doi.org/10.1212/WNL.0b013e318248de9b.

28. Akers A, Al-Shahi Salman RA, Awad I, et al. Synopsis of guidelines for the clinical management of cerebral cavernous malformations: consensus recommendations based on systematic literature review by the Angioma Alliance Scientific Advisory Board Clinical Experts Panel. Neurosurgery. 2017;80:665–80. https://doi.org/10.1093/neuros/nyx091.

29. Ardelt AA, Deveikis JP, Harrigan MR. Handbook of cerebrovascular disease and neurointerventional technique. New York: Springer; 2013.

30. Poorthuis M, Samarasekera N, Kontoh K, et al. Comparative studies of the diagnosis and treatment of cerebral cavernous malformations in adults: systematic review. Acta Neurochir. 2013;155:643–9. https://doi.org/10.1007/s00701-013-1621-4.

31. Moultrie F, Horne M, Josephson C, et al. Outcome after surgical or conservative management of cerebral cavernous malformations. Neurology. 2014;83:582–9. https://doi.org/10.1212/WNL.0000000000000684.

32. Pasqualin A, Meneghelli P, Giammarusti A, et al. Results of surgery for cavernomas in critical supratentorial areas. Acta Neurochir Suppl. 2014;119:117.

33. Bilginer B, Narin F, Hanalioglu S, et al. Cavernous malformations of the central nervous system (CNS) in children: clinico-radiological features and management outcomes of 36 cases. Childs Nerv Syst. 2014;30:1355–66. https://doi.org/10.1007/s00381-014-2442-3.

34. von der Brelie C, Kuczaty S, von Lehe M. Surgical management and long-term outcome of pediatric patients with different subtypes of epilepsy associated with cerebral cavernous malformations. J Neurosurg Pediatr. 2014;13:699–705. https://doi.org/10.3171/2014.2.PEDS13361.

35. Cohen DS, Zubay GP, Goodman RR. Seizure outcome after lesionectomy for cavernous malformations. J Neurosurg. 1995;83:237–42. https://doi.org/10.3171/jns.1995.83.2.0237.

36. Hemphill JC, Greenberg SM, Anderson CS, et al. Guidelines for the management of spontaneous intracerebral hemorrhage: a guideline for healthcare professionals from the American Heart Association/American Stroke Association. Stroke. 2015;46:2032–60. https://doi.org/10.1161/STR.0000000000000069.

# Chapter 8
# Cavernoma-Related Epilepsy


**Philipp Dammann, Carlos M. Quesada, Taku Sato, and Ulrich Sure**


## 8.1 Definitions

To avoid terminological ambiguities the following definitions should be used both clinically and scientifically when we talk about epilepsy and cavernous malformations:

An epilepsy definitely or probably related to a cavernous malformation (CCM) should be called **cavernoma-related epilepsy (CRE)**.

The definitions of "definite" and "probable" CRE were proposed by the surgical task force of the ILAE commission on therapeutic strategies [1]:

**Definite CRE** epilepsy in patients with at least one CCM and evidence of a seizure-onset zone in the immediate vicinity of the CCM.

**Probable CRE** epilepsy in patients with one CCM and evidence that the epilepsy is **focal** and arises from the **same hemisphere** as the CCM. At the same time, there is no evidence of other causes of epilepsy.

In other scenarios an epilepsy would be regarded as unrelated to a CCM.


P. Dammann (✉) · U. Sure
Department of Neurosurgery, University Hospital Essen, University of Duisburg-Essen, Essen, Germany
e-mail: Philipp.Dammann@uk-essen.de

C. M. Quesada
Department of Neurology, University Hospital Essen, University of Duisburg-Essen, Essen, Germany

T. Sato
Department of Neurosurgery, Fukushima Medical University, Fukushima, Japan



© Springer Nature Switzerland AG 2020

O. Bradáč, V. Beneš (eds.), *Cavernomas of the CNS*,
https://doi.org/10.1007/978-3-030-49406-3_8

## 8.2   Pathophysiological Background

Cavernous malformations consist of enlarged vascular spaces with a single-layer endothelium and no tigh junctions, muscular layer or embedded brain tissue (when cerebral) [2]. They resemble a capillary lesion without specifical arterious or venous proportion. Their size varies between a few millimeters and several centimeters and can be found not only in the brain and meninges but in many other organs including liver [3] and orbit [4].

CCM are considered highly epileptogenic lesions [1]. The cortical localization of cavernomas has been shown to be critical for the development of seizures, especially when affecting the mesiotemporal structures [5]. Other possible factors which may be related with the occurrence of seizures are the number or size of the CCMs or of the hemosiderin rim, although different studies show contradictory results regarding these variables [6–8].

The exact mechanisms leading to the development of an neural aggregate capable of generating spontaneous seizures are not well understood, but may involve hypoxia, microbleedings and local reorganization [9]. The deposit of hemosiderin caused by repetitive bleeding has been classically regarded as the main epileptogenic factor, although the deposit of iron in brain cortex has only been related to the occurrence of epileptogenic discharges [10]. The astrogliosis found around most cavernomas, as in some other epileptogenic lesions, might be the necessary precipitating factor leading to seizures [11, 12]. The presence of hypoxia inducible factor (HIF-1alpha) and metalloproteasa (MMP-9) in brain tissue and endothelium adjacent to CCMs have been related to the occurrence of seizures [9]. Gene mutations related to the occurrence of CCMs, like CCM1, CCM2 and CCM3, have been known to play a role in the abnormal vascular proliferation, but not in the epileptogenesis [13].

## 8.3   Clinical Aspects

### 8.3.1   Epidemiology and Natural History of a CRE

While most CCM are diagnosed incidentally (approx. 50%), a seizure is the second most common initial clinical presentation of a CCM (approx. 25%) [14]. A population-based prospective observational study revealed that the majority of patients (>90%) with an initial seizure related to a CCM will experience further seizures and develop a CRE [8]. Most of the adult patients in clinical series are relatively young at the age of diagnosis (median age around 20 years [15, 16]) or surgery (median age around 35 years [6, 16]), respectively. While most patients present with a solitary, sporadic CCM, 15–20% present with multiple CCM [14], which is, in most cases [17], suggestive for a familial disease [1].

## 8.3.2   Indicators for a CRE

In view of the prevalence of CCM in the population (approx. 0.5% [2, 18]), the chance of seeing a patient with a seizure and an *incidental* CCM is relatively low, however such a situation may occur. Indicative for a CRE are supratentorial localization and cortical involvement of the CCM [1] as well as archicortical/mesiotemporal localization [5, 19]. If the size of the CCM and the extent of the hemosiderin rim are correlated with the presence of a CRE is discussed controversially [5, 7, 8]. To note, seizures may occur during a symptomatic hemorrhage but also in the absence of a symptomatic hemorrhage [6, 20]. See Fig. 8.1.

## 8.3.3   The "Typical" Patient with a CRE

Nowadays, most patients with CRE will be admitted to a neurosurgical consultation after the first (few) seizure (s). In view of the widespread availability of MRI, patients with chronic epilepsy in which a CCM was initially overlooked and not diagnosed will only rarely present at your consultation, except in specialized epilepsy centers. Most patients will be young and otherwise relatively healthy. Most of the times, the lesion will be located in the (mesio-) temporal lobe. Approx. in a third of the cases the first seizure will be accompanied by signs of an acute hemorrhage

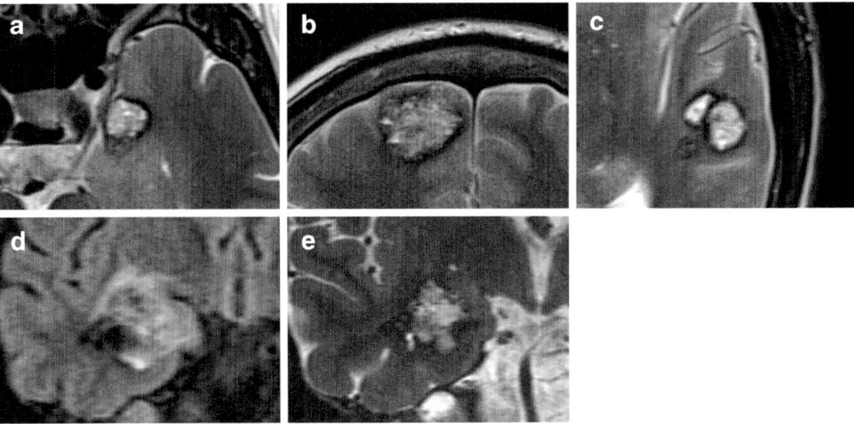


**Fig. 8.1** Typical initial MRI findings in patients with CRE. (**a**) and (**b**) showing "silent" CCM without symptomatic hemorrhage events accompanying the first seizure. (**c**) showing a "chronic" state several weeks after a symptomatic hemorrhage/seizure event. Note the bleeding cavity adjacent to the CCM lesion (arrow). (**d**) showing the acute state of a symptomatic hemorrhage with accompanying seizure two days after the event. Note the acute blood signal and perifocal edema. (**e**) showing the same patient several weeks later, prior to surgery, with resolved edema

on MRI (seizure as a manifestation of a first symptomatic hemorrhage (SH)). Typically, the patients are not significantly impaired by the hemorrhage, as supratentorial SHs usually have a relatively benign clinical course regarding local space occupying effects [21].

In most regions of the world, sporadic solitary CCM will contribute for the majority of cases. Multiple CCM are rare, however identifying the epileptogenic lesion (s) may be complex.


### 8.3.4 Baseline Diagnostics

All patients with CRE should receive a cranial MRI with at least: a thin-sliced T2 weighted sequence, a thin-sliced T1 weighted sequence with/without contrast enhancement, hemo-sequences (t2*, SWI).

The baseline MRI should depict the CCMs ultrastructure and adjacent hemosiderin deposits (T2, T1), age and ultrastructure of intra- or extra-lesional hemorrhage (T2, T1), presence/absence of an associated developmental venous anomaly DVA (T1_CE) and presence/absence of further CCM not visible on conventional imaging (spot-like lesions) indicating e.g. a familial disease (T2*, SWI). Adequate neuroimaging is crucial for surgical decision making and the epileptological work-up of the patient. To properly consult the patient you should clarify:

1. did the patient experience a symptomatic hemorrhage (increasing the risk for further symptomatic hemorrhages over the next 5 years [21, 22]),
2. what is the extent of hemosiderin deposits around the lesion (incomplete resection (e.g. occurring in eloquent regions) may impair the postoperative seizure control [23]),
3. is a DVA associated with the CCM (may increase risk of surgery/accessability of lesion due to potential venous infarction [24]),
4. does the patient have multiple CCM? If yes, which CCM(s) cause(s) the CRE?

All patients with CRE should receive anamnesis of epilepsy-specific history, analysis of ictal symptomatology and at least one routine electroencephalography (EEG). A careful history taking might reveal the prior occurrence of seizures after supposed first seizures [25]. *The EEG can help to elucidate if the epileptic seizures are related to the CCM but mostly help to detect an epilepsy not related to CCM (for instance if generalized epileptic discharges occur or focal discharges in other location not close to the CCM are detected).* The combined evaluation of seizure semiology, EEG and MRI can confirm the existence of a CRE. In patients with inconsistent findings, multiple CCM, or medically refractory epilepsy a meticulous epileptological work-up is recommended. See Fig. 8.2.

In general, patients with a potential CRE should be consulted by an interdisciplinary team of neurosurgeons and epileptologists to interpret clinical, MRI and EEG data.

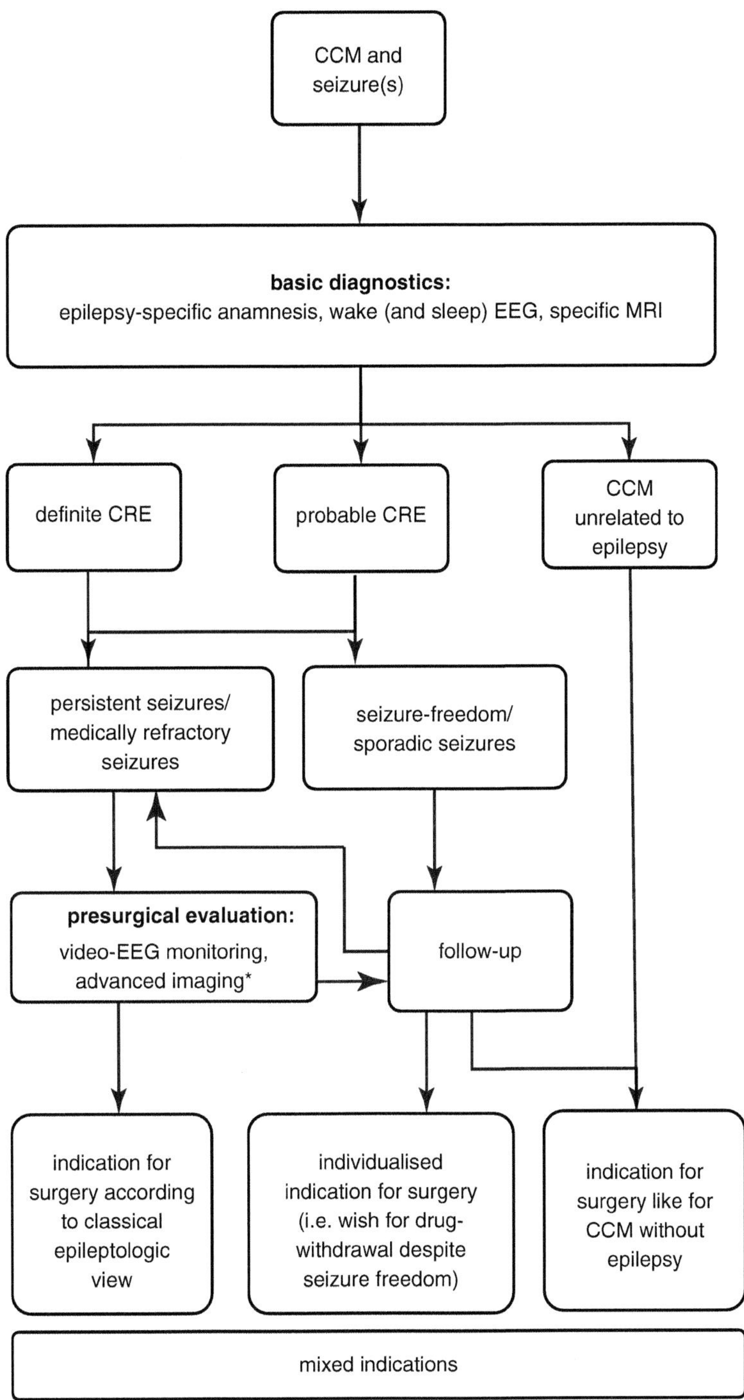


**Fig. 8.2** Treatment algorithm for CRE

## 8.3.5 Baseline Treatment

The current definition of epilepsy requires the occurrence of two unprovoked seizures (more than 24 h apart) or one unprovoked seizure plus a >60% probability of further seizures [26]. This probability is usually given in the presence of specific epileptic activity in EEG or a potentially epileptogenic lesion in MR. Since the risk of further unprovoked seizures in patients with CCM can be up to 94% [8], a diagnosis of epilepsy can be done after the first seizure and antiepileptic treatment should be initiated. The type of AED should be chosen according to the individual patient characteristics by the treating neurologist. The decision about treatment withdrawal after years of seizure-freedom must be individualized, since many factors may play a role in the risk of seizure recurrence [27]. In our experience most patients will receive AEDs permanently once the AED treatment has started. This is also based on medico-legal issues (driving license).

The chance of staying seizure free under initial AED therapy in CRE is roughly 50% in the first 5 years according to the relatively sparse data available [6]. This means most people with an initial CCM related seizure will develop further seizures even under AED treatment. Further seizures may or may not be associated with a SH.

A smaller proportion of patients with CRE may develop persisting seizures or medically refractory epilepsy and should be treated accordingly (AED dose increase, double/triple AED treatment, surgical treatment).

## 8.3.6 Indication for Surgery

In general, the indication for surgery should be posed by the interdisciplinary team (neurosurgery/epileptology)!

We should define three different groups of patients here:

1. Patients with new-onset single or multiple seizures.
2. Patients with controlled CRE under AED treatment
3. Patients with persisting seizures (or even medically refractory epilepsy) under AED treatment.

According to ILAE recommendation [1], surgery for CRE after the first (few) seizure(s) can be performed if a patient (a) wants to withdrawal AED, (b) is presumably not compliant with AED medication or (c) has a high risk of CCM re-bleeding (more or less only accounting for patients that present with a symptomatic hemorrhage at the time of CRE diagnosis). While pros and cons of AED treatment can be discussed with the patient, the risk for re-bleeding of CCM remains difficult to estimate in the first place. We know that there is a 20–30% risk of re-bleeding after an initial hemorrhage within the first 5 years. Main risk factor for a SH of a supratentorial CCM is a previous SH. Other risk factors (such as DVA) are at least discussed controversial. Generally speaking, SH seem to cluster when they occur but we don't know the initial stimulus of this "active phase". However, we know also, that supra-tentorial SHs oftentimes show a benign course. This is why, we normally recommend a watch and wait strategy for patients with an initial SH of a supra-tentorial CCM. Except for, well, patients with an accompanying CRE.

While ILAE sees an *absolute* indication for surgery only in patients with *persisting* seizures under AED treatment (however, without a mandatory need to fulfill the rigorous criteria of a **medically refractory** CRE [28], we have a more "pro-active" position in this regard. In surgically accessible lesions (which accounts for most lesions), we recommend surgery relatively early. Even after an initial unprovoked seizure (new-onset single or multiple seizures) or in patients that are for a certain time seizure-free under AED treatment, surgery may be justified in our opinion. This is for multiple reasons:

- As mentioned earlier nearly all patients with an initial unprovoked seizure related to a CCM will develop CRE. Consequently, patients will receive AEDs from then on.
- Most patients are young, facing many years with a CRE, being under AED treatment.
- There is some evidence that seizure outcome is worse the longer a CRE is present before surgery (see below).
- Hemosiderin deposits around the CCM will enlarge over time due to recurrent micro-hemorrhages and possible SH. Following the principle of a lesionectomy the hemosiderin deposits should be removed with the CCM (otherwise seizure outcome may be impaired, see below) what will then become more invasive/difficult or even impossible (e.g. in eloquent regions).
- Seizure outcome is significantly better with surgery compared to standard AED treatment (80–90% complete seizure freedom vs. 40–50% [6], no level 1–2 evidence).
- Chance to stop AED treatment is much higher after surgery [6]. In our department patients undergo a standardized AED withdrawal protocol.
- Patients will have no risk for SH after CCM removal

Those patients who are surgically treated without fulfilling the criteria for drug resistant epilepsy but whose epilepsy or risk of (further) seizure might benefit from it should be regarded as being treated after a mixed "neurosurgical" and "epileptological" indication. Until a prospective randomized controlled trial will give us a definite answer, both early surgical treatment and conservative treatment will, however, stay as treatment options in a new-onset CRE.

In patients with multiple CCM (not if epileptological focus was clearly identified by routine EEG), persisting seizures under AED treatment ("chronic epilepsy") or medically refractory epilepsy a meticulous epileptological work-up is recommended to ensure the proper identification of the seizure onset zone. To note, in some, but rather few, patients an extended lesionectomy may be helpful [29].

## 8.3.7 Specific Epileptological Work-Up

The specific epileptological work-up is performed in-hospital in a specialized epilepsy center. It contains the anamnesis of epilepsy-specific history and the analysis of ictal symptomatology as well as video-EEG monitoring. The goal is to confirm the electro-clinical correlation of the habitual seizures with the presumed epileptogenic CCM [1]. At the same time the risk of neurological or neuropsychological deficits after the withdrawal of the presumed epileptogenic lesion should be assessed. A careful presurgical evaluation should end with a detailed and comprehensive conversation with the patient, during which the estimated chance of long-term seizure freedom as well as the risk and nature of probable operative complications or the risks of "non surgical treatment strategy" are to be discussed.

## 8.3.8 Surgical Strategy

### 8.3.8.1 Lesionectomy

The main goal of the surgery is the safe and complete resection of the CCM and the adjacent hemosiderin deposits (so called **lesionectomy**). The incomplete resection of the CCM is associated with risk for recurrence and impaired seizure outcome [30]. There is also evidence that the seizure outcome is impaired when the hemosiderin is not completely resected [23]. Of course, hemosiderin resection may be limited in eloquent areas. In this case, pre- and intraoperative mapping (awake surgery) and monitoring to define the resectable tissue should be performed.

The access to the CCM can be reached via the typical trans-sulcal, trans-cisternal or trans-cerebral approaches. It should be common sense now, that any associated DVA must be preserved to avoid venous infarction [24]. The microsurgical technique is standard. Hemosiderin deposits can be identified as yellowish, gliotic tissue directly adjacent to the CCM. Especially in complex configured or localized CCM, intraoperative ultrasound helps to ensure the complete resection. Hemosiderin typically shows a hyper-echoic signal on ultrasound. Normally, vascularization of the CCM itself is sparse without larger feeders and drainer. We recommend postoperative MRI control, confirming the complete resection including the hemosiderin deposits. Due to early postoperative imaging artefacts, the MRI should be routinely performed after 3 months [31].

As a rule, in patients with new-onset single or multiple seizures a lesionectomy is sufficient for excellent seizure control. As an exception, in patients with a temporo-mesial CCM with CRE and an additional ipsilateral hippocampal sclerosis, simultaneous removal of *both lesions* is recommended [1, 32, 33].

### 8.3.8.2 Extended Resections

Extended resections (lesionectomy and resection of epileptogenic onset zone) may be considered in patients with *persisting seizures after* an initial lesionectomy and the suspicion of a residual seizure onset zone. The specific epileptological work-up may than identify the epileptogenic zone for which a tailored removal can be performed. Such a 2-step strategy has been e.g. proposed by Ferroli et al. [34].

Patients that present a history of longstanding or frequent seizures or that fulfil the criteria of a medically refractory CRE should mandatorily undergo a specific epileptological work-up before any surgery is performed. These patients may show a worse seizure outcome compared to patients with a short seizure history [35]. Video EEG monitoring should be performed to identify the epileptogenic zone and tailor the resection. Magnetencephalography (MEG), electrical source imaging (ESI) and ictal SPECT may provide further helpful information in this regard but should be considered optional at present [1]. As a rule, patients that show a discordance between EEG video monitoring localization of the epileptogenic zone and the localization of the suspected CCM are at risk for incomplete seizure control after sole lesionectomy [32]. In such a situation ILAE proposes a preoperative *invasive* EEG evaluation (deep electrodes, grid).

## 8.3.9 Surgical Outcome

### 8.3.9.1 General Surgical Outcome

General risks of surgery are comparable to those in other neurosurgical procedures. Main risks are infection and postoperative complications necessitating any medical intervention. They are reported around 3% and around 10%, respectively [36, 37]. Specific surgical risks are mainly related to the anatomic localization of the lesion. However, even the resection of lesions in eloquent regions can normally be safely performed under brain mapping/monitoring.

### 8.3.9.2 General Seizure Outcome

Overall seizure outcome after surgery based on the current body of literature is difficult to interpret. Missing or fragmentary data on rates of withdrawal from AEDs and on functional outcome, along with varying definitions of seizure freedom and medically refractory CRE are the most common drawbacks [38]. The series of Baumann et al. is still the largest series published so far, including 168 patients from different centers. The authors reported 70% Engel class 1 at 1-year follow-up, declining to 65% at the third year follow-up. Smaller series including mainly new-onset seizures report seizure freedom in around 80–90% [19, 39]. In our own comparative observational series of 79 patients (data from 2002 to 2011) we found 88% with new-onset seizure and 79% with "chronic" seizures seizure free for at least 2 years at the last follow-up. The 5-year cumulative probability to stay completely seizure free after surgery was 73% and 68%, respectively. Under conservative treatment this probability was only 22%. 78%, 58% and 8% were off AEDs at the last follow-up, respectively [6].

### 8.3.9.3 Predictors for Seizure Outcome

Many series have analyzed specific predictors for seizure outcome in their data. Naturally, all results are significantly limited by the mostly retrospective, non-controlled, non-randomized study designs. Some predictors accordingly showed a controversial impact (sex, age). However, one predictor showed a constant impact on outcome throughout multiple studies: the duration of epilepsy is negatively correlated with seizure outcome [15, 16, 19, 32, 39–41]. Most authors found this negative correlation after CRE duration of >2 years.

## 8.4 Summary

While a watch and wait strategy for patients with CCM is advisable in many cases, especially in supratentorial (asymptomatic) CCM, patients with a CRE represent a special subgroup. Being of relatively young age at the time of diagnosis and being at a high risk for future seizure events, they may significantly profit from an early control of their epilepsy and the potential withdrawal of AEDs. Although high level evidence is still missing, due to the lack of randomized controlled trials, it seems that a surgical treatment of the lesions is relatively safe and effective compared to a conservative approach. In general, the interdisciplinary consultation of these patients should be aspired and will lead to additive positive effects for both, the patients and the doctors.

## References


1. Rosenow F, et al. Cavernoma-related epilepsy: review and recommendations for management-report of the surgical task force of the ILAE Commission on Therapeutic Strategies. Epilepsia. 2013;54(12):2025–35.
2. Otten P, et al. 131 cases of cavernous angioma (cavernomas) of the CNS, discovered by retrospective analysis of 24,535 autopsies. Neurochirurgie. 1989;35(2):82–3. 128–31.
3. Choi J, et al. Hepatic cavernous hemangiomas: long-term (> 5 years) follow-up changes on contrast-enhanced dynamic computed tomography or magnetic resonance imaging and determinant factors of the size change. Radiol Med. 2018;123(5):323–30.

4. Calandriello L, et al. Cavernous venous malformation (cavernous hemangioma) of the orbit: current concepts and a review of the literature. Surv Ophthalmol. 2017;62(4):393–403.
5. Menzler K, et al. Epileptogenicity of cavernomas depends on (archi-) cortical localization. Neurosurgery. 2010;67(4):918–24.
6. Dammann P, et al. Outcome after conservative management or surgical treatment for new-onset epilepsy in cerebral cavernous malformation. J Neurosurg. 2017;126(4):1303–11.
7. Moriarity JL, et al. The natural history of cavernous malformations: a prospective study of 68 patients. Neurosurgery. 1999;44(6):1166–71. discussion 1172–3.
8. Josephson CB, et al. Seizure risk from cavernous or arteriovenous malformations: prospective population-based study. Neurology. 2011;76(18):1548–54.
9. Alvarez de Eulate-Beramendi S, et al. Pathogenetic bases of epileptogenesis in cerebral cavernomas. Rev Neurol. 2012;55(12):718–24.
10. Willmore LJ, et al. Chronic focal epileptiform discharges induced by injection of iron into rat and cat cortex. Science. 1978;200(4349):1501–3.
11. Fedele DE, et al. Astrogliosis in epilepsy leads to overexpression of adenosine kinase, resulting in seizure aggravation. Brain. 2005;128(Pt 10):2383–95.
12. Seifert G, Schilling K, Steinhauser C. Astrocyte dysfunction in neurological disorders: a molecular perspective. Nat Rev Neurosci. 2006;7(3):194–206.
13. Cox EM, Bambakidis NC, Cohen ML. Pathology of cavernous malformations. Handb Clin Neurol. 2017;143:267–77.
14. Al-Shahi Salman R, et al. Untreated clinical course of cerebral cavernous malformations: a prospective, population-based cohort study. Lancet Neurol. 2012;11(3):217–24.
15. Moran NF, et al. Supratentorial cavernous haemangiomas and epilepsy: a review of the literature and case series. J Neurol Neurosurg Psychiatry. 1999;66(5):561–8.
16. Baumann CR, et al. Seizure outcome after resection of supratentorial cavernous malformations: a study of 168 patients. Epilepsia. 2007;48(3):559–63.
17. Dammann P, et al. Correlation of the venous angioarchitecture of multiple cerebral cavernous malformations with familial or sporadic disease: a susceptibility-weighted imaging study with 7-Tesla MRI. J Neurosurg. 2017;126(2):570–7.
18. Vernooij MW, et al. Incidental findings on brain MRI in the general population. N Engl J Med. 2007;357(18):1821–8.
19. Casazza M, et al. Supratentorial cavernous angiomas and epileptic seizures: preoperative course and postoperative outcome. Neurosurgery. 1996;39(1):26–32. discussion 32–4.
20. Al-Shahi Salman R, et al. Hemorrhage from cavernous malformations of the brain: definition and reporting standards. Angioma Alliance Scientific Advisory Board. Stroke. 2008;39(12):3222–30.
21. Dammann P, et al. Solitary sporadic cerebral cavernous malformations: risk factors of first or recurrent symptomatic hemorrhage and associated functional impairment. World Neurosurg. 2016;91:73–80.
22. Horne MA, et al. Clinical course of untreated cerebral cavernous malformations: a meta-analysis of individual patient data. Lancet Neurol. 2016;15(2):166–73.
23. Dammann P, Schaller C, Sure U. Should we resect peri-lesional hemosiderin deposits when performing lesionectomy in patients with cavernoma-related epilepsy (CRE)? Neurosurg Rev. 2017;40(1):39–43.
24. Buhl R, et al. Therapeutical considerations in patients with intracranial venous angiomas. Eur J Neurol. 2002;9(2):165–9.
25. King MA, et al. Epileptology of the first-seizure presentation: a clinical, electroencephalographic, and magnetic resonance imaging study of 300 consecutive patients. Lancet. 1998;352(9133):1007–11.
26. Fisher RS, et al. ILAE official report: a practical clinical definition of epilepsy. Epilepsia. 2014;55(4):475–82.
27. Lamberink HJ, et al. Individualised prediction model of seizure recurrence and long-term outcomes after withdrawal of antiepileptic drugs in seizure-free patients: a systematic review and individual participant data meta-analysis. Lancet Neurol. 2017;16(7):523–31.

28. Kwan P, et al. Definition of drug resistant epilepsy: consensus proposal by the ad hoc task force of the ILAE commission on therapeutic strategies. Epilepsia. 2010;51(6):1069–77.
29. Rocamora R, et al. Epilepsy surgery in patients with multiple cerebral cavernous malformations. Seizure. 2009;18(4):241–5.
30. Kim DS, et al. An analysis of the natural history of cavernous malformations. Surg Neurol. 1997;48(1):9–17. discussion 17–8.
31. Chen B, et al. Reliable? The value of early postoperative magnetic resonance imaging after cerebral cavernous malformation surgery. World Neurosurg. 2017;103:138–44.
32. Hammen T, et al. Prediction of postoperative outcome with special respect to removal of hemosiderin fringe: a study in patients with cavernous haemangiomas associated with symptomatic epilepsy. Seizure. 2007;16(3):248–53.
33. Stefan H, Hammen T. Cavernous haemangiomas, epilepsy and treatment strategies. Acta Neurol Scand. 2004;110(6):393–7.
34. Ferroli P, et al. Cerebral cavernomas and seizures: a retrospective study on 163 patients who underwent pure lesionectomy. Neurol Sci. 2006;26(6):390–4.
35. Stavrou I, et al. Long-term seizure control after resection of supratentorial cavernomas: a retrospective single-center study in 53 patients. Neurosurgery. 2008;63(5):888–96. discussion 897.
36. Young RF, Lawner PM. Perioperative antibiotic prophylaxis for prevention of postoperative neurosurgical infections. A randomized clinical trial. J Neurosurg. 1987;66(5):701–5.
37. Sarnthein J, et al. A patient registry to improve patient safety: recording general neurosurgery complications. PLoS One. 2016;11(9):e0163154.
38. von der Brelie C, Schramm J. Cerebral cavernous malformations and intractable epilepsy: the limited usefulness of current literature. Acta Neurochir. 2011;153(2):249–59.
39. Yeon JY, et al. Supratentorial cavernous angiomas presenting with seizures: surgical outcomes in 60 consecutive patients. Seizure. 2009;18(1):14–20.
40. Cappabianca P, et al. Supratentorial cavernous malformations and epilepsy: seizure outcome after lesionectomy on a series of 35 patients. Clin Neurol Neurosurg. 1997;99(3):179–83.
41. Cohen DS, Zubay GP, Goodman RR. Seizure outcome after lesionectomy for cavernous malformations. J Neurosurg. 1995;83(2):237–42.

# Chapter 9
# Surgery of Deep-Seated Cavernous Malformations

Petr Skalický, Vladimír Beneš, and Ondřej Bradáč

## 9.1 Thalamic Cavernomas

The number of reports in the literature of natural history, treatment and outcomes of thalamic CMs is low. The first reported cases particularly by Becker et al. [1] and Roda et al. [2] were associated with poor surgical outcome. The patients most commonly present with contralateral sensoric and motor deficits [3], however the relation of thalamus to many functions of the brain predisposes the lesions to cause other symptoms on the location such as hemianopsia, thalamic pain [4] or even an obstructive hydrocephalus after bleeding in the proximal areas to the third ventricle [5]. Thalamic CMs therefore share many similarities with the brainstem cavernomas, but are further complicated by a close relationship with the deep venous drainage of the brain [6]. The mass effect or haemorrhage of the lesion could cause conspicuous deficits due to the sensitivity of the important thalamic structures to even micromorphological changes [7]. Stereotactic surgery has been used by Kondziolka et al. [8] in nine thalamic cases. It was indicated after two small volume haemorrhages. Reduction of haemorrhagic risk after 2-year latency period was observed but 26% of patients had permanent or transient neurologic worsening due to the rebleeding, radionecrosis and prolonged cerebral edema. For other deep seated lesions, the use of intraoperative neuronavigation [9, 10] or auto-navigating operating microscope [11] may be beneficial in the hands of a well experienced neurosurgeon, although objective benefits for neurological outcomes are not yet validated. In cases where the motor and somatosensory pathways are in proximity, monitoring of evoked potentials can be expected [12].


P. Skalický · V. Beneš · O. Bradáč (✉)
Department of Neurosurgery and Neurooncology, First Medical Faculty, Military University Hospital and Charles University, Prague, Czech Republic
e-mail: ondrej.bradac@uvn.cz



© Springer Nature Switzerland AG 2020
O. Bradáč, V. Beneš (eds.), *Cavernomas of the CNS*,
https://doi.org/10.1007/978-3-030-49406-3_9

### 9.1.1 Natural History

The natural history of thalamic cavernomas is difficult to elucidate. In the study of 27 patients by Li et al. [13] the preoperative annual haemorrhage rate was 5.2%. However, in the study of the clinical course of untreated thalamic CMs in 121 patients, the overall annual haemorrhage rate (subsequent to the initial presentation—93.4% of patients with prior haemorrhage) was 9.7% with initial presentation with FND (hazard ratio (HR) 2.767, 95% CI 1.336–5.731) and associated DVA (HR 2.510, 95% CI 1.275–4.942) to be independent haemorrhage risk factors [14]. However, given the low haemorrhage mortality rate in this study (2.5%) and relatively low percentage of patients with worsened clinical condition during the follow-up (20.7%) (mean follow-up duration 3.6 years) observation was adequate in the absence of a surgical indication, although haemorrhage during the follow-up with altered clinical condition justify surgery [14]. The observed haemorrhage rate in this study is comparable to 11.0% reported for basal ganglia CMs but substantially lower than the 21.5% reported for brainstem CMs in the same study as for the basal ganglia CMs [15]. Although this is lower than the numbers reported for brainstem CMs, the mentioned estimates for brainstem CMs in the natural history paragraph are derived from a meta-analysis.

### 9.1.2 Surgical Approach

Due to the close relation to important neurovascular structures it is difficult to select an appropriate surgical approach. Rangel-Castilla and Spetzler [16] divided the thalamus into six regions and matched them with the corresponding approach (Table 9.1) with excellent surgical outcomes. Out of 46 reported patients 4 (9%) of them were worse relative to their preoperative condition. Out of 27 reported patients in the study by Li et al. [13] 2 (7.4%) of them were worse relative to their preoperative state.

**Table 9.1** Proposed classification of thalamic regions for surgical approach decision for thalamic CMs based on the study by Rangel-Castilla and Spetzler [16]

| Region | Location | Approach[a] |
|---|---|---|
| 1 | Anteroinferior | OZ |
| 2 | Lateral | AIT |
| 3 | Medial | ACT |
| 4 | Posterosuperior | PIT |
| 5 | Lateral Posteroinferior | POT |
| 6 | Medial Posteroinferior | SCIT |

[a]Abbreviations: *ACT* anterior contralateral interhemispheric transcallosal, *AIT* anterior ipsilateral interhemispheric transcallosal, *OZ* orbitozygomatic, *PIT* posterior interhemispheric transcallosal, *POT* parietooccipital transventricular, *SCIT* suboccipital supracerebellar infratentorial

Region 1 consists of inferior parts of anterior and ventral anterior nuclei of the thalamus, and lies next to the Regions 2 and 3 which form the superior and posterior margins. Region 2 contains the superior part of anterior nucleus, medial and median nuclei. Region 3 consists of the superior and posterior part of ventral anterior nucleus, ventral and lateral nuclei. The margin between the Regions 2 and 3 is made of internal medullary lamina. Regions 4, 5 and 6 house different parts of pulvinar—Region 4: superior part, Region 5: lateral inferior part and Region 6: medial inferior part. This division is due to the 3 different compartments of the surrounding structures making the surgical approach more challenging. Region 4 is facing the upper part of the ambient and quadrigeminal cisterns, is inferiorly to the lateral ventricle and the corpus callosum and medially to the posterior limb of the internal capsule. Region 5 projects to the anterior wall of the atrium, medially is limited by the choroid plexus and laterally by the tail of the caudate nucleus and posterior limb of the internal capsule. Region 6 is next to the ambient cistern and close to the pineal gland, habenular commissure and lateral habenular nucleus making the paramedian supracerebellar infrantentorial approach most reasonable option. Both Regions 5 and 6 continue inferiorly to the midbrain [16]. On the other hand, every patient is unique and a particular lesion often can be reached via more than one corridor. The choice of approach depends on the anatomy of the lesion and the principle of lowest possible damage of adjacent eloquent areas. Some examples of resected cavernomas together with approach description is depicted in Figs. 9.1, 9.2, 9.3, 9.4, 9.5, 9.6, 9.7, 9.8, 9.9, and 9.10.

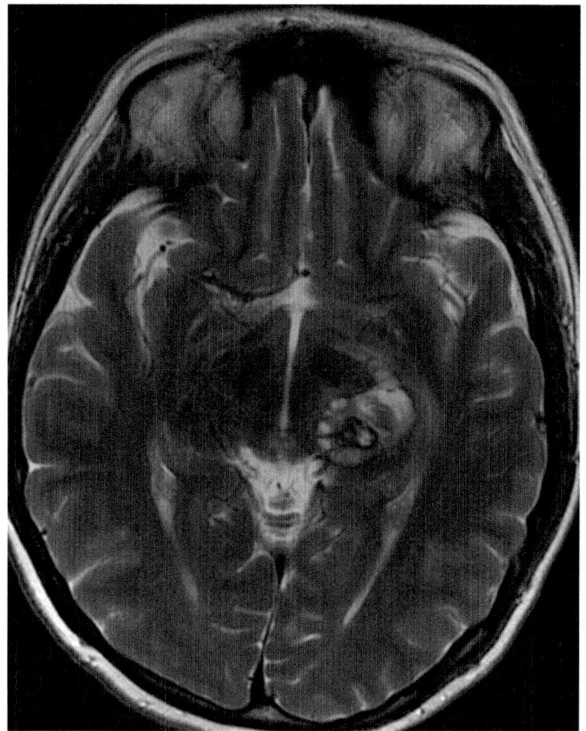

**Fig. 9.1** Thalamic cavernoma. Supracerebellar-infratentorial approach was used. Preop MR axial scan

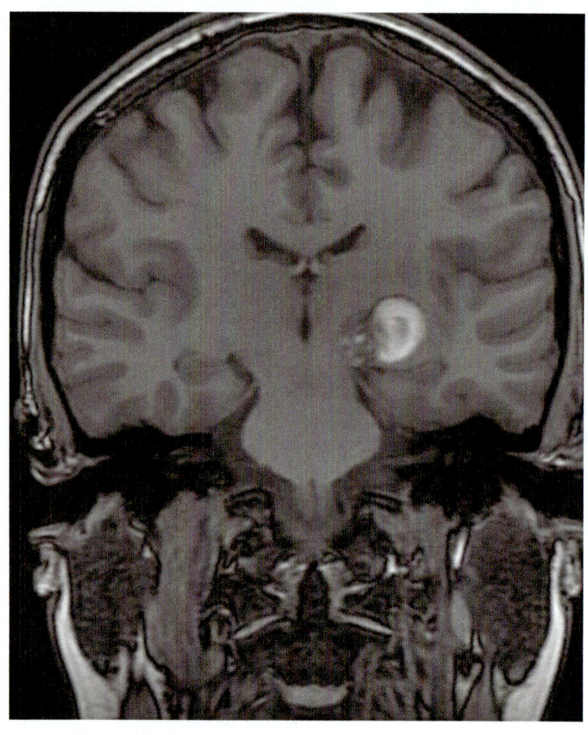

**Fig. 9.2** Thalamic cavernoma. Supracerebellar-infratentorial approach was used. Preop MR coronal scan

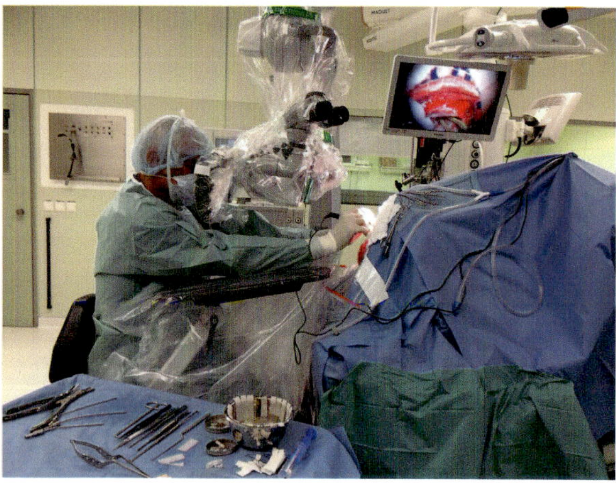

**Fig. 9.3** Supracerebellar-infratentorial approach. Intraop setup

**Fig. 9.4** Thalamic cavernoma. Supracerebellar-infratentorial approach was used. Entry point between vessels

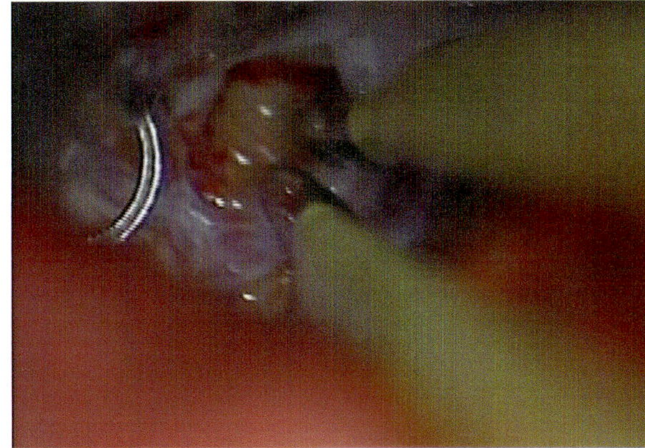

**Fig. 9.5** Thalamic cavernoma. Supracerebellar-infratentorial approach was used. Cavernoma resection

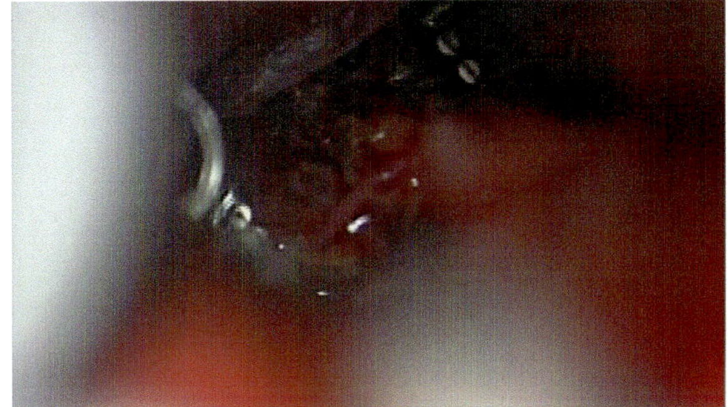

**Fig. 9.6** Thalamic cavernoma. Supracerebellar-infratentorial approach was used. Resection cavity with intact vessels around thalamus entry

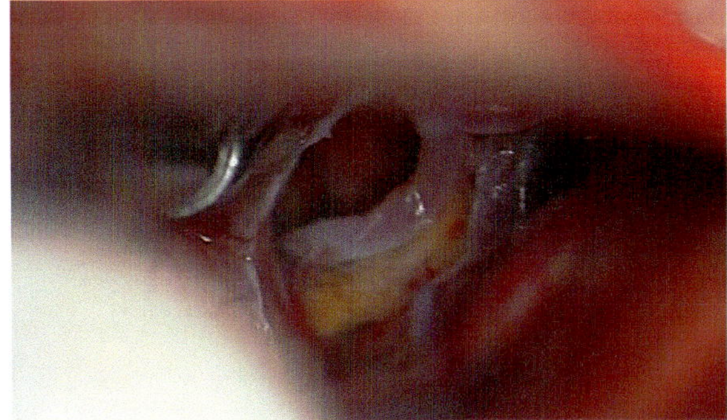

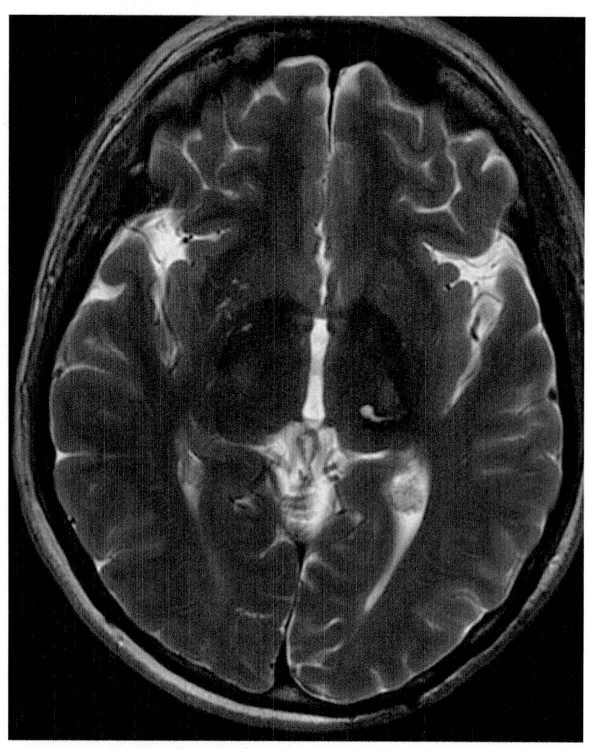

**Fig. 9.7** Thalamic cavernoma. Supracerebellar-infratentorial approach was used. Postop MR axial scan

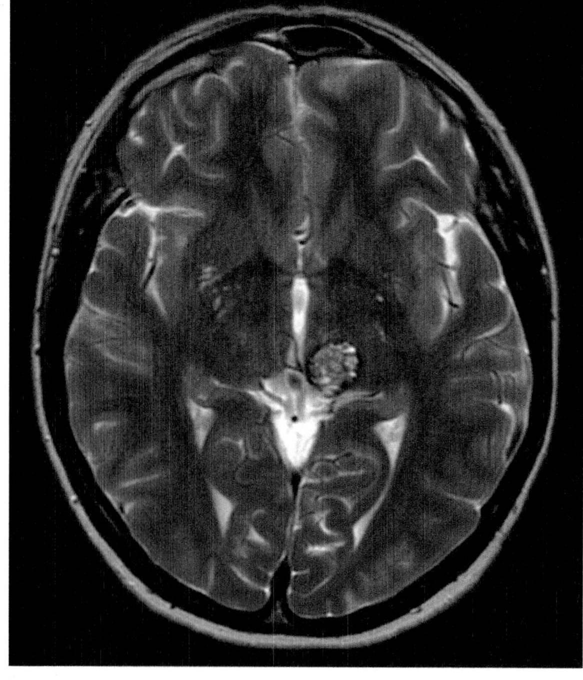

**Fig. 9.8** Case of a 52 years old woman with a left thalamic cavernoma in Region 6—according to a classification by Rangel-Castilla and Spetzler. After 9 years of observation she presented with acute onset of hemihypestesia, mild hemiparesis and cephalea. MRI (axial T2WI image) revealed enlargement of the lesion due to a haemorrhage. She was operated via supracerebellar infratentorial approach 2 weeks after bleeding with intraoperative neurophysiological monitoring of MEPs and SEPs which remained unchanged during the resection

**Fig. 9.9** Postoperative MRI (axial T2WI image) confirmed gross total resection with residual hemosiderin deposits in the cavity walls

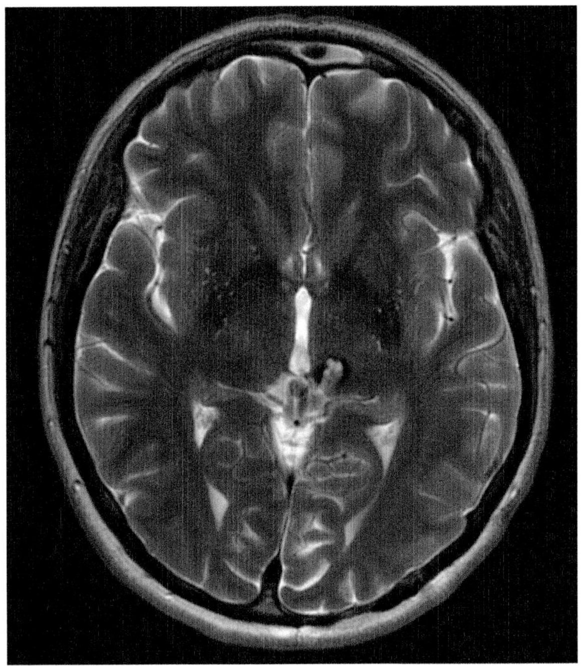

**Fig. 9.10** MRI (axial T2WI image) showing no changes in the cavity after 9 months of follow-up while the woman's hemiparesis and hemihypestesia slightly improved

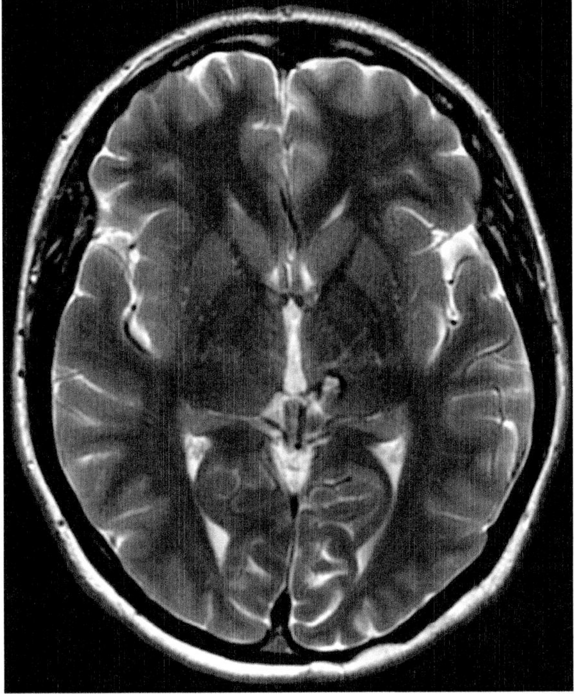

**Keypoints**
- Symptomatic thalamic lesions that have bled at least once and reach the pial or ependymal surface should be surgically resected with careful consideration of the case specific anatomy and usage of relatively safe surgical approaches to different parts of thalamus.
- Gross total resection should be achieved without an inadequate traction and over-aggressive resection of the surrounding parenchyma. The risks of damage to the surrounding tissue must be weighed against the risks of leaving residual cavernous malformation with a risk of delayed haemorrhage.
- Timing of surgery, natural history of cavernomas in this specific location as well as the effects of radiosurgical therapy remains unclear. The management of particular cases depends on the specific bias of the lesion and patient, in concordance with the surgeon's expertise.

## 9.2 Basal Ganglia Cavernomas

Gross et al. [3] provided a review of CMs of both basal ganglia and thalamus. The annual bleeding rates for these lesions were 2.8–4.1% in the included natural history studies. The resection rate in surgical series was 89% with 10% risk of long-term surgical morbidity and 1.9% risk of surgical mortality. Most of the patients presented with sensorimotor deficits. For basal ganglia CMs specifically, patients may present with parkinsonism [17] and other extrapyramidal symptoms such as hemichorea [18] with possible improvement of hemichorea with medication, for instance sodium valproate in a patient with a putaminal CM who declined surgery [19] or pimozide in a patient with caudostriatal CM [20]. Some of the studies where surgery completely relieved hemichorea [18] or ballismus [21] proposed a mechanism of release phenomena caused by interruption of striatal projections. Dystonia is another less common presentation for both thalamic and basal ganglia CMs [22]. Lorenzana et al. [23] reported focal hand dystonia in a patient with a lentiform CM with resolution of symptoms after surgical excision. As the radiosurgical therapeutic effects are unclear in the treatment of CMs in all locations due to the lack of prospective studies, its use for basal ganglia CMs should be reserved for the symptomatic cases with two or more haemorrhages where surgical resection is contraindicated. This is despite the fact that most of the retrospective studies reported significant reduction of rebleeding after 2 year latency period with a permanent radiation induced complication ranging from 0 to 75% [3].

### 9.2.1 Surgical Approach

Surgical approaches to the basal ganglia comprise of four possible safe routes (Table 9.2). The CMs in the head of the caudate nucleus can be reached by the anterior transsylvian-transinsular approach if the lesions are located in the lateral aspect of the nucleus/anterior limb of the internal capsule, are thinning the overlying

**Table 9.2**  Surgical approaches to different parts of basal ganglia based on Chang et al. and Potts et al. [24, 25]

| Location | Approach |
| --- | --- |
| Head of the caudate nucleus | Anterior transsylvian-transinsular |
| Claustrum, extreme capsule, lentiform nucleus | Posterior transsylvian-transinsular |
| Lentiform nucleus, anterior limb of internal capsule | Supracarotid-infrafrontal |
| Medial aspect of the caudate nucleus | Contralateral transcallosal |

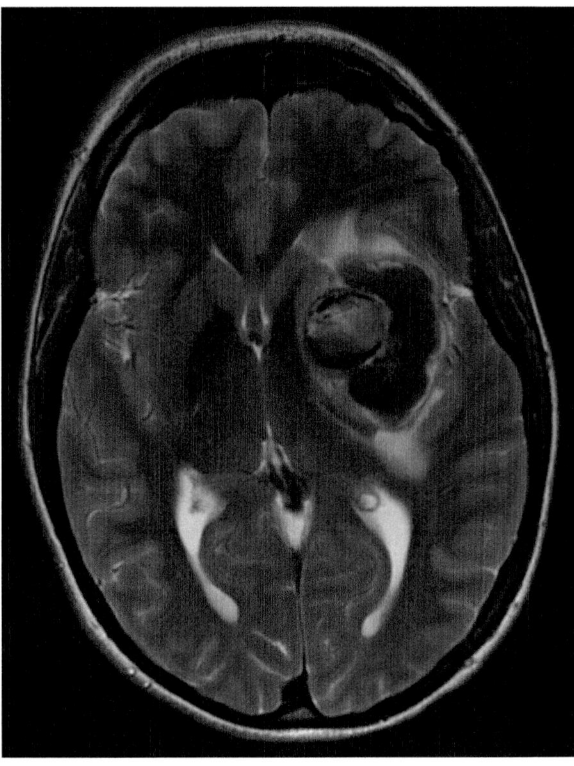

**Fig. 9.11**  Case of a 29 years old woman presenting with acute onset of mild aphasia and cephalea. MRI (axial T2WI image) showed an intracerebral haematoma in the left caudate nucleus. She was operated 10 days after onset of symptoms via posterior transsylvian transinsular approach. Haematoma was aspirated, cavernoma was revealed on the medial wall of the cavity and totally resected. Postoperatively she developed dyscalculia. Degree of aphasia remained unchanged, showing slight improvement during the follow-up (53 months)

insular cortex, and displace the caudate head medially. If these structures are displaced laterally and the lesion has an ependymal projection on the ventricular wall, the contralateral transcallosal approach is optimal. This is applicable for the lesions in the head of the caudate nucleus and the anterior part of its body due to the proximity to the ventricular wall. The claustrum, extreme capsule, globus pallidus and putamen can be reached via the posterior transsylvian-transinsular approach especially if the overlying insular cortex is thinned by the CM or haematoma. The posterior limb or the genu of internal capsule define the medial extent of the exposure. The supracarotid-infrafrontal approach can be used in occasions when there is thinned medial orbital gyrus and the normal basal ganglia structures are displaced posterosuperiorly [24]. Again, some examples of resected cavernomas together with approach description are depicted in Figs. 9.11, 9.12, 9.13, 9.14, 9.15, 9.16, 9.17, 9.18, 9.19, 9.20, 9.21, 9.22, and 9.23.

**Fig. 9.12** Postoperative images (axial T2WI image) showed no residuum of the cavernoma in the resection cavity during whole follow-up

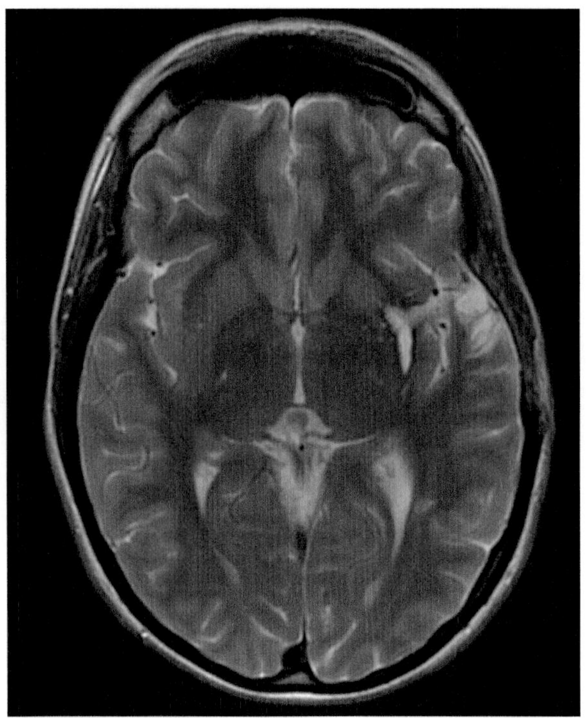

**Fig. 9.13** Deep seated cavernoma. Axial MR scan. Approach via middle temporal gyrus was chosen

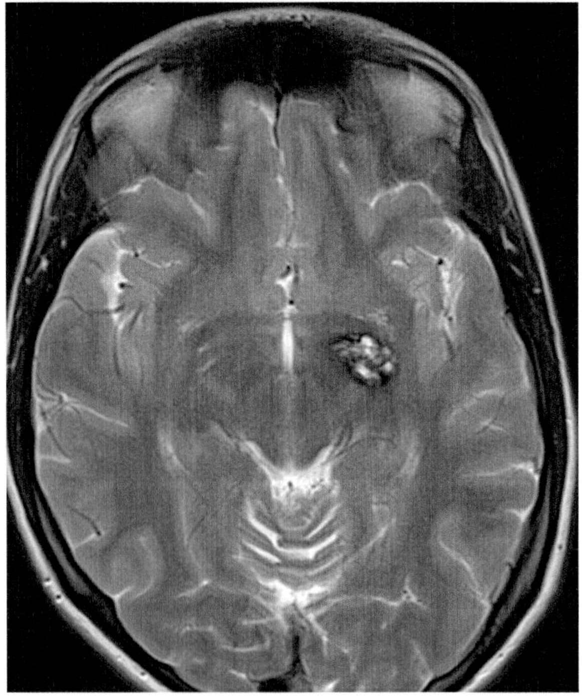

**Fig. 9.14** Deep seated cavernoma. Sagittal MR scan. Approach via middle temporal gyrus was chosen

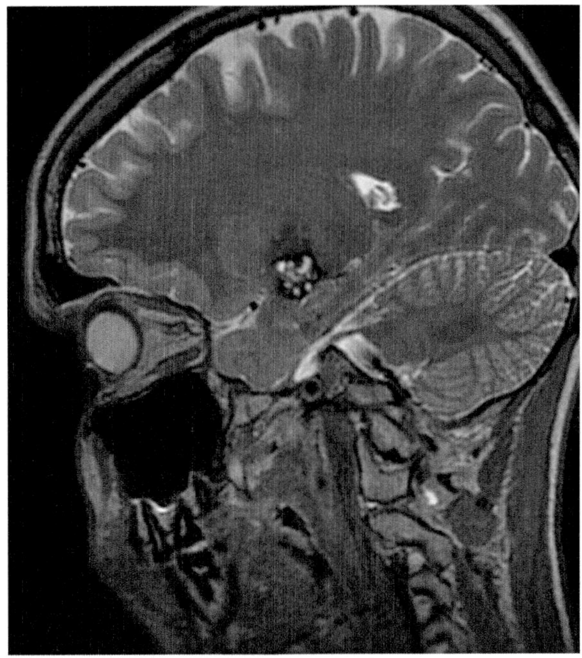

**Fig. 9.15** Deep seated cavernoma. Coronal MR scan. Approach via middle temporal gyrus was chosen

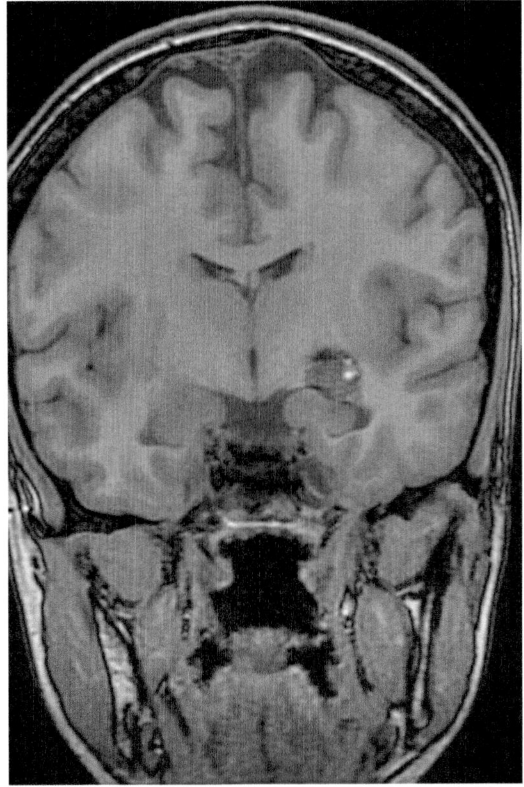

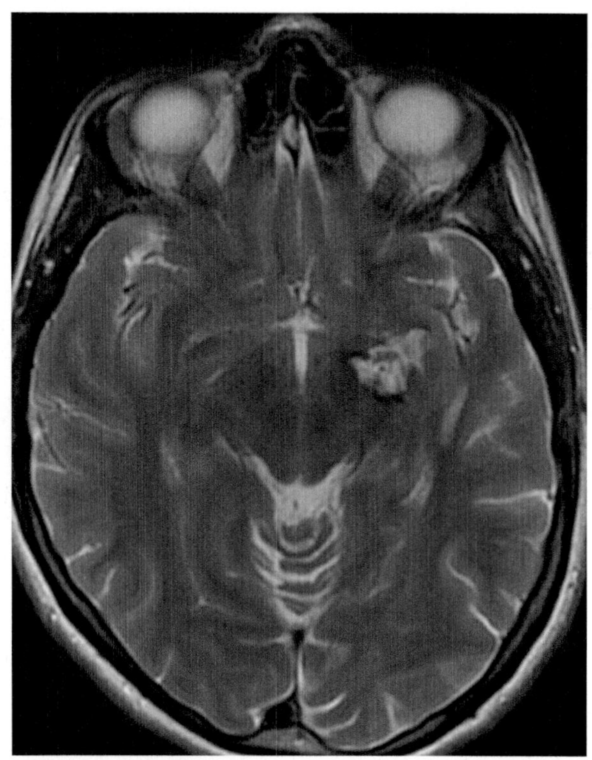

**Fig. 9.16** Deep seated cavernoma. Postop axial MR scan. Approach via middle temporal gyrus was chosen

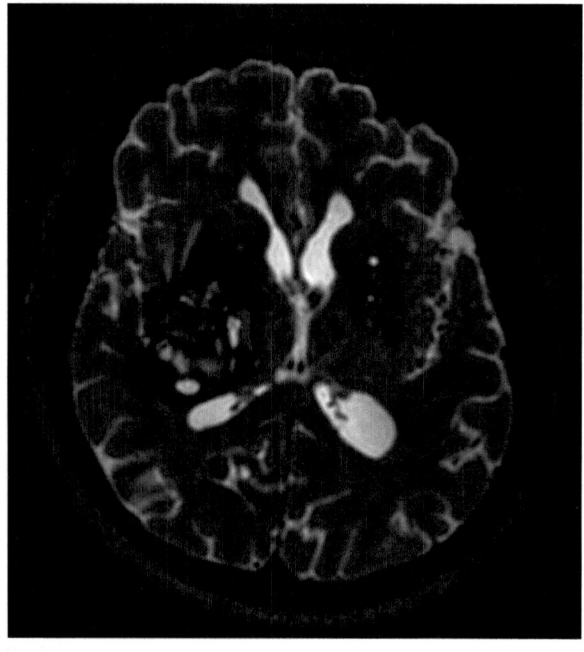

**Fig. 9.17** Cavernoma of basal ganglia, insula and thalamus with signs of bleeding. Axial T2WI scan. Corticospinal tract depicted. Patient presented with hemiparesis and hemidysesthesia. Approach via Sylvian fissure was chosen

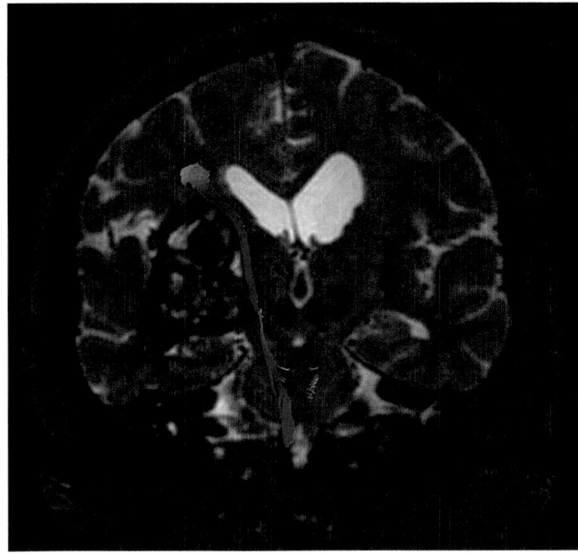

**Fig. 9.18** Cavernoma of basal ganglia, insula and thalamus with signs of bleeding. Coronal T2WI scan. Corticospinal tract depicted. Approach via Sylvian fissure was chosen

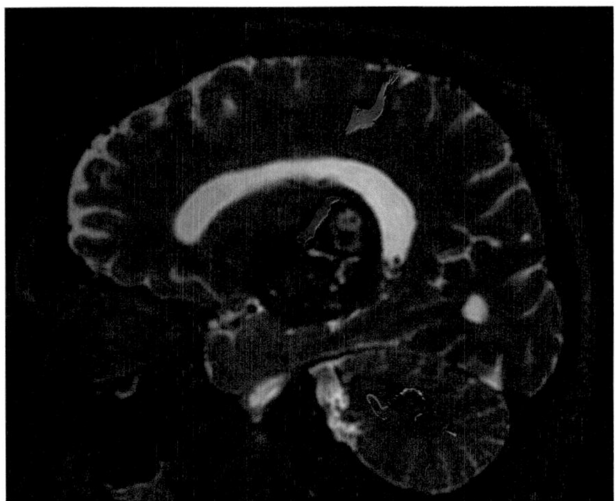

**Fig. 9.19** Cavernoma of basal ganglia, insula and thalamus with signs of bleeding. Sagittal T2WI scan. Corticospinal tract depicted. Approach via Sylvian fissure was chosen

## Key Points

- The annual bleeding rates for these lesions are 2.8–4.1%.
- The resection rate in surgical series is reported 89% with 10% risk of long-term surgical morbidity and 1.9% risk of surgical mortality.
- Most of the patients present with sensorimotor deficits. For basal ganglia CMs specifically, patients may present with parkinsonism and other extrapyramidal symptoms such as hemichorea.
- Surgical approach is strictly individual tailored to lesion.

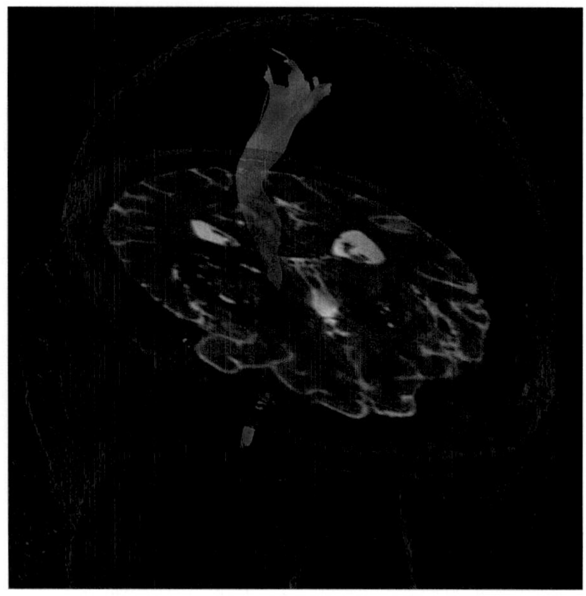

**Fig. 9.20** Cavernoma of basal ganglia, insula and thalamus with signs of bleeding. 3D reconstruction of corticospinal tract and T2WI scan. Approach via Sylvian fissure was chosen

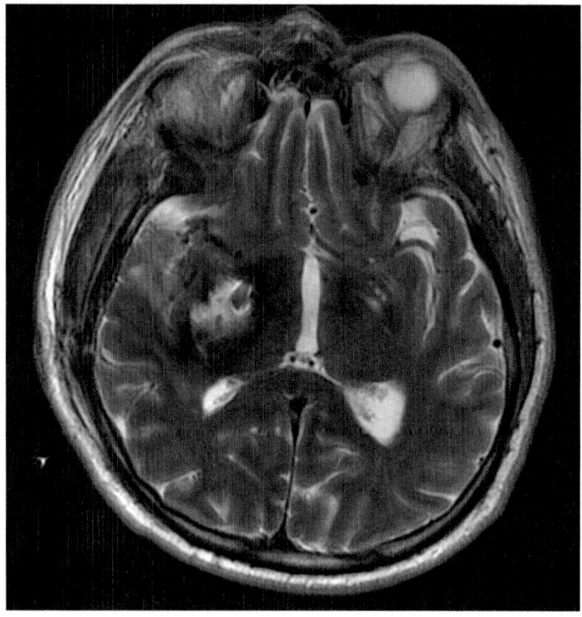

**Fig. 9.21** Cavernoma of basal ganglia, insula and thalamus with signs of bleeding. Post-op axial T2WI scan. Corticospinal tract depicted. Approach via Sylvian fissure was chosen

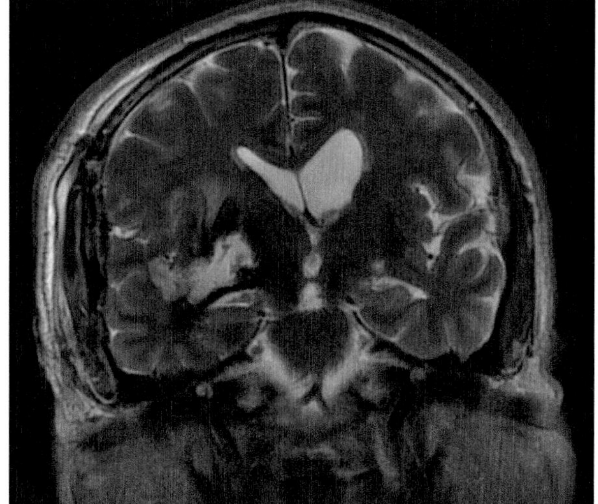

**Fig. 9.22** Cavernoma of basal ganglia, insula and thalamus with signs of bleeding. Post-op coronal T2WI scan. Corticospinal tract depicted. Approach via Sylvian fissure was chosen

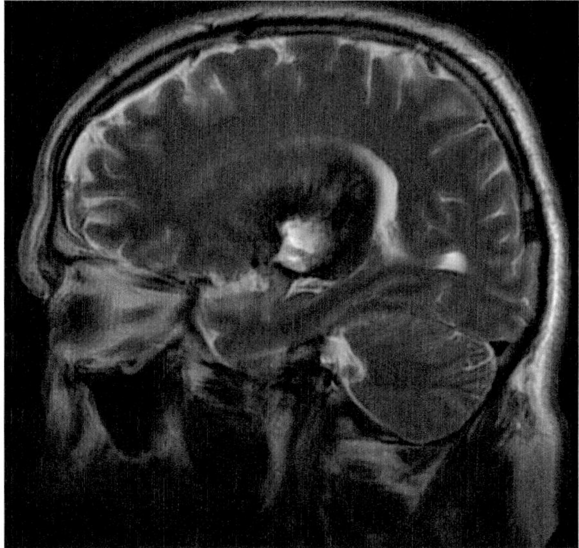

**Fig. 9.23** Cavernoma of basal ganglia, insula and thalamus with signs of bleeding. Post-op sagittal T2WI scan. Corticospinal tract depicted. Approach via Sylvian fissure was chosen

## 9.3   Third Ventricle Cavernomas

Beechar et al. [26] provided a review of 39 symptomatic cases with third ventricle CMs. Most of the patients (66.7%) presented with headaches, and memory disturbances were seen in 30.8% of patients due to a mass effect on fornices. According to the location of the lesions, hydrocephalus was common in these cases and developed in 59% of patients due to the obstruction of foramen Monroi or cerebral aqueduct. As CMs are prone to bleeding, intraventricular haemorrhage may manifest as well (seen in 15.4% of patients). Due to the low blood flow in CMs, none of the intraventricular haemorrhages was catastrophic. Seizures are common symptom of cerebral cavernomas but they were not seen in any of the presented cases of third ventricle CMs. Of the patients (84.6%) that had total resection of the lesion 81.8% had favourable outcomes. Kivelev et al. [27] grouped IVCMs into 3 categories: A—"true" intraventricular lesions attached either to the choroid plexus or ependymal border, B—lesions with <50% volume of intraparenchymal component and C—paraventricular lesions with minimal intraventricular component. In the presented study of 12 patients with group A and B CMs in all of the ventricles, 5 of them had 8 rehaemorrhages soon after primary haemorrhage. This indicates a higher tendency of intraventricular CMs to raehemorrage than CMs in other locations. However, majority of the overall reported rebleeding caused no significant permanent neurological deficits and thus did not require emergency treatment. It was also suggested that the treatment strategy for group C cavernomas should be similar to the intraparenchymal ones. There is not much information about the natural history of intraventricular CMs, however it is believed that these lesions are capable of rapid growth and as suggested by Longatti et al. [28] it may be due to the lower resistance from CSF compared to the parenchyma, and due to intralesional bleeding. This might be more frequent than in other locations, which is in concordance with extensive thrombosis and connective tissue proliferation seen in surgical specimens [29]. As the hemosiderin rim in group A CMs is thinner or absent, special consideration may be important in terms of differential diagnostics of intraventricular lesions [27]. Despite the limited data on third ventricle CMs, gross total resection leads to optimal outcomes in the majority of symptomatic cases without need for permanent CSF diversion in most of the cases that presented with hydrocephalus or intraventricular haemorrhage [26]. However, there is lack of literature for asymptomatic or radiosurgically treated third ventricle CMs, creating inconsistency in the management of these cases.

### 9.3.1 Surgical Approach

The CMs at the foramen of Monroi and lateral walls of the third ventricle are most commonly resected with transcallosal approach. CMs of the ventricular floor could be resected with transcortical transventricular, transcallosal or trans-lamina terminal approaches. Transcortical transventricular and transcallosal approaches are preferred if the lesion is extending laterally and the transcallosal is preferred in patients without hydrocephalus. Trans-lamina terminalis approach is good for resection of the lesions in the floor of the third ventricle and suprachiasmatic region but care must be taken to critical structures to avoid endocrine and visual side effects of the surgery. Another suitable surgical approach to the suprachiasmatic region is interhemispheric transforaminal transchoroidal approach [26]. CMs in the posterior part of the third ventricle can be resected through supracerebellar infratentorial or occipital-transtentorial approaches. The occipital-transtentorial approach carries a higher risk of neurological sequelae due to potential damage to the visual pathway, internal cerebral veins or basal vein of Rosenthal. The supracerebellar infrantetorial approach is safer in terms of surgical corridor, but patient must be in the sitting position [30, 31]. Table 9.3 shows potential options according to the location of the lesion from anterior to posterior parts of the third ventricle. Knowledge of anatomical and pathological consequences is needed for the decision about surgical approach, in order to decrease the potential risk of morbidity, just as it is in other deep seated locations. Figs. 9.24, 9.25, 9.26, 9.27, 9.28, 9.29, 9.30, 9.31, 9.32, 9.33, 9.34, 9.35, 9.36, 9.37, 9.38, 9.39, 9.40, 9.41, and 9.42.

**Table 9.3** Surgical approaches to the third ventricle based on the location of the lesion by Beechar et al. [26]

| Location | Approach |
|---|---|
| Anterior | Subfrontal trans-lamina terminalis |
| => | Transcortical transventricular |
| => | Interhemispheric transforaminal transchoroidal |
| <= | Posterior interhemispheric transcallosal |
| <= | Occipital transtentorial |
| Posterior | Supracerebellar infratentorial |

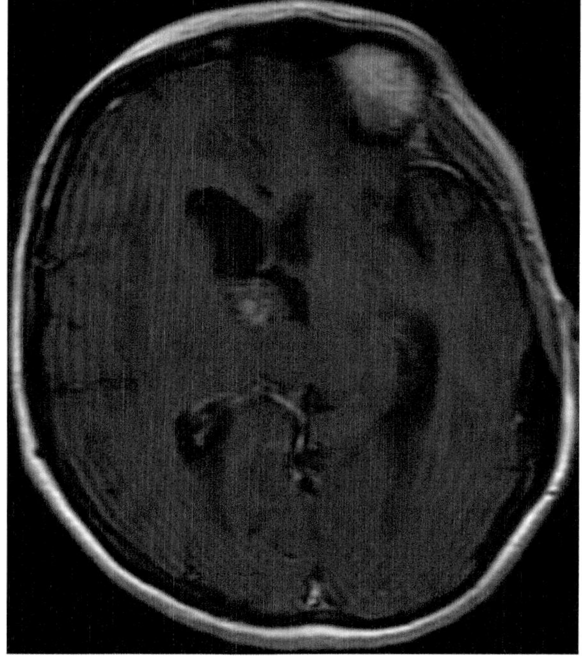

**Fig. 9.24** Cavernoma of the IIIrd ventricle. Axial MR scan. Ipsilateral transcortical approach was chosen

**Fig. 9.25** Cavernoma of the IIIrd ventricle. Coronal MR scan. Ipsilateral transcortical approach was chosen

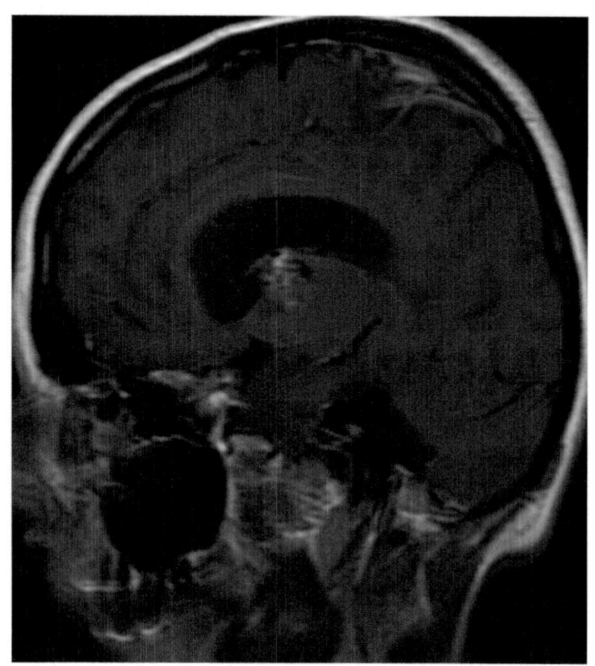

**Fig. 9.26** Cavernoma of the IIIrd ventricle. Coronal MR scan. Ipsilateral transcortical approach was chosen

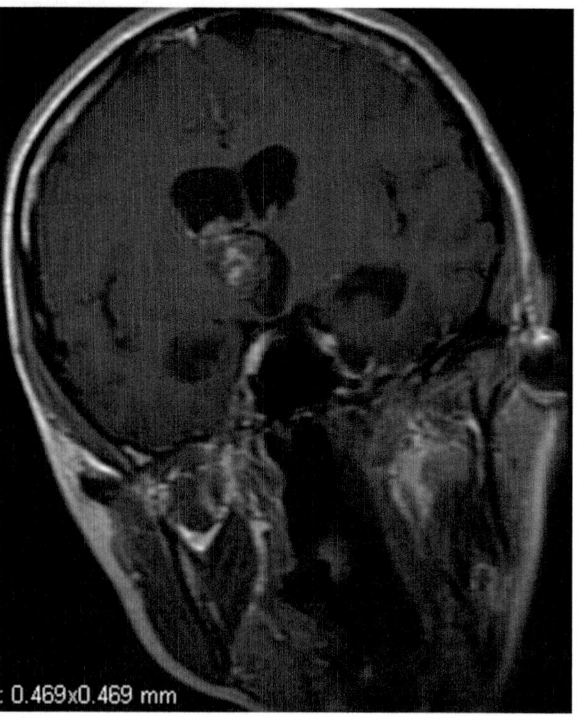

**Fig. 9.27** Cavernoma of the IIIrd ventricle. Postop coronal MR scan. Ipsilateral transcortical approach was chosen

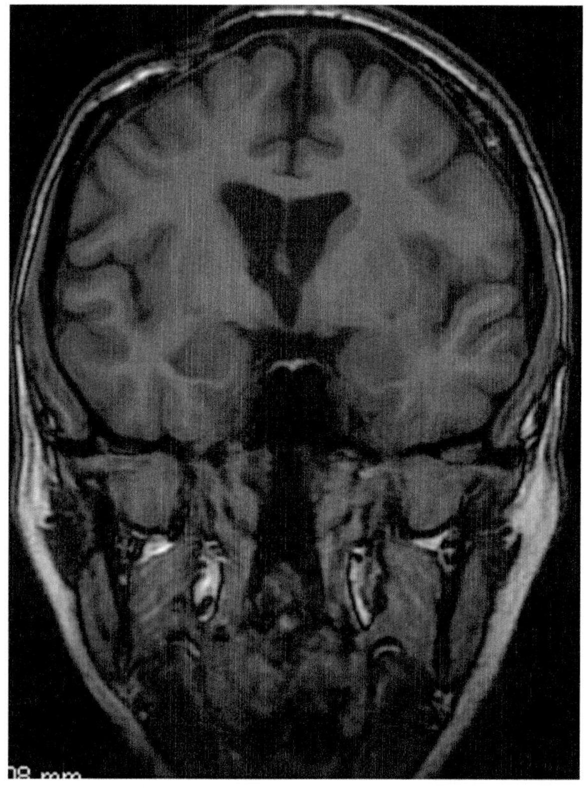

**Fig. 9.28** Cavernoma of the IIIrd ventricle in 6 months old boy. Axial MR scan. Most suitable for transcallosal approach

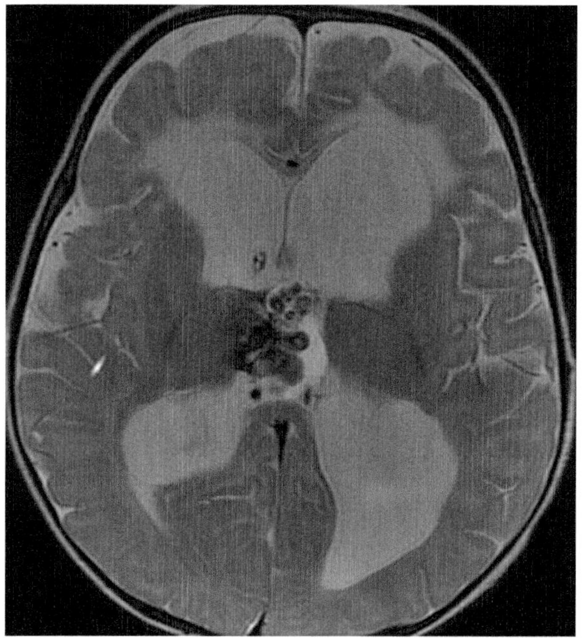

**Fig. 9.29** Cavernoma of the IIIrd ventricle in 6 months old boy. Coronal MR scan. Most suitable for transcallosal approach

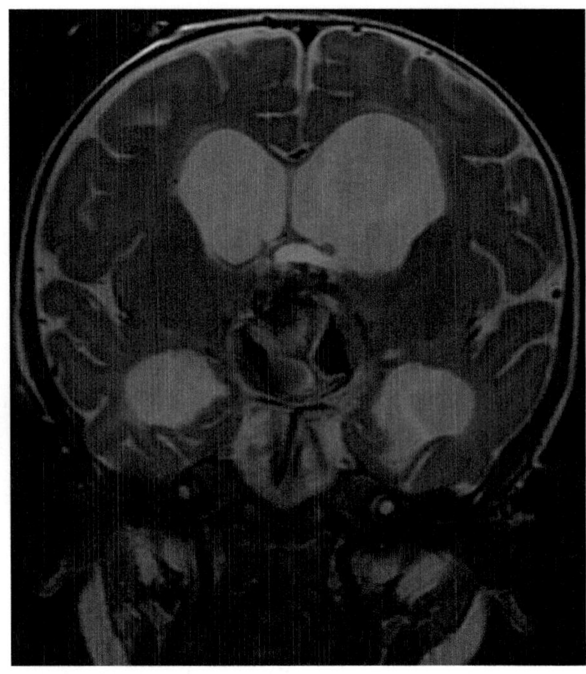

**Fig. 9.30** Cavernoma of the IIIrd ventricle in 6 months old boy. Sagittal MR scan. Most suitable for transcallosal approach

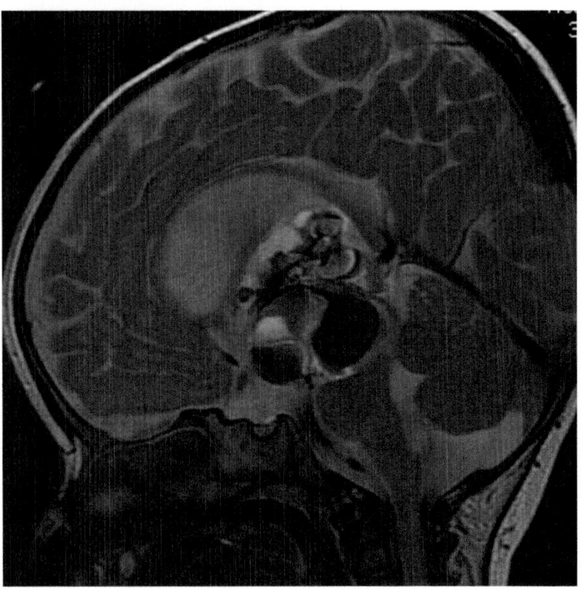

**Fig. 9.31** Cavernoma of the IIIrd ventricle in 6 months old boy. Postop axial MR scan

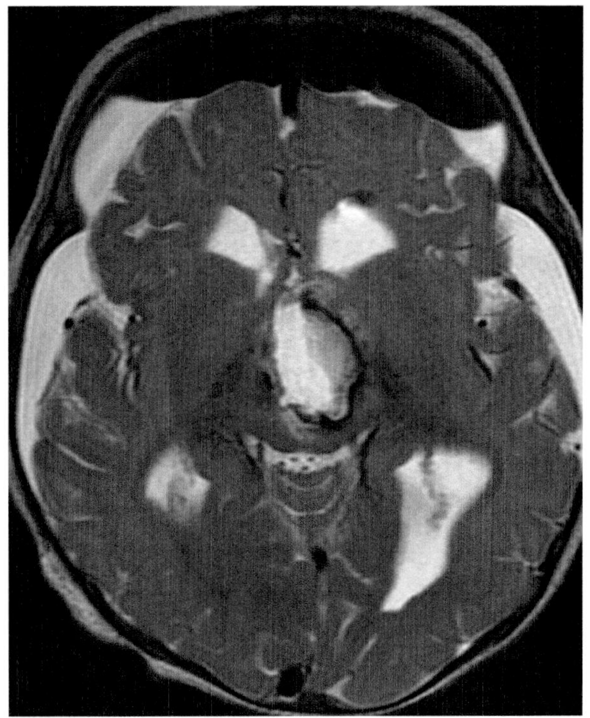

**Fig. 9.32** Cavernoma of the IIIrd ventricle in 6 months old boy. Postop coronal MR scan

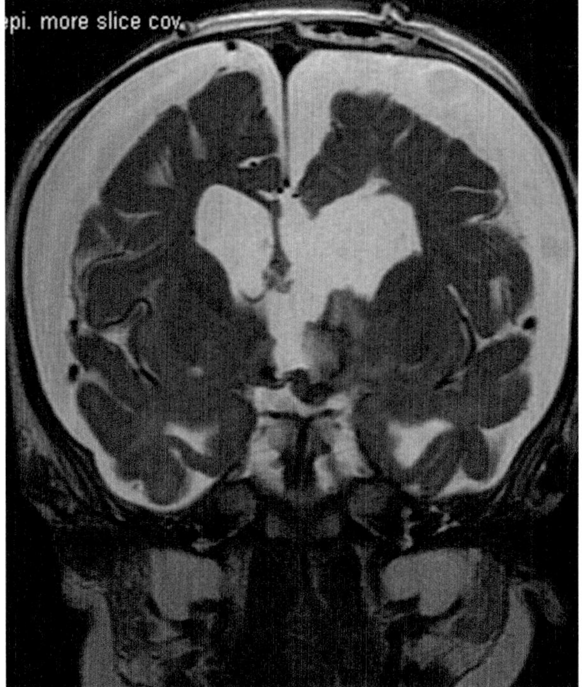

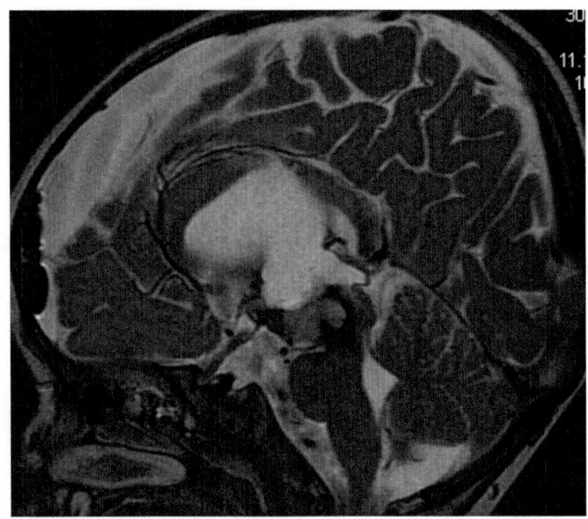

**Fig. 9.33** Cavernoma of the IIIrd ventricle in 6 months old boy. Postop sagittal MR scan

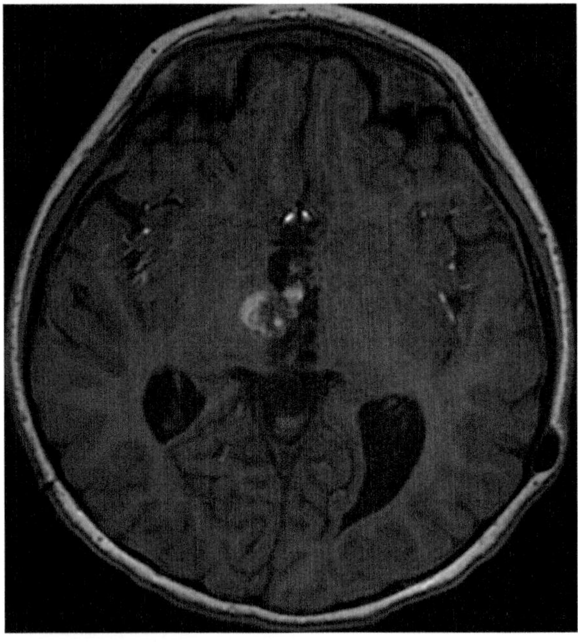

**Fig. 9.34** Cavernoma of the IIIrd ventricle, recurrence of cavernoma at the age of 3 years. Axial MR scan. Transcallosal approach used again

**Fig. 9.35** Cavernoma of the IIIrd ventricle, recurrence of cavernoma at the age of 3 years. Coronal MR scan. Transcallosal approach used again

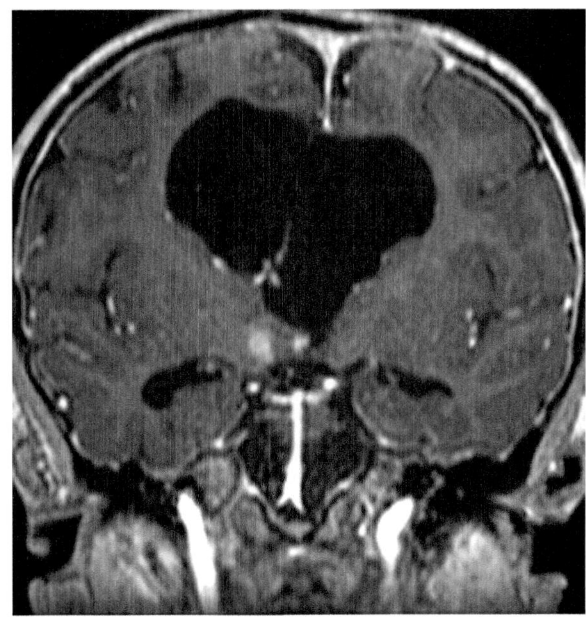

**Fig. 9.36** Cavernoma of the IIIrd ventricle, recurrence of cavernoma at the age of 3 years. Sagittal MR scan. Transcallosal approach used again

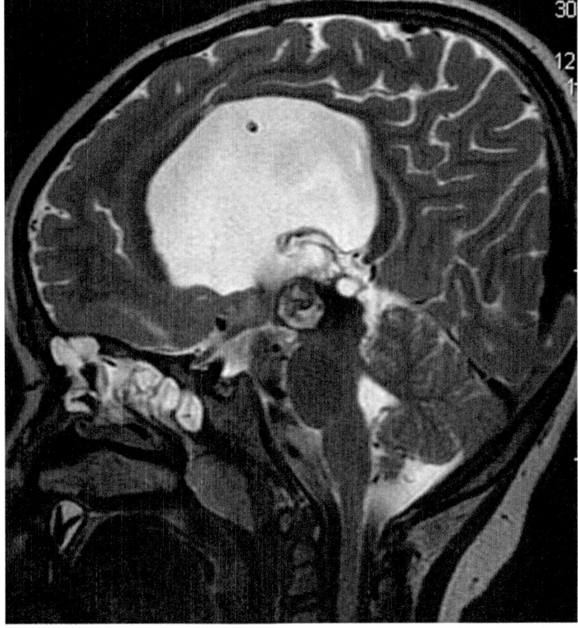

**Fig. 9.37** Cavernoma of the IIIrd ventricle, recurrence of cavernoma at the age of 3 years. Postop coronal MR scan

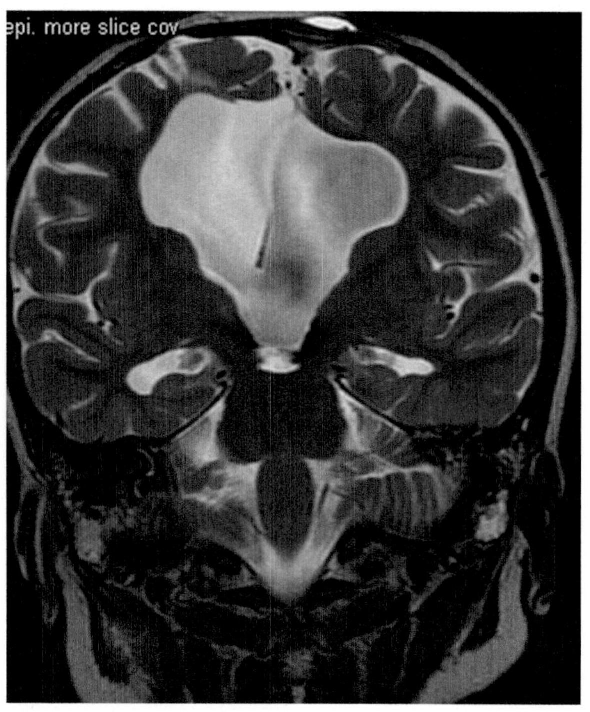

**Fig. 9.38** Cavernoma of the IIIrd ventricle, recurrence of cavernoma at the age of 3 years. Postop sagittal MR scan

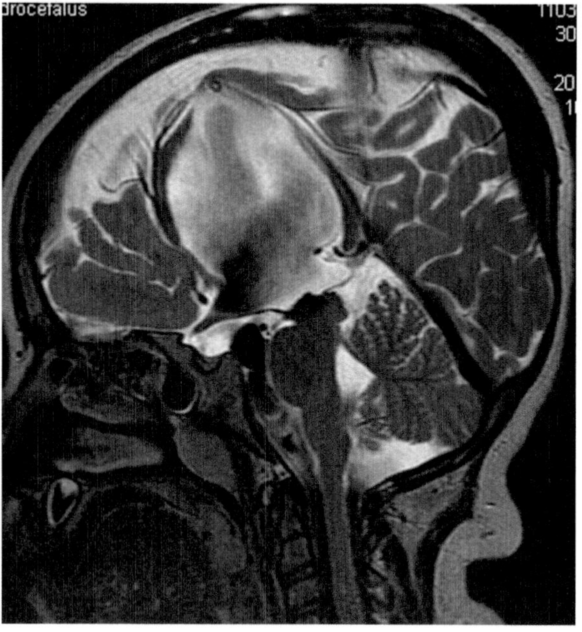

**Fig. 9.39** Case of a 53 years old woman with a 3rd ventricle CM incidentally found in the MRI (axial T2WI image) indicated for hypacusis on the left side. Because of the proximity to the left foramen of Monroi and risk of its obstruction and potential risk of bleeding she was offered surgery. The lesion was totally resected via transcortical transventricular approach

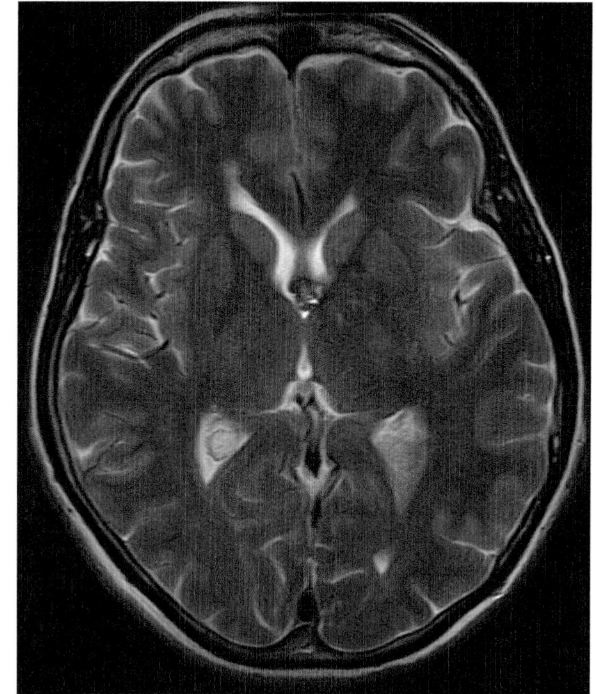

**Fig. 9.40** Case of a 53 years old woman with a 3rd ventricle CM incidentally found in the MRI (sagittal T2WI image)

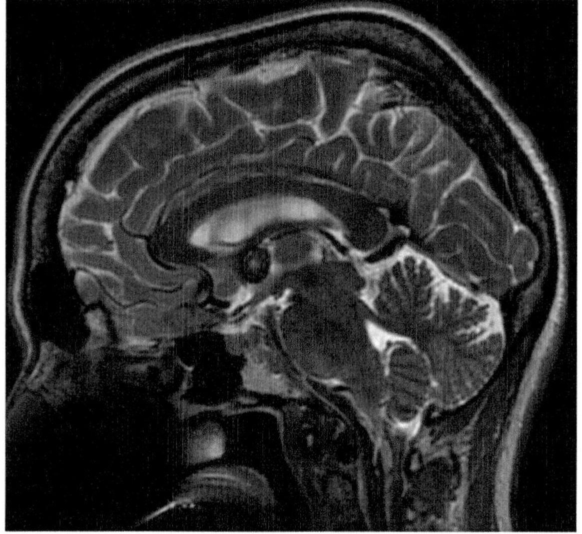

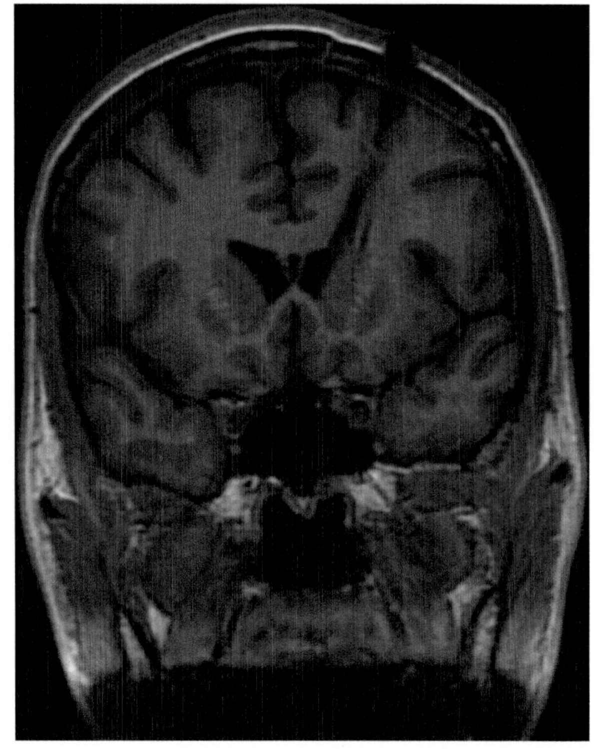

**Fig. 9.41** Case of a 53 years old woman with a 3rd ventricle CM incidentally found in the MRI. Postoperatively she was without any new neurological deficit which remained unchanged during the follow up. MRI 4 months after surgery did not reveal any residual (coronal T1WI image)

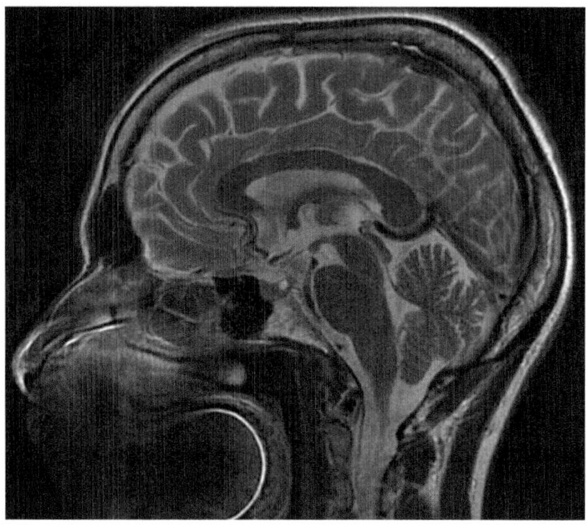

**Fig. 9.42** Case of a 53 years old woman with a 3rd ventricle CM incidentally found in the MRI. Postoperatively she was without any new neurological deficit which remained unchanged during the follow up. MRI 4 months after surgery did not reveal any residual (sagittal T2WI image)

**Key Points**
- Most of the patients present with headaches and memory disturbances.
- According to the location of the lesion, hydrocephalus is common in these cases and develops in 59% of patients due to the obstruction of foramen Monroi or cerebral aqueduct.
- It is believed that these lesions are capable of rapid growth, which be due to the lower resistance from CSF compared to the parenchyma, and due to intralesional bleeding.
- Despite the limited data on third ventricle CMs, gross total resection leads to optimal outcomes in the majority of symptomatic cases without need for permanent CSF diversion in most of the cases that presented with hydrocephalus or intraventricular haemorrhage.
- Surgical approach is strictly individual tailored to lesion.

# References


1. Becker DH, Townsend JJ, Kramer RA, Newton TH. Occult cerebrovascular malformations: a series of 18 histologically verified cases with negative angiography. Brain. 1979;102:249–87.
2. Roda JM, Alvarez F, Isla A, Blazquez MG. Thalamic cavernous malformation. Case Rep J Neurosurg. 1990;72:647–9. https://doi.org/10.3171/Jns.1990.72.4.0647.
3. Gross BA, Batjer HH, Awad IA, Bendok BR. Cavernous malformations of the basal ganglia and thalamus. Neurosurgery. 2009;65:7–19. https://doi.org/10.1227/01.NEU.0000347009.32480.D8.
4. Otani N, Fujioka M, Oracioglu B, Muroi C, Khan N, Roth P, Yonekawa Y. Thalamic cavernous angioma: Paraculminar supracerebellar infratentorial transtentorial approach for the safe and complete surgical removal. Acta Neurochir Suppl. 2008;103:29–36.
5. Mathiesen T, Edner G, Kihlstrom L. Deep and brainstem cavernomas: a consecutive 8-year series. J Neurosurg. 2003;99:31–7. https://doi.org/10.3171/Jns.2003.99.1.0031.
6. Sarris CE, Atwal GS, Nakaji P. Thalamic cavernous malformations. In: Handbook of clinical neurology, vol. 143. Amsterdam: Elsevier; 2017. p. 297–302.
7. Porter PJ, Willinsky RA, Harper W, Wallace MC. Cerebral cavernous malformations: natural history and prognosis after clinical deterioration with or without hemorrhage. J Neurosurg. 1997;87:190–7. https://doi.org/10.3171/Jns.1997.87.2.0190.
8. Kondziolka D, Lunsford LD, Flickinger JC, Kestle JRW. Reduction of hemorrhage risk after stereotactic radiosurgery for cavernous malformations. J Neurosurg. 1995;83:825–31. https://doi.org/10.3171/Jns.1995.83.5.0825.
9. Winkler D, Lindner D, Strauss G, Richter A, Schober R, Meixensberger J. Surgery of cavernous malformations with and without navigational support - a comparative study. Minim Invasive Neurosurg. 2006;49:15–9. https://doi.org/10.1055/S-2005-919163.
10. Zhao J, Wang Y, Kang S, Wang S, Wang J, Wang R, Zhao Y. The benefit of neuronavigation for the treatment of patients with intracerebral cavernous malformations. Neurosurg Rev. 2007;30:313–9. https://doi.org/10.1007/S10143-007-0080-X.
11. Bohl MA, Oppenlander ME, Spetzler R. A prospective cohort evaluation of a robotic, auto-navigating operating microscope. Cureus. 2016;8:e662.
12. Steinberg GK, Chang SD, Gewirtz RJ, Lopez JR. Microsurgical resection of brainstem, thalamic, and basal ganglia angiographically occult vascular malformations. Neurosurgery. 2000;46:260–70. Discussion 270–261.

13. Li D, Zhang J, Hao S, Tang J, Xiao X, Wu Z, Zhang L. Surgical treatment and long-term outcomes of thalamic cavernous malformations. World Neurosurg. 2013;79:704–13. https://doi.org/10.1016/J.Wneu.2012.01.037.

14. Tian K-B, Zheng J-J, Ma J-P, Hao S-Y, Wang L, Zhang L-W, Wu Z, Zhang J-T, Li D. Clinical course of untreated thalamic cavernous malformations: hemorrhage risk and neurological outcomes. J Neurosurg. 2017;127:480–91. https://doi.org/10.3171/2016.8.JNS16934.

15. Aiba T, Tanaka R, Koike T, Kameyama S, Takeda N, Komata T. Natural history of intracranial cavernous Malformations. J Neurosurg. 1995;83:56–9. https://doi.org/10.3171/Jns.1995.83.1.0056.

16. Rangel-Castilla L, Spetzler RF. The 6 thalamic regions: surgical approaches to thalamic cavernous malformations, operative results, and clinical outcomes. J Neurosurg. 2015;123:676–85.

17. Ertan S, Benbir G, Tanriverdi T, Alver I, Uzan M. Parkinsonism caused by cavernoma located in basal ganglion. Parkinsonism Relat Disord. 2005;11:517–9. https://doi.org/10.1016/J.Parkreldis.2005.07.003.

18. Carpay HA, Arts WF, Kloet A, Hoogland PH, Van Duinen SG. Hemichorea reversible after operation in a boy with cavernous angioma in the head of the caudate nucleus. J Neurol Neurosurg Psychiatry. 1994;57:1547–8. https://doi.org/10.1136/Jnnp.57.12.1547.

19. Donmez B, Cakmur R, Uysal U, Men S. Putaminal cavernous angioma presenting with hemichorea. Mov Disord. 2004;19:1379–80. https://doi.org/10.1002/Mds.20207.

20. Yakinci C, Durmaz Y, Korkut M, Aladag A, Onal C, Aydinli M. Cavernous hemangioma in a child presenting with hemichorea: response to pimozide. J Child Neurol. 2001;16:685–8. https://doi.org/10.1177/088307380101600912.

21. Hidaka M, Shimoda M, Sato O, Watabe T, Tsugane R, Ohsuga H, Araki G. Case report: hemiballism due to a putaminal cavernous hemangioma. No To Shinkei. 1989;41:1135–9.

22. Akbostancı MC, Yiğit A, Ulkatan S. Cavernous angioma presenting with hemidystonia. Clin Neurol Neurosurg. 1998;100:234–7. https://doi.org/10.1016/S0303-8467(98)00046-8.

23. Lorenzana L, Cabezudo JM, Porras LF, Polaina M, Rodriguez-Sanchez JA, Garcia-Yague LM. Focal dystonia secondary to cavernous angioma of the basal ganglia: case report and review of the literature. Neurosurgery. 1992;31:1108–11;. Discussion 1111–1102. https://doi.org/10.1227/00006123-199212000-00019.

24. Chang EF, Gabriel RA, Potts MB, Berger MS, Lawton MT. Supratentorial cavernous malformations in eloquent and deep locations: surgical approaches and outcomes. J Neurosurg. 2011;114:814–27. https://doi.org/10.3171/2010.5.JNS091159.

25. Potts MB, Chang EF, Young WL, Lawton MT. Transsylvian-transinsular approaches to the insula and basal ganglia: operative techniques and results with vascular lesions. Neurosurgery. 2012;70:824–34. https://doi.org/10.1227/NEU.0b013e318236760d.

26. Beechar VB, Srinivasan VM, Reznik OE, Sen A, Klisch TJ, Ropper AE, Mandel JJ, Heck KA, Seipel TJ, Patel AJ. Intraventricular cavernomas of the third ventricle: report of 2 cases and a systematic review of the literature. World Neurosurg. 2017;105:935–43. https://doi.org/10.1016/J.Wneu.2017.06.109.

27. Kivelev J, Niemelä M, Kivisaari R, Hernesniemi J. Intraventricular cerebral cavernomas: a series of 12 patients and review of the literature. J Neurosurg. 2010;112:140–9. https://doi.org/10.3171/2009.3.JNS081693.

28. Longatti P, Fiorindi A, Perin A, Baratto V, Martinuzzi A. Cavernoma of the foramen of monro: case report and review of the literature. Neurosurg Focus. 2006;21:1–4.

29. Pozzati E. Thalamic cavernous malformations. Surg Neurol. 2000;53:30–40. https://doi.org/10.1016/S0090-3019(99)00164-0.

30. Behari S, Garg P, Jaiswal S, Nair A, Naval R, Jaiswal AK. Major surgical approaches to the posterior third ventricular region: a pictorial review. J Pediatr Neurosci. 2010;5:97–101. https://doi.org/10.4103/1817-1745.76093.

31. Qiao N, Ma Z, Song J, Wang Y, Shou X, Zhang X, Shen M, Qiu H, Ye Z, He W, Li S, Fu C, Zhao Y. A systematic review and meta-analysis of surgeries performed for treating deep-seated cerebral cavernous malformations. Br J Neurosurg. 2015;29:493–9. https://doi.org/10.3109/02688697.2015.1023773.

# Chapter 10
# Surgery of Brainstem and Cerebellar Cavernous Malformations

Ondřej Bradáč, Petr Skalický, and Vladimír Beneš

## 10.1   Introduction

Cavernous malformations (CMs) (also known as cavernomas, cryptic vascular malformations, cavernous angiomas or cavernous hemanigomas) are vascular hamartomas that have a multi-lobulated, mulberry-like appearance. These lesions are comprised of grossly dilated blood vessels lined with a single layer of endothelial cells that lack tight junctions. There is no elastic lamina or smooth muscle in the lining of these vessels and little or no intervening neural tissue [1]. The vessels are filled with blood at various stages of thrombosis and usually surrounded by gliosis and hemosiderine [2]. Although the brain is the most common site for these lesions, CMs may occur in any organ. The prevalence of cerebral cavernomas is approximately around 0.5% of the general population [3]. Lesion distribution reflects the distribution of CNS tissue. 76% of CMs are supratentorial, 23% infratentorial and 1% both supra- and infratentorial. 19% of patients harbour multiple intracranial CMs [4]. At least 80% of the multiple lesion cases are familial [5]. Hereditary forms have an autosomal dominant pattern of transmission and are caused by loss-of-function mutations in one of three CCM genes (CCM1, CCM2 and CCM3) [6]. Individuals with CMs may present with seizures (23–50%), focal neurological deficits (20–45%), headaches (6–52%) or haemorrhages (9–56%) [1]. Patients with infratentorial lesions are more likely to present with focal neurological deficits than the patients with supratentorial lesions (64% of infratentorial CM cases vs. 41% of supratentorial CM cases in a study by Moriarity et al.) [7] and the presence of seizures is higher in individuals with lesions in cortical supratentorial regions [8]. Developmental venous anomalies (DVAs) are radiographically present in 9% of

O. Bradáč (✉) · P. Skalický · V. Beneš
Department of Neurosurgery and Neurooncology, First Medical Faculty, Military University Hospital and Charles University, Prague, Czech Republic
e-mail: ondrej.bradac@uvn.cz

© Springer Nature Switzerland AG 2020
O. Bradáč, V. Beneš (eds.), *Cavernomas of the CNS*,
https://doi.org/10.1007/978-3-030-49406-3_10

cases overall and may play a role in CM development [4]. CMs associated with DVAs also tend to be more aggressive [9]. In the study of 104 surgically treated patients with brainstem CM by Garcia et al. [10] 54.8% had an associated DVA. Understanding the anatomy of the brainstem is essential for devising a surgical strategy. Deep location makes approaches to this region challenging. The neurosurgeon must think over the risks of surgical treatment to prevent the subsequent complications it may produce. We have therefore decided to discuss the published data on brainstem and deep-seated cavernomas.

## 10.1.1 Brainstem Cavernomas

### 10.1.1.1 Natural History

Understanding the natural history of cavernous malformations is vital for patient management, particularly when considering of radiosurgical therapy. Taslimi et al. [2] reviewed natural history studies and concluded that rough estimate of the annual incidence of symptomatic haemorrhage with radiological evidence is 2.8% (95% CI 2.5–3.3%) per person in brainstem lesions with an annual rehaemorrhage rate of 32.3% (95% CI 19.8–52.7%)) per person year, and is considerably more common during the first 2 years after bleeding (incidence rate ratio of 1.8 (95% CI 1.5–2.0) for all CNS cavernomas). Natural history studies of familial cases have suggested that familial cavernomas might tend to have a higher risk of haemorrhage [5, 11], but this finding could be attributable to inclusion of asymptomatic haemorrhage in concordance with imaging surveillance in familial series as opposed to the imaging performed while the patient was symptomatic in sporadic cases [2, 12]. Other possible risk factors for haemorrhage are female sex, younger age, perilesional edema, large lesion size, and presence of DVA. However the role of these factors is still discussed and inconsistently concluded among the studies [13].

### 10.1.1.2 Timing of Surgery

The surgical intervention should be performed after at least one haemorrhage and pial or ependymal projection of the lesion [14]. Although the brainstem location is not generally a risk factor for haemorrhage by itself, the clinical course is clearly more malignant than in non-eloquent lobar location [15]. On reviewing our results we advocate performing the intervention after the first symptomatic haemorrhage. Given that the brainstem CM may have a relatively benign natural history, surgery for asymptomatic and incidental lesions is not recommended [16]. In preparation for surgery, in accordance with our previously published 10.5% morbidity and mortality rate and 18.4% rate of early tracheostomy and/or PEG, [17] we assume that the early postoperative outcome may imitate a haemorrhagic event, as expected by other groups [18]. According to other authors [19–21] we prefer postponed surgery in 4–8 weeks after haemorrhagic event, ideally after 6 weeks. This allows a better resection plane and better identification of the cavernous malformation because of the liquefaction of the haematoma and presence of a haemorrhagic cavity [22]. The "two-point" method advocated by Brown et al. [23] is used to select the best surgical approach, however safe entry zone to the brainstem should be chosen from a number of potential options after thorough study of preop images as demonstrated in following the subchapter. Surgical approach is selected according to the chosen brainstem entry.

### 10.1.1.3 Surgical Approach

Regardless of the surgical approach, care must be taken to preserve an associated DVA to lower the risk of consequent venous infarction [24]. After the initial drainage of haematoma, complete resection of cavernoma should be achieved without an undue traction of adjacent brainstem tissue, as 62% of residual lesions demonstrated in meta-analysis by Gross et al. bled postoperatively [14]. Garcia et al. [10] proposed a grading scale for brainstem CMs (Table 10.1). In this grading system based on 104 surgically treated patients the risk of unfavourable outcome (mRS 3–6) increases with the number of points and 100% of patients with 0 or 1 point (14 patients) had a favourable outcome (mRS 0–2). The scale may be useful for selection of surgical candidates but in our opinion should not be used as the only selection of factors worth considering before the potential surgery. Lastly, Flores et al. in 2015 [25] suggested to use diffusion tensor imaging/diffusion tensor tractography in preoperative planning as it may be beneficial for choosing a surgical approach and brainstem entry especially for those lesions without pial or ependymal projection.

In Figs. 10.1, 10.2, 10.3, 10.4, 10.5, 10.6, 10.7, 10.8, 10.9, 10.10, 10.11, 10.12, 10.13, 10.14, 10.15, 10.16, 10.17, 10.18, 10.19, 10.20, 10.21, 10.22, 10.23, 10.24, 10.25 are depicted selected cases with comments on surgical approaches.

**Table 10.1** Proposed brainstem CMs grading scale by Garcia et al.

| Predictor | Criteria | Points |
| --- | --- | --- |
| Size (cm) | ≤2 | 0 |
| | >2 | 1 |
| Crossing axial midpoint | No | 0 |
| | Yes | 1 |
| DVA present | No | 0 |
| | Yes | 1 |
| Age (years) | ≤40 | 0 |
| | >40 | 1 |
| Haemorrhage | (0–3 weeks ago) | 0 |
| | (3–8 weeks ago) | 1 |
| | (>8 weeks ago) | 2 |
| Total | | 7 |

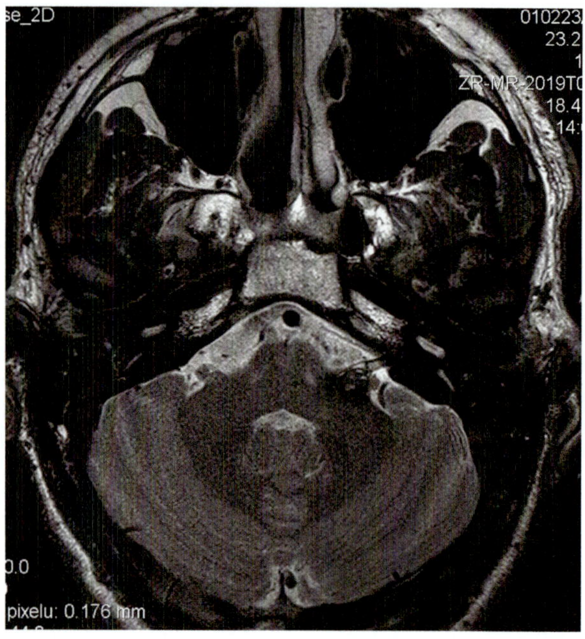

**Fig. 10.1** Cavernoma of VII/VIIIth nerve presenting with hearing loss. Retrosigmoid approch was used

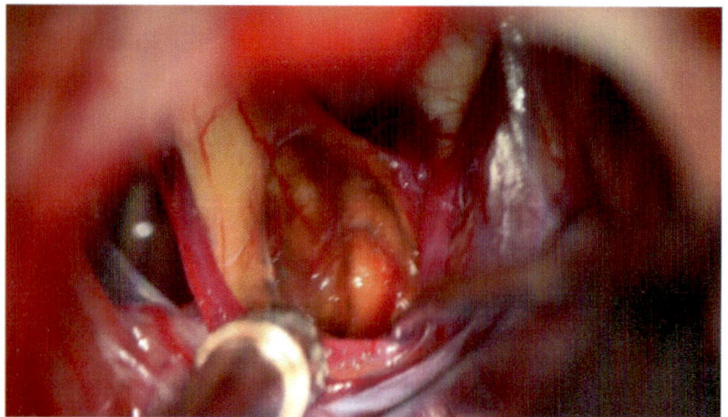

**Fig. 10.2** Cavernoma of VII/VIIIth nerve. Intraop image after resection. Both nerves in continuity

### 10.1.1.4 Outcomes of Surgery

The postoperative morbidity (8.5%) and mortality (3.4%) rate in our series of 58 patients (59 operations; Jan 1998–Aug 2019) is comparable to the published larger series. We have published our results of 37 cases in 2013 with postoperative morbidity 10.5% and mortality 5.3% [17]. We believe that the improvement of results is due to a learning curve of the operating surgeon. In the given tables (Tables 10.2, 10.3, 10.4, and 10.5) we summarize the cases in the same manner as in our previously published article [17]. Garcia et al. [10] reports 10.6% postoperative morbidity and 0.96% mortality in his series of 104 patients. Zhang et al. [26] reports a series of 120 cases with 10.4% postoperative morbidity and 1.7% mortality.

**Fig. 10.3** Cavernoma of VII/VIIIth nerve. Post-op scan. Hearing loss improved

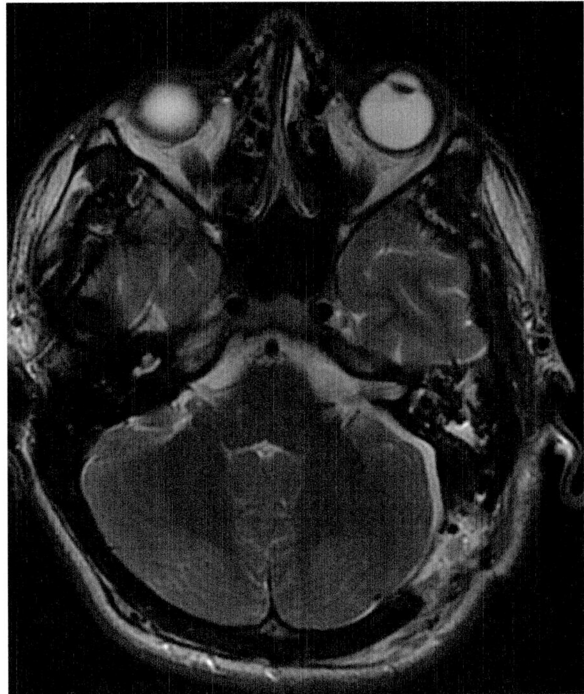

**Fig. 10.4** Mesencephalic cavernoma. Supracerebellar-infratentorial approach was used. Axial scan

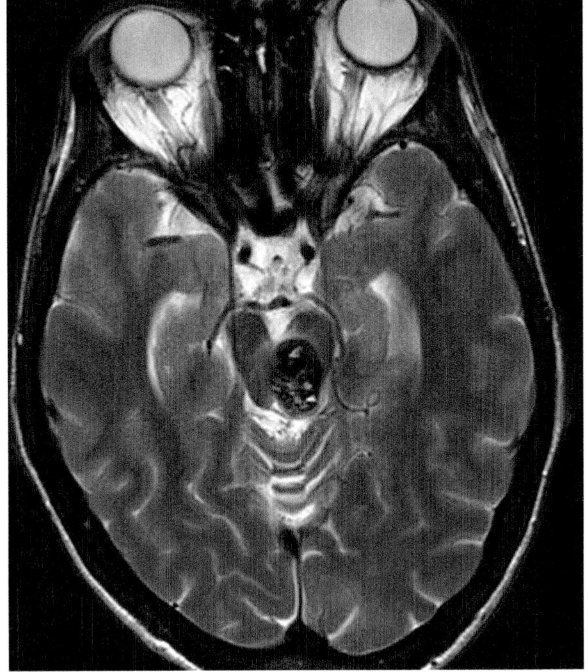

**Fig. 10.5** Mesencephalic cavernoma. Supracerebellar-infratentorial approach was used. Coronal scan

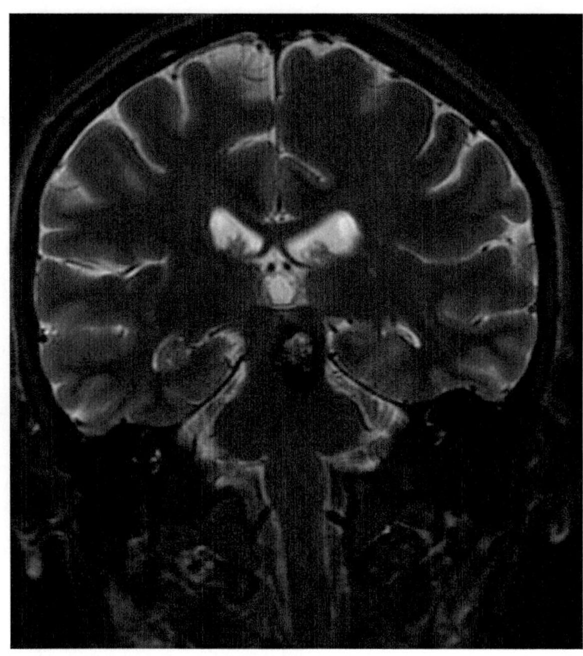

**Fig. 10.6** Lower pontine cavernoma. Axial scan

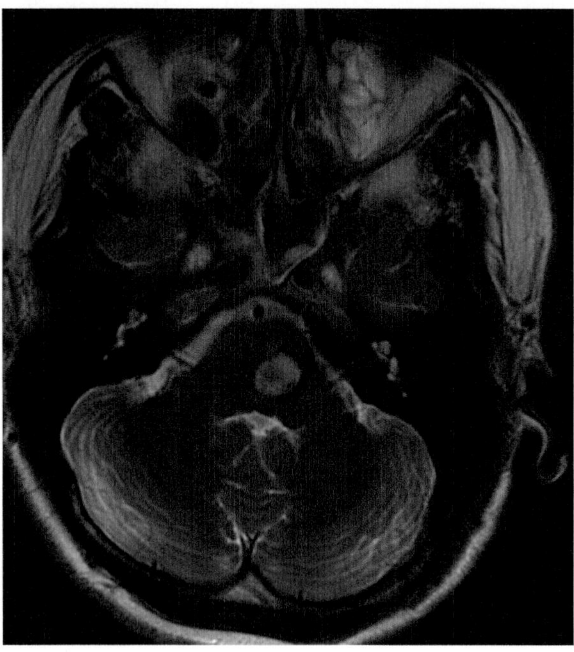

**Fig. 10.7** Lower pontine cavernoma. Sagittal scan

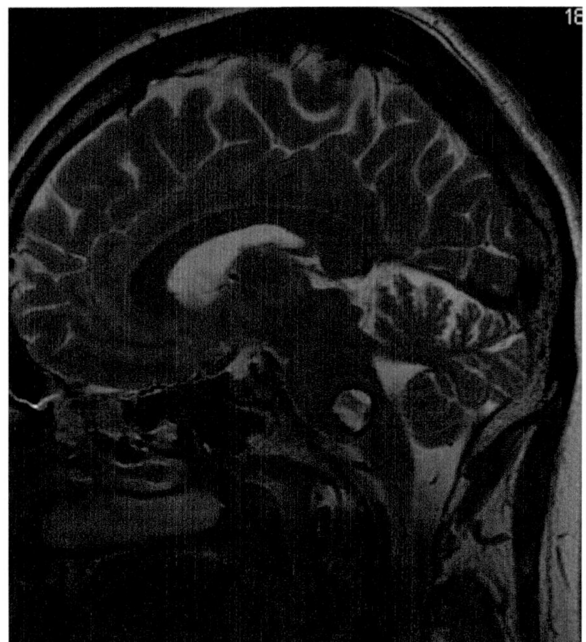

**Fig. 10.8** Lower pontine cavernoma. Coronal scan. This scan dictates the far lateral approach

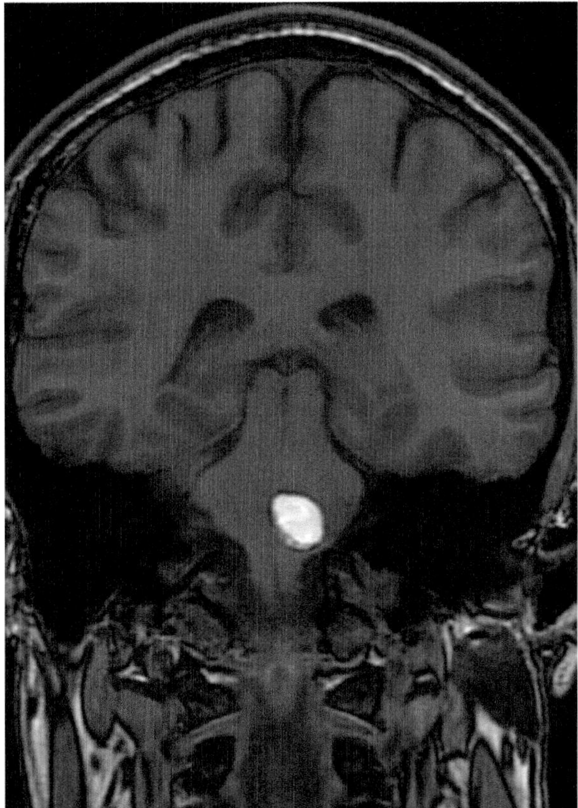

**Fig. 10.9** Lower pontine cavernoma. Postop scan

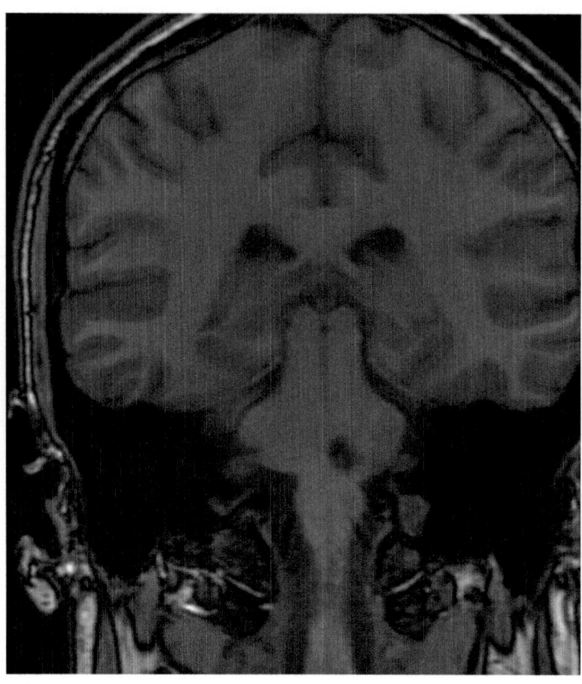

**Fig. 10.10** Another example of far lateral approach. Patient with multiple lesions, brainstem lesion recently bled. Axial scan

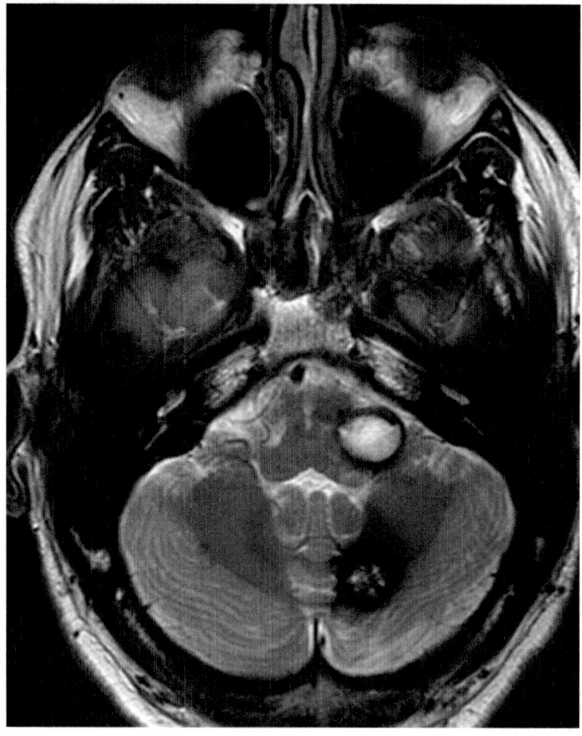

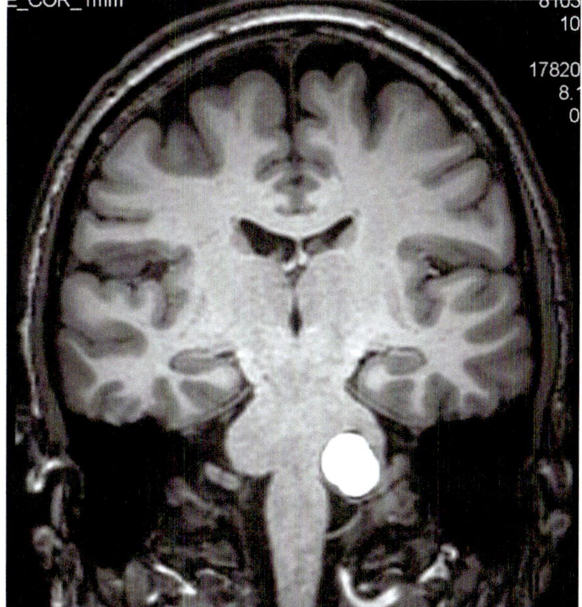

**Fig. 10.11** Another example of far lateral approach. Patient with multiple lesions, brainstem lesion recently bled. Coronal scan

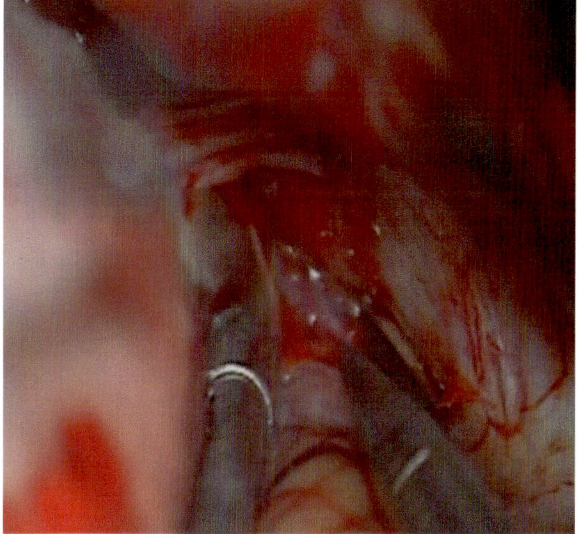

**Fig. 10.12** Another example of far lateral approach. Patient with multiple lesions, brainstem lesion recently bled. Cavernoma projection on brainstem surface

**Fig. 10.13** Another example of far lateral approach. Patient with multiple lesions, brainstem lesion recently bled. Cavernoma resection

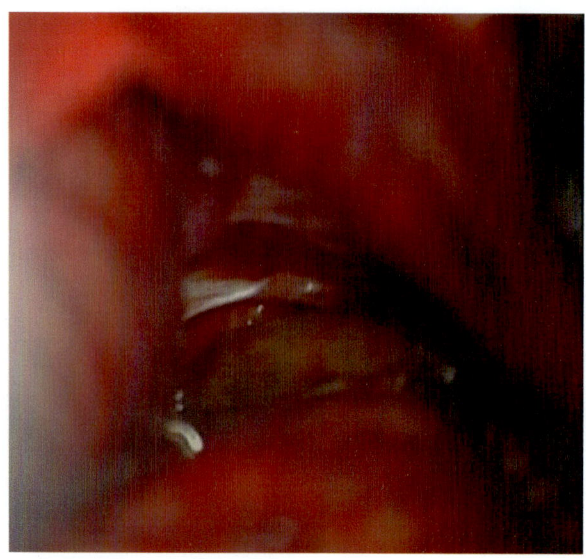

**Fig. 10.14** Another example of far lateral approach. Patient with multiple lesions, brainstem lesion recently bled. Postop MR axial scan

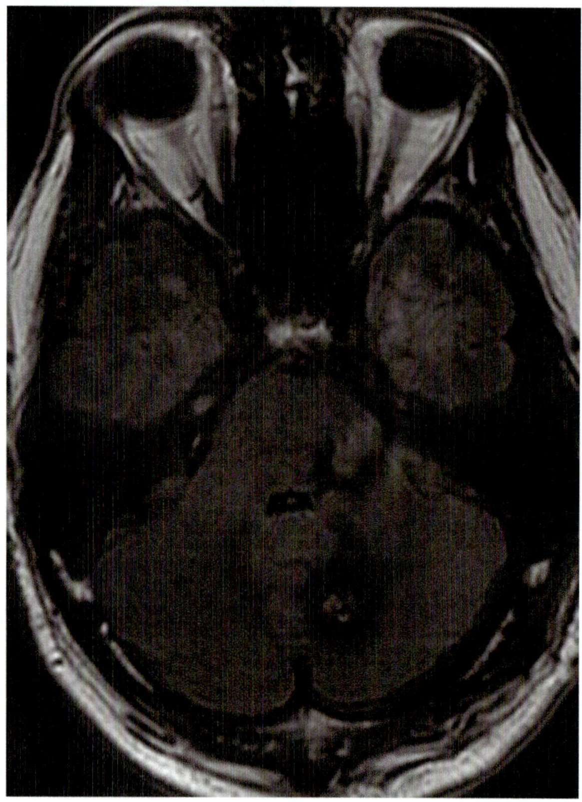

**Fig. 10.15** Another example of far lateral approach. Patient with multiple lesions, brainstem lesion recently bled. Postop MR coronal scan

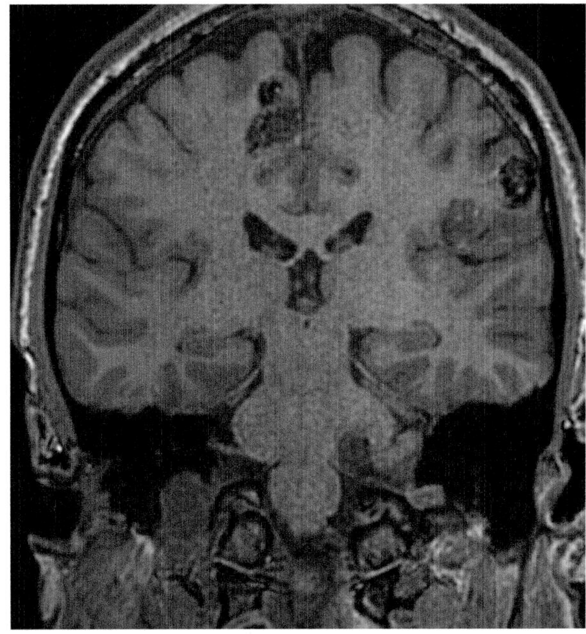

**Fig. 10.16** Mesencephalic cavernoma. Supracerebellar-infratentorial approach was used. Preop MR scan

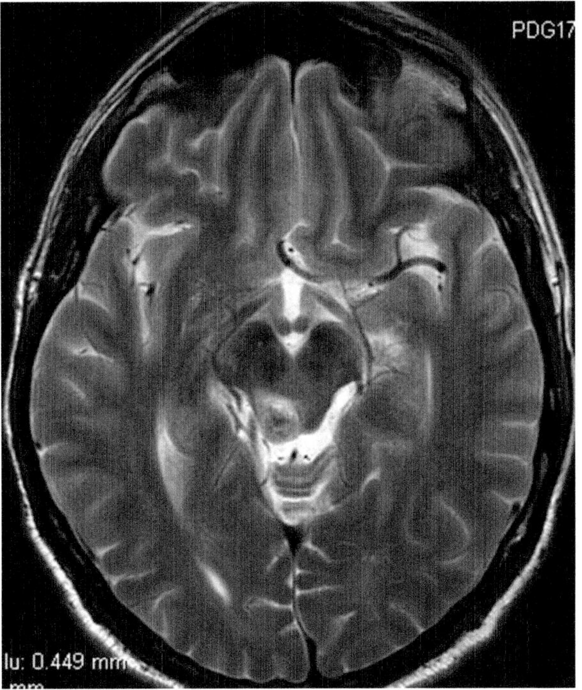

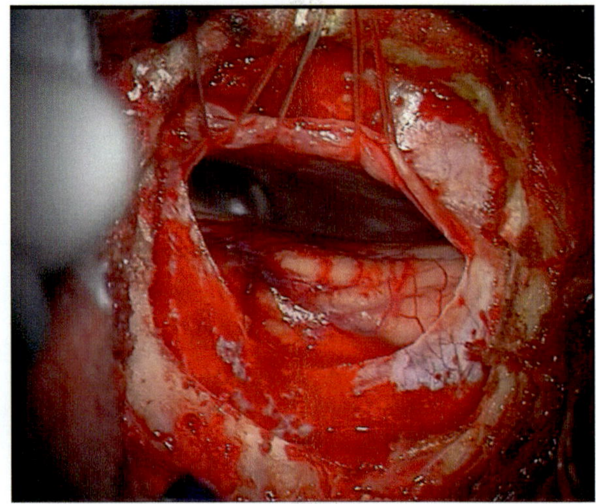

**Fig. 10.17** Mesencephalic cavernoma. Supracerebellar-infratentorial approach was used. Intraop picture showing extent of unilateral approach

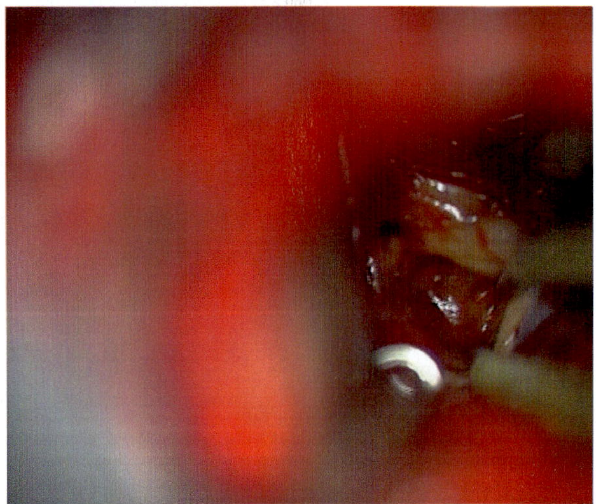

**Fig. 10.18** Mesencephalic cavernoma. Supracerebellar-infratentorial approach was used. Intraop picture showing cavernoma resection

Pandey et al. [16] reports worsening of the symptoms in 11.2% in his series of brainstem (136), thalamic (27) and basal ganglia CMs (16), and reports delayed hypertrophic olivary degeneration in 6.7% of cases occurring months after predominantly pontine lesions (9/10 cases). The largest series of 397 patients published by Zaidi et al. [22] shows a permanent neurological morbidity in 35.3% of cases. Gross et al. [14] in his meta-analysis of 1390 surgical cases found permanent worsening of the symptoms in 15% of patients and 1.5% mortality rate. In a report by Wostrack et al. [27] the surgical morbidity in patients with brainstem lesions was significantly higher than for those with a CM in supratentorial eloquent regions (37.5% vs 10.5%).

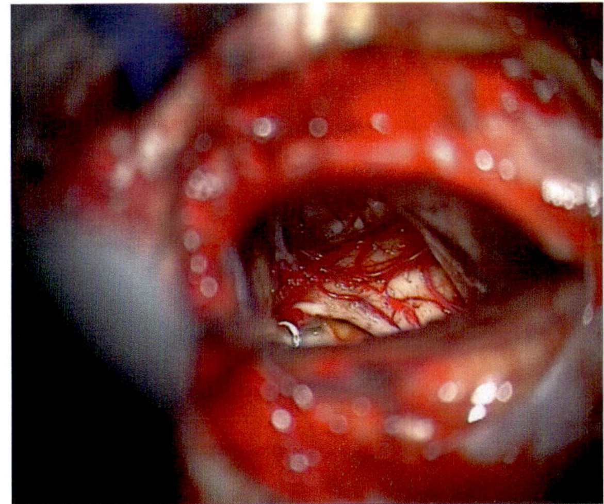

**Fig. 10.19** Mesencephalic cavernoma. Supracerebellar-infratentorial approach was used. Intraop picture showing end of cavernoma resection

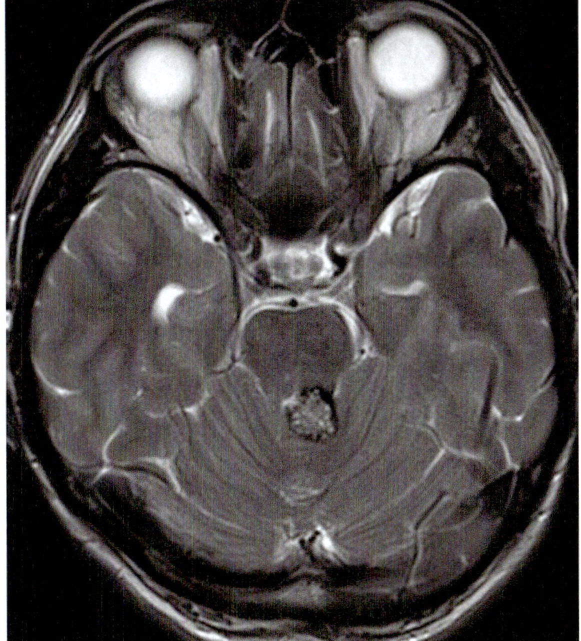

**Fig. 10.20** Mesencephalic cavernoma filling upper part of IVth ventricle. Supracerebellar-infratentorial approach with paravermian incision was used. Preop MR axial scan

### 10.1.1.5  Radiosurgery

Radiosurgical therapy of cavernous malformations for controlling rehaemorrhage of cavernomas has been reported by many authors [28, 29]. Pathologic effect of stereotactic radiosurgery (SRS) can include sclerosis and thrombotic obliteration of the vessels but also the recurrence of haemorrhage due to incomplete sclerosis and

**Fig. 10.21** Mesencephalic cavernoma filling upper part of IVth ventricle. Supracerebellar-infratentorial approach with paravermian incision was used. Preop MR sagittal scan

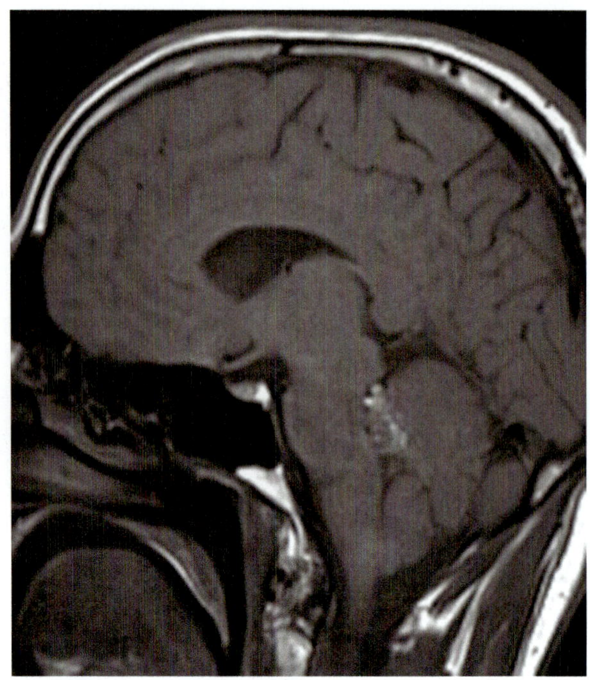

**Fig. 10.22** Mesencephalic cavernoma filling upper part of IVth ventricle. Supracerebellar-infratentorial approach with paravermian incision was used. Intraop picture of paravermian incision with cavernoma clearly visible

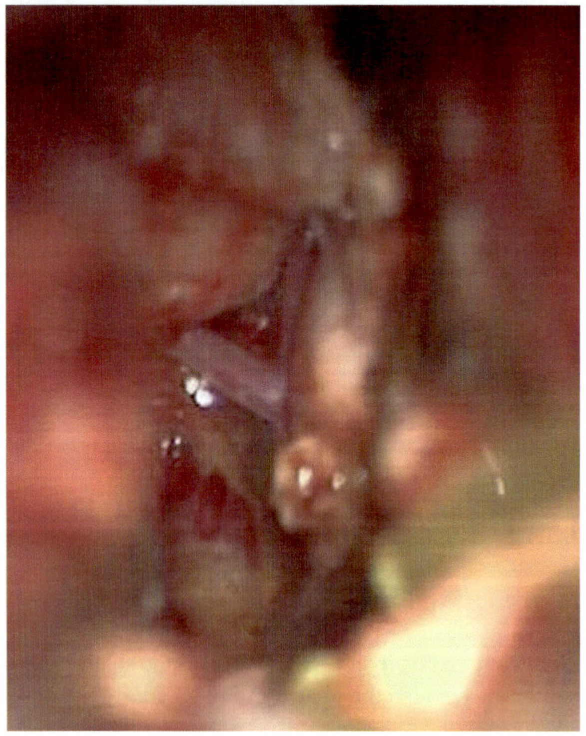

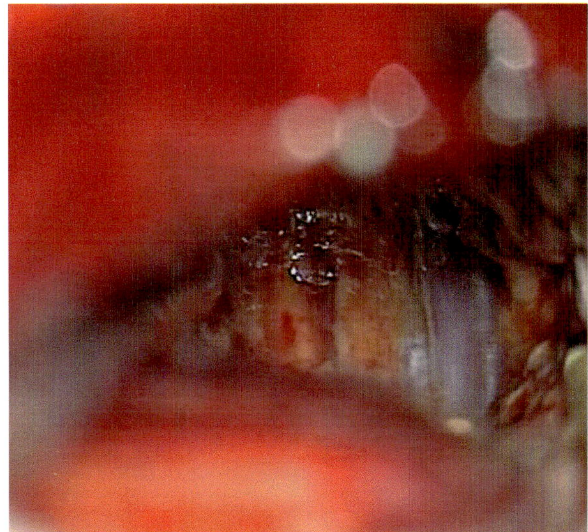

**Fig. 10.23** Mesencephalic cavernoma filling upper part of IVth ventricle. Supracerebellar-infratentorial approach with paravermian incision was used. Intraop picture after resection with all veins in continuity

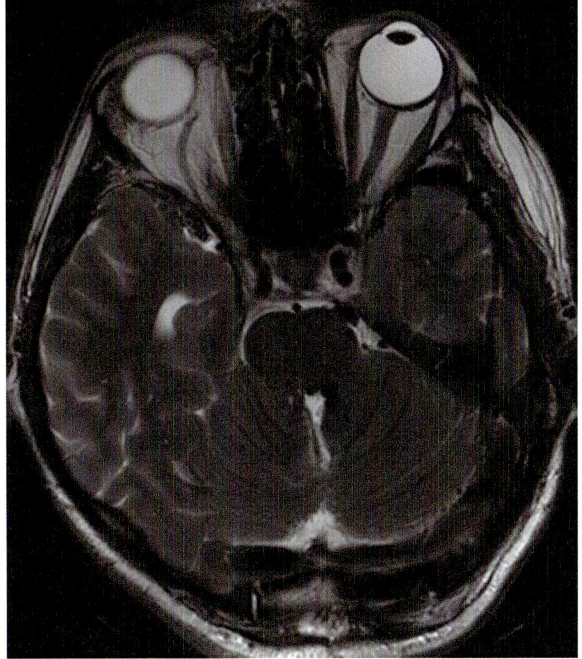

**Fig. 10.24** Mesencephalic cavernoma filling upper part of IVth ventricle. Supracerebellar-infratentorial approach with paravermian incision was used. Postop MR axial scan

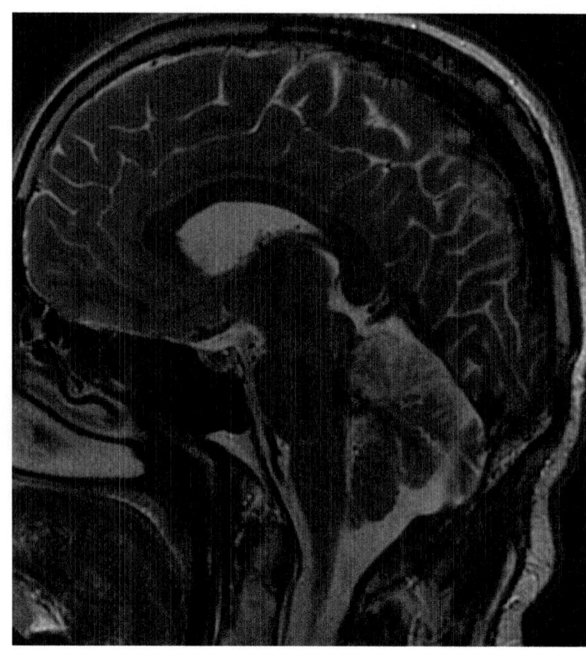

**Fig. 10.25** Mesencephalic cavernoma filling upper part of IVth ventricle. Supracerebellar-infratentorial approach with paravermian incision was used. Postop MR sagittal scan

**Table 10.2** Neurological symptoms prior to surgery

| Pre-op symptoms | Count |
| --- | --- |
| Limb paresis | 15 |
| Facial paresis | 12 |
| Limb numbness | 13 |
| Facial numbness | 6 |
| Diplopia | 11 |
| Dysfagia | 11 |

**Table 10.3** Summary of patients showing GOS deterioration after surgery

| Patient no. | Location | Decrease on GOS scale | Neurological outcome | Perioperative complication |
| --- | --- | --- | --- | --- |
| 1 | Pons | 3 | Exitus | Operation in urgent fashion, air embolism |
| 2 | Pons IV. Ventricle | 4 | Exitus | Venous anomaly, air embolism |
| 3 | Pons IV. Ventricle | 1 | Onset of myoklonus | |
| 4 | Medulla oblongata | 1 | Bulbar paresis, ataxia | |
| 5 | Midbrain posterior | 1 | Upper extremity and facial paresis | |

**Table 10.4** Summary of perioperative complications

| Perioperative complications | Count |
| --- | --- |
| Limb paresis | 8 |
| Facial paresis | 16 |
| Diplopia | 16 |
| Dysfagia | 8 |
| Cerebellar symptoms | 8 |
| Hydrocephalus | 2 |
| Tracheostomy | 8 |
| Air embolism | 5 |

**Table 10.5** Lesion distribution

| Cavernoma location | Count | Pial projection[a] |
| --- | --- | --- |
| Midbrain anterior/anterolateral | 5 | 0 |
| Midbrain posterior | 9 | 4 |
| Pons anterior/anterolateral | 14 | 5 |
| Pons IV. Ventricle | 27 | 6 |
| Medulla oblongata | 4 | 2 |

[a]according to intraoperative findings

neovascularisation [30]. Histopathologic examination of surgically resected cavernoma 1 year after 40-Gy irradiation found endothelial cell destruction and fibrosis with scar tissue formation [31]. Given the experience with stereotactic radiosurgery, the expected complete obliteration is after a 2 year latency period [32]. However other examinations of eight cavernous malformations with prior radiosurgery or conventional radiation therapy (mean 3.5 years) did not find complete histologic vascular obliteration. These findings are not representative of all irradiated patients, and rehaemorrhage may relate to poor radiation response in some patients [33]. Higher marginal doses and bigger lesion sizes were reported, corresponding to neurological complications [34]. Marginal dose of 12–15 Gy together with conformal treatment planning makes the treatment safer as Nagy et al. [35] reported only 7.2% of permanent adverse radiation effects. The positive effects of radiosurgical treatment for CMs are however further compromised by reports of CM development in the area of prior radiation years after the therapeutic intervention [36]. Radiosurgery for CMs is associated with higher morbidity after previous surgery and therefore its use after subtotal resection is controversial [37]. Despite the inconclusive studies about the effects of radiosurgery on CMs Wen et al. [38] in the recent meta-analysis of 9 studies suggested that the annual haemorrhage rate is reduced not only after 2 years after the procedure (12.13 risk ratio of haemorrhage rate comparing pre-GKRS with 2 years after GKRS (95%CI 1.73–85.07)) but even in the first 2 years (3.3 risk ratio (95% CI 2.65–4.11). However, these estimates might not differ much from natural course itself. Barker et al. [39] statistically modelled haemorrhage clustering. Over the first year after bleeding, a cumulative re-bleed rate was 14% and 56% over 5 years. The probability of bleeding during first 2.5 years was 2% per month and only 0.8% per month thereafter. In the retrospective study of 210 radiosurgically treated patients with brainstem and thalamic/basal ganglia CMs by Nagy et al. [35] the lifetime annual bleed rate of CMs having a single haemorrhage prior to treatment was 2.4% per lesion. The haemorrhage rate stabilized at 1.1% after a temporary increase of 4.3% within the first 2 years after RS. The annual pretreatment haemorrhage rate was 2.8% for the lesions having multiple bleeds prior to RS with a pretreatment rehaemorrhage rate of 20.7% and with a modest gradual decrease within the first 5 years, remaining stable at 11.55% thereafter. As the pretreatment haemorrhages resulted in permanent deficits in 48.8% of the cases with a single bleed and in 77.1% of the cases with multiple bleeds, we agree with the more aggressive approach to treat the patients after single haemorrhage but with the preference of surgery if the criteria mentioned above are met. Finally, as the prospective multicentre studies comparing radiosurgery with natural course for brainstem cavernomas are still missing it should serve as an alternative to observation but not to surgery and should be reserved for lesions which are surgically inaccessible [40].

**Keypoints**
- The annual haemorrhage rate for brainstem CMs is estimated to be 2.5–3.3% given the fact that these lesions are congenital. However some of these may develop throughout life and this rate might be different.
- Familial CMs have a higher risk of haemorrhage and are prone to be multiple.
- After haemorrhage there is an increased risk of subsequent rehaemorrhage. The annual rehaemorrhage rate was estimated to be 19.8–52.7%.
- Radiosurgical therapy is not as effective as it is for AVMs. The benefit is unclear, however some studies show reduction of bleeding after a latent period of 2 years. Currently it should only serve as an alternative to observation, and the risk of complications must be considered.
- Surgery should be done in 4–8 weeks after first or second haemorrhage because the resection is facilitated by firmness of cavity walls and liquefaction of haematoma.
- Criteria for surgical resection also include: Safe surgical approach and corridor to the lesion, symptomatic cases, and pial or ependymal projection of the lesion. The two point method should be used in planning for surgical access and the DVA should be preserved.
- Worsening of the symptoms after surgery is approximately in 15% of cases and the mortality is 1.5%. Excellent results may be achieved with profound selection of surgical candidates and operation has to be performed by an expert surgeon.
- Neuronavigation may be beneficial for planning a surgical approach and for tracking the lesion intraoperatively. Electrophysiologic monitoring is useful to guide the surgeon to a safe entry point in the brainstem. Selection of the methods depends on anatomical localization of the CM.

## *10.1.2   Cerebellar Cavernomas*

Data on haemorrhage risk and outcomes of cerebellar CMs are limited. Wu et al. [41] presented a study of 58 patients with cerebellar CMs, 93.1% of patients presented with haemorrhage and 36% with focal neurological deficits. The annual haemorrhage rate was 2.9% and the annual rehaemorrhage rate was 25.6%. Knerlich-Lukoschus et al. [42] in a study of paediatric patients found that these individuals commonly presented with sudden onset headaches, vomiting, double-vision and gait ataxia. Zhang et al. [43] analyzed a series of 41 patients with cerebellar cavernomas with or without an associated DVA (26.8% of patients) and found no statistically significant difference between the outcomes of both groups after coagulating and dissecting distal radices of a DVA associated with a cavernoma. Although there is a lack of data on cerebellar CMs, we believe that it is appropriate to follow the general rules for neurosurgical management of CMs.

# References


1. Batra S, Lin D, Recinos PF, Zhang J, Rigamonti D. Cavernous malformations: natural history, diagnosis and treatment. Nat Rev Neurol. 2009;5:659–70. https://doi.org/10.1038/nrneurol.2009.177.
2. Taslimi S, Modabbernia A, Amin-Hanjani S, Barker FG, Macdonald RL. Natural history of cavernous malformation: systematic review and meta-analysis of 25 studies. Neurology. 2016;86:1984–91. https://doi.org/10.1212/WNL.0000000000002701.
3. Atwal GS, Sarris CE, Spetzler RF. Brainstem and cerebellar cavernous malformations. In: Handbook of clinical neurology, vol. 143. Amsterdam: Elsevier; 2017. p. 291–5.
4. Gross BA, Lin N, Du R, Day AL. The natural history of intracranial cavernous malformations. Neurosurg Focus. 2011;30:E24. https://doi.org/10.3171/2011.3.FOCUS1165.
5. Zabramski JM, Wascher TM, Spetzler RF, Johnson B, Golfinos J, Drayer BP, Brown B, Rigamonti D, Brown G. The natural history of familial cavernous malformations: results of an ongoing study. J Neurosurg. 1994;80:422–32. https://doi.org/10.3171/jns.1994.80.3.0422.
6. Cavalcanti DD, Kalani MY, Martirosyan NL, Eales J, Spetzler RF, Preul MC. Cerebral cavernous malformations: from genes to proteins to disease. J Neurosurg. 2012;116:122–32. https://doi.org/10.3171/2011.8.JNS101241.
7. Moriarity JL, Wetzel M, Clatterbuck RE, Javedan S, Sheppard J-M, Hoenig-Rigamonti K, Crone NE, Breiter SN, Lee RR, Rigamonti D. The natural history of cavernous malformations: a prospective study of 68 patients. Neurosurgery. 1999;44:1166–73.
8. Menzler K, Chen X, Thiel P, Iwinska-Zelder J, Miller D, Reuss A, Hamer HM, Reis J, Pagenstecher A, Knake S, Bertalanffy H, Rosenow F, Sure U. Epileptogenicity of cavernomas depends on (archi-) cortical localization. Neurosurgery. 2010;67:918–24. https://doi.org/10.1227/NEU.0b013e3181eb5032.
9. Wurm G, Schnizer M, Fellner FA. Cerebral cavernous malformations associated with venous anomalies: surgical considerations. Operative Neurosurg. 2005;57:42–58.
10. Garcia RM, Ivan ME, Lawton MT. Brainstem cavernous malformations: surgical results in 104 patients and a proposed grading system to predict neurological outcomes. Neurosurgery. 2015;76:265–78. https://doi.org/10.1227/NEU.0000000000000602.
11. Labauge P, Brunereau L, Lévy C, Laberge S, Houtteville JP. The natural history of familial cerebral cavernomas: a retrospective MRI study of 40 patients. Neuroradiology. 2000;42:327–32. https://doi.org/10.1007/s002340050893.
12. Labauge P, Brunereau L, Laberge S, Houtteville J-P. Prospective follow-up of 33 asymptomatic patients with familial cerebral cavernous malformations. Neurology. 2001;57:1825–8. https://doi.org/10.1212/WNL.57.10.1825.
13. Xie M-G, Li D, Guo F-Z, Zhang L-W, Zhang J-T, Wu Z, Meng G-L, Xiao X-R. Brainstem cavernous malformations: surgical indications based on natural history and surgical outcomes. World Neurosurg. 2018;110:55–63. https://doi.org/10.1016/j.wneu.2017.10.121.
14. Gross BA, Batjer HH, Awad IA, Bendok BR, Du R. Brainstem cavernous malformations: 1390 surgical cases from the literature. World Neurosurg. 2013;80:89–93. https://doi.org/10.1016/j.wneu.2012.04.002.

15. Porter PJ, Willinsky RA, Harper W, Wallace MC. Cerebral cavernous malformations: natural history and prognosis after clinical deterioration with or without hemorrhage. J Neurosurg. 1997;87:190–7. https://doi.org/10.3171/jns.1997.87.2.0190.
16. Pandey P, Westbroek EM, Gooderham PA, Steinberg GK. Cavernous malformation of brainstem, thalamus, and basal ganglia: a series of 176 patients. Neurosurgery. 2013;72:573–89;. discussion 588-579. https://doi.org/10.1227/NEU.0b013e318283c9c2.
17. Bradac O, Majovsky M, de Lacy P, Benes V. Surgery of brainstem cavernous malformations. Acta Neurochir. 2013;155:2079–83. https://doi.org/10.1007/s00701-013-1842-6.
18. Abla AA, Lekovic GP, Turner JD, de Oliveira JG, Porter R, Spetzler RF. Advances in the treatment and outcome of brainstem cavernous malformation surgery: a single-center case series of 300 surgically treated patients. Neurosurgery. 2011;68:403–14.; discussion 414–405. https://doi.org/10.1227/NEU.0b013e3181ff9cde.
19. Bruneau M, Bijlenga P, Reverdin A, Rilliet B, Regli L, Villemure JG, Porchet F, de Tribolet N. Early surgery for brainstem cavernomas. Acta Neurochir. 2006;148:405–14. https://doi.org/10.1007/s00701-005-0671-7.
20. Sola RG, Pulido P, Pastor J, Ochoa M, Castedo J. Surgical treatment of symptomatic cavernous malformations of the brainstem. Acta Neurochir. 2007;149:463–70. https://doi.org/10.1007/s00701-007-1113-5.
21. Wang CC, Liu A, Zhang JT, Sun B, Zhao YL. Surgical management of brain-stem cavernous malformations: report of 137 cases. Surg Neurol. 2003;59:444–54. discussion 454.
22. Zaidi HA, Mooney MA, Levitt MR, Dru AB, Abla AA, Spetzler RF. Impact of timing of intervention among 397 consecutively treated brainstem cavernous malformations. Neurosurgery. 2017;81:620–6. https://doi.org/10.1093/neuros/nyw139.
23. Brown AP. The two-point method: evaluating brain stem lesions. BNI Quart. 1996;12:20–4.
24. Asaad WF, Walcott BP, Nahed BV, Ogilvy CS. Operative management of brainstem cavernous malformations. Neurosurg Focus. 2010;29:E10. https://doi.org/10.3171/2010.6.FOCUS10134.
25. Flores BC, Whittemore AR, Samson DS, Barnett SL. The utility of preoperative diffusion tensor imaging in the surgical management of brainstem cavernous malformations. J Neurosurg. 2015;122:653–62. https://doi.org/10.3171/2014.11.JNS13680.
26. Zhang S, Li H, Liu W, Hui X, You C. Surgical treatment of hemorrhagic brainstem cavernous malformations. Neurol India. 2016;64:1210–9. https://doi.org/10.4103/0028-3886.193825.
27. Wostrack M, Shiban E, Harmening K, Obermueller T, Ringel F, Ryang Y-M, Meyer B, Stoffel M. Surgical treatment of symptomatic cerebral cavernous malformations in eloquent brain regions. Acta Neurochir. 2012;154:1419–30. https://doi.org/10.1007/s00701-012-1411-4.
28. Frischer JM, Gatterbauer B, Holzer S, Stavrou I, Gruber A, Novak K, Wang W-T, Reinprecht A, Mert A, Trattnig S, Mallouhi A, Kitz K, Knosp E. Microsurgery and radiosurgery for brainstem cavernomas: effective and complementary treatment options. World Neurosurg. 2014;81:520–8. https://doi.org/10.1016/j.wneu.2014.01.004.
29. Liu HB, Wang Y, Yang S, Gong FL, Xu YY, Wang W. Gamma knife radiosurgery for brainstem cavernous malformations. Clin Neurol Neurosurg. 2016;151:55–60. https://doi.org/10.1016/j.clineuro.2016.09.018.
30. Shin SS, Murdoch G, Hamilton RL, Faraji AH, Kano H, Zwagerman NT, Gardner PA, Lunsford LD, Friedlander RM. Pathological response of cavernous malformations following radiosurgery. J Neurosurg. 2015;123:938–44. https://doi.org/10.3171/2014.10.JNS14499.
31. Nyary I, Major O, Hanzely Z, Szeifert GT. Histopathological findings in a surgically resected thalamic cavernous hemangioma 1 year after 40-Gy irradiation. J Neurosurg. 2005;102. Suppl:56–8.
32. Nagy G, Razak A, Rowe JG, Hodgson TJ, Coley SC, Radatz MW, Patel UJ, Kemeny AA. Stereotactic radiosurgery for deep-seated cavernous malformations: a move toward more active, early intervention. Clinical article. J Neurosurg. 2010;113:691–9. https://doi.org/10.3171/2010.3.JNS091156.

33. Gewirtz RJ, Steinberg GK, Crowley R, Levy RP. Pathological changes in surgically resected angiographically occult vascular malformations after radiation. Neurosurgery. 1998;42:738–41. https://doi.org/10.1097/00006123-199804000-00031.
34. Kida Y, Kondoh T, Satoh M, Shuto T, Hasegawa T, Hayashi M, Iwai Y. Radiosurgery for symptomatic cavernous malformations: a multi-institutional retrospective study in Japan. Surg Neurol Int. 2015;6:249. https://doi.org/10.4103/2152-7806.157071.
35. Nagy G, Burkitt W, Stokes SS, Bhattacharyya D, Yianni J, Rowe JG, Kemeny AA, Radatz MWR. Contemporary radiosurgery of cerebral cavernous malformations: part 1. Treatment outcome for critically located hemorrhagic lesions. J Neurosurg. 2019;130:1817–25. https://doi.org/10.3171/2017.5.JNS17776.
36. Jain R, Robertson PL, Gandhi D, Gujar SK, Muraszko KM, Gebarski S. Radiation-induced cavernomas of the brain. Am J Neuroradiol. 2005;26:1158–62.
37. Liscak R, Vladyka V, Simonova G, Vymazal J, Novotny J Jr. Gamma knife surgery of brain cavernous hemangiomas. J Neurosurg. 2005;102(Suppl):207–13.
38. Wen R, Shi Y, Gao Y, Xu Y, Xiong B, Li D, Gong F, Wang W. The efficacy of gamma knife radiosurgery for cavernous malformations: a meta-analysis and review. World Neurosurg. 2019;123:371–7. https://doi.org/10.1016/j.wneu.2018.12.046.
39. Barker FG 2nd, Amin-Hanjani S, Butler WE, Lyons S, Ojemann RG, Chapman PH, Ogilvy CS. Temporal clustering of hemorrhages from untreated cavernous malformations of the central nervous system. Neurosurgery. 2001;49:15–24. discussion 24–15.
40. Lu X-Y, Sun H, Xu J-G, Li Q-Y. Stereotactic radiosurgery of brainstem cavernous malformations: a systematic review and meta-analysis. J Neurosurg. 2014;120:982–7. https://doi.org/10.3171/2013.12.JNS13990.
41. Wu H, Yu T, Wang S, Zhao J, Zhao Y. Surgical treatment of cerebellar cavernous malformations: a single-center experience with 58 cases. World Neurosurg. 2015;84:1103–11. https://doi.org/10.1016/j.wneu.2015.05.062.
42. Knerlich-Lukoschus F, Steinbok P, Dunham C, Cochrane DD. Cerebellar cavernous malformation in pediatric patients: defining clinical, neuroimaging, and therapeutic characteristics. J Neurosurg Pediatr. 2015;16:256–66. https://doi.org/10.3171/2015.1.PEDS14366.
43. Zhang P, Liu L, Cao Y, Wang S, Zhao J. Cerebellar cavernous malformations with and without associated developmental venous anomalies. BMC Neurol. 2013;13:134. https://doi.org/10.1186/1471-2377-13-134.

# Chapter 11
# Stereotactic Radiosurgery of Cavernous Malformations

Gábor Nagy and Matthias W. R. Radatz

## 11.1 Introduction

We attempt to summarize in this chapter the clinical experience treating cerebral cavernous malformations (CCMs) with stereotactic radiosurgery (SRS) in Sheffield, in the context of our recent knowledge on natural history and of the published radiosurgical series applying modern treatment protocols.

Earlier and more reliable radiological detection due to the wide availability of magnetic resonance imaging (MRI), as well as our better understanding of their natural history due to accumulation of large population based data, has significantly changed management strategy of cerebral cavernous malformations (CCMs, also known as "cavernomas", "cavernous angiomas", or "cavernous hemangiomas") during the last two decades. However, due to their heterogeneity and the lack of high quality evidence, their optimal management is still controversial. While the management of deep and eloquent lesions in the brainstem, thalamus and basal ganglia, especially for those after one or no hemorrhage is still a matter of intensive debate due to their more aggressive behavior and a higher risk of any intervention, consensus seems to exist in the treatment of hemispheric (superficial) CCMs: observation for incidental and microsurgery for symptomatic lesions in eligible patients [1].

Due to the higher morbidity of microsurgical resection of the more aggressive deep-seated CCMs [2, 3], seeking treatment alternative was warranted especially in

G. Nagy
Department of Functional Neurosurgery, National Institute of Clinical Neurosciences, Budapest, Hungary

M. W. R. Radatz (✉)
Department of Neurosurgery, Royal Hallamshire Hospital, Sheffield, UK

National Centre for Stereotactic Radiosurgery, Royal Hallamshire Hospital, Sheffield, UK

Thornbury Radiosurgery Centre, Sheffield, UK
e-mail: radatz@blueyonder.co.uk

© Springer Nature Switzerland AG 2020
O. Bradáč, V. Beneš (eds.), *Cavernomas of the CNS*,
https://doi.org/10.1007/978-3-030-49406-3_11

the surgically challenging cases. SRS appeared a good idea, and was introduced for the treatment of CCMs based on the assumption that their pathological vessels would respond similarly to arteriovenous malformations (AVMs), which were known to undergo thrombo-obliteration after SRS [4]. However, the role of SRS in the management of CCMs has been being intensively criticized for two reasons. Firstly, neither MRI nor catheter angiography can demonstrate their cure after SRS [5], therefore its beneficial effect is assumed based on statistical analysis of the outcomes of treated patient populations [6]. Thus, its critics from the neurosurgical community raised the question, whether it was a real alternative to microsurgery in terms of effectiveness. Secondly, early attempts of SRS often resulted in high rate of complications [7], leading to the other question raised by the critics, whether it was safe enough to be offered instead of observation. During the last decade, however, increasing numbers of publications reporting good clinical outcome from all over the world created the baseline definition of modern CCMs SRS resulting in reliably low and mild morbidity [6]. Due to initial skepticism based on uncertain clinical outcome, SRS was first recommended as a treatment option for surgically inaccessible CCMs with repeated hemorrhages [8]. However, based on promising early results [9, 10], some large centers encouraged the radiosurgical community to treat CCMs with SRS early soon after the first presentation [11, 12]. The argument behind this policy was to avoid the stepwise neurological deterioration caused by repeated hemorrhages, especially in deep-seated lesions that carry higher morbidity. This policy seemed to gain wider acceptance amongst the neurovascular community more recently [1]. In order to adopt this proactive policy we need to answer the two major critical questions regarding SRS. It was easier to first answer the concern regarding safety with the increasing number of published outcomes with low and mild morbidity of large contemporary radiosurgical series [6]. The question of efficacy, however, is harder to answer due to the heterogeneous quality of evidence regarding natural history and long-term outcome of SRS. It is probably the last 5 years that have brought the first reliable data to answer this question both with the publication of larger observed and treated patient populations that were followed up for sufficient time. This has shifted a pure speculative debate that dominated the field 10 years ago [13, 14] to a more fact-based debate [15–17]. The Sheffield group, accumulating massive data on large patient population treated by SRS over the last 20 years, is in the frontier of this ongoing intensive debate [18]. In this chapter we update our current knowledge on the natural history of CCMs, define their state-of-the art radiosurgical treatment, and review outcomes of contemporary CCM SRS that reassured us to continue our proactive treatment policy.

## 11.2   Natural History of CCMs

Understanding of natural history of CCMs is the key in the definition of management strategy and proper interpretation of results of SRS. These lesions, with an estimated prevalence of 0.15–0.9% [19–22] compose a large proportion of the previously described angiographically occult vascular malformations (AOVM) [23–25]. 76% of CCMs are located supratentorially, 8% in the basal ganglia/thalamus, and 18% in the brainstem [26]. Approximately 19% of the patients harbor multiple lesions [26], more frequently in familiar forms that comprise at least 6% of all cases [27]. Of the 6 cases detected per million per year, 47–60% are asymptomatic at detection [28]. When patients become symptomatic, typically in their 30s, 37% present with seizures, 36% with hemorrhage, 23% with headaches, and 22% with focal neurological deficits [26].

## *11.2.1   Hemorrhage from CCMs*

The primary aim of CCM treatment is to prevent hemorrhages and consequential neurological deterioration. It is the last decade that brought consensus in the definition of clinical hemorrhage that was far from obvious. Not all clinical events (acute neurological deterioration) are associated with evidence of concurrent hemorrhage [29], while hemosiderin ring is always present even in asymptomatic cases [24]. The latter is explained by ultrastructural studies suggesting a compromised blood-brain barrier at the site of a CCM that may lead to a chronic erythrocyte diapedesis into the surrounding brain and to consequential deposition of hemosiderin even in the absence of clinically significant hemorrhage [30, 31]. The definition of clinical hemorrhage described by Al-Shahi Salman et al. [25] has gained wide acceptance recently [1]: it is a clinical event with acute or subacute onset symptoms with radiological, pathological, surgical, or cerebrospinal fluid evidence of recent extra- or intralesional hemorrhage, whereas the mere existence of a hemosiderin ring or the sole increase in diameter are not considered as clinical hemorrhage.

Despite evidence of de novo CCM formation [24, 32], both retrospective studies assuming lesion presence since birth and prospective studies gave similar estimates for first ever hemorrhage rates, 0.1–2.7%/lesion/year [19, 20, 33–35]. Hemorrhagic presentation was found to be the most significant risk factor for further bleeding, indicating destabilization of CCMs by the first bleed [36–38]. While annual bleed rate was found 0.4–0.6% after non-hemorrhagic presentation [37], the annual rebleed rate was estimated between 4.5 and 33.77% [39, 40], giving rise to a cumulative incidence of rebleed of 16–57% at 5 and up to 72% at 10 years after hemorrhagic presentation [15, 41]. Several studies suggest that elevated rebleed risk decreases a few years after the first hemorrhage ("temporal clustering"), which is a matter of intensive debate since its first description [41]. In the original study a 2.4 fold decline of the annual rebleed rate from 25.2 to 9.6% was found 2.5 years after hemorrhagic presentation. Whilst such a 1.65–2.3 fold decline of rebleed rate after 2 years have been confirmed by several subsequent observational studies, in all except one studies rebleed rate did not return to baseline (defined as the annual rate of first hemorrhage) even 5 years after the first bleed [15, 38]. Brainstem location was found to be a significant risk factor for rebleed with an annual rebleed rate of

32.3% as compared to 6.3% in other locations [38], and the estimated risk of first hemorrhage within 5 years of diagnosis was 30.8 and 8% with or without hemorrhagic presentation, respectively [15]. Another study found even lower 5-year hemorrhage free survival of brainstem CMs, estimating 53% with median hemorrhage free survival times of 5–6 and 9 years for cases of hemorrhagic and non-hemorrhagic presentation, respectively [42]. Similarly, the annual rebleed rate of deep supratentorial CMs was found to be higher (14.1%) with 55.3% 5-year overall hemorrhage free survival [43]. The 5-year morbidity of unselected cases was found to be 37% [44], and up to 40–60% of the cases are left with persisting morbidity after a single bleed from the brainstem [45], with a substantial risk of mortality [33]. Moreover, each subsequent bleeding episodes carry the chance of cumulatively increase of permanent disability in deep-seated lesions [16, 46], and only 19% of pediatric patients harboring hemorrhagic brainstem CCM recovered fully at 4 years [47]. However, such a cumulative increase of permanent disability caused by subsequent bleeding in superficial hemispheric lesions is not clearly demonstrated [17, 46]. The morbidity of the latter CCMs after a bleed usually manifests in epilepsy and only rarely in focal neurological deficit [48, 49].

It is, therefore, fundamental for informed therapeutic decision-making to consider the difference between first and repeated hemorrhages and also the distinct behavior of superficial and deep-seated lesions. It is also possible, that there are even more distinct subpopulations, some lesions behaving aggressively with a high risk of rebleeding (temporarily or for a much longer period after a first hemorrhage), whilst others are more quiescent. This is supported by immunohistochemical studies demonstrating proliferation of abnormal endothelial cells in CCMs with recurrent bleeds [31]. Lesions with the complete absence of tight junction immunoreactivity have also been found to have significantly higher propensity to develop major hemorrhages and perilesional edema [50]. However, the proportion of these more unstable lesions is unknown and currently we are unable to predict from clinical or radiological signs which pattern of behavior a CCM would follow, but can only rely on lesion location and prior hemorrhage in our clinical judgment.


### 11.2.2   CCMs and Seizures

Seizures are the other clinically significant events related to CCMs, which are thought to be induced by surrounding hemosiderin deposition, perilesional gliosis, and inflammation [51]. Supratentorial location seems exclusive for seizure development, with a rate of 13% in the thalamus or basal ganglia and 55% in hemispheric location, 42% of the latter with hemorrhagic presentation [17]. The 5-year risk of first unprovoked seizure is relatively low, 6% in CCMs presented with hemorrhage or focal neurological deficit and 4% in incidental lesions [52]. However, the 5-year risk of developing epilepsy after a single seizure reaches 94%. Moreover, despite the fact that 97% of the patients were prescribed AEDs and 46% receiving polytherapy, only 53% of them achieved 2-year seizure freedom [52].

## 11.3  Treatment Modalities for CCMs

Currently there is no consensus for the role of the three management options for CCMs—microsurgical removal, SRS and observation—due to the lack of quality evidence [1]. It seems, however, that despite the overlap between indications, these three are not competitive but complementing each other. While incidental hemispheric lesions can be observed due to the low chance of resulting persisting morbidity, intervention is generally only advocated for symptomatic hemispheric lesions. Surgery is the treatment of choice in most of these cases due to its low morbidity combined with high effectiveness [53]. Large series report a rate of surgical morbidity of around 5%, with negligible mortality, and with a rate of complete resection of 98% [54–56]. Surgery is generally also recommended for CCMs causing epilepsy resistant to conservative management. Favorable outcome is achieved in 71% after resection of a single lesion, with the highest chance of medically controlled seizures, and if the CCM is resected within 1 year after presentation (81% in each) [57]. Knowing the fact that nearly all patients harboring CCMs presented with seizures go on to develop epilepsy within 5 years and only half of them can be controlled medically, some surgeons advocate early surgical intervention [58]. Thus, the question is whether RS may be a treatment alternative for microsurgical resection in selected patients under some circumstances, such as eloquent location, the patient's medical condition, or the patient's preference.

Due to the risk of intervention, the role of the three management options in the management of deep-seated CCMs is more controversial [53, 59]. For these lesions surgical removal is generally recommended only in limited circumstances in experienced hands. Lesions with the history of repeated hemorrhages causing progressive neurological deficit or significant mass effect should either reach the pial or ependymal surface or should be approachable through a non-eloquent surgical corridor [60]. Admittedly, the risk of microsurgery has decreased recently with increasing experience and with the introduction of safer techniques [60, 61]. However, it is still substantial, resulting in at best 10–14% persisting morbidity and 1.5–1.9% mortality. Although it offers a definitive cure, the rate of complete resection is only 89–91%, and the rebleed rate never goes to zero: 62% of residual lesions rebleed with an annual rate of 0.5–2% and with 6% mortality [2, 3]. Thus, prophylactic surgical removal of deep-seated CCMs in patients with no or minimal neurological deficit is not a common practice [62, 63].

## 11.4  Radiosurgery of CCMs: Past and Present

The lack of radiological proof of cure after treatment is the major pitfall of CCM SRS that keeps skepticism alive. For AVMs we are able to define the cure as obliteration that prevents further bleeding and the rate lies between 90 and 45% depending on size and treatment parameters [64]. We are also able to define cure for tumors as lack of growth and thereby to give local control rate of metastases 81–96%) [65], or the 5-year tumor control of benign tumors (around 95%) [66, 67]. In the case of CCMs the problem is not only the fact that these lesions are angiographically occult, but MRI also fails to demonstrate a definite change in the appearance of the lesion after SRS (Figs. 11.1, 11.2 and 11.3). Although the proportion of true growth is somewhat higher in untreated population [24, 32, 49, 68–70], MRI-appearance of CCMs after SRS is statistically as heterogeneous as without treatment. Approximately half of the lesions shrink [14, 69], but post-radiosurgery shrinkage may in part be due to resolution of intra-lesional hematomas. Thus, we can only rely on statistical evaluation of retrospective clinical data based on standardized modern SRS treatment protocols (Tables 11.1 and 11.2) [6, 10, 14, 16, 17, 49, 68, 69, 71–83] and put them into context of outcomes of other management modalities.

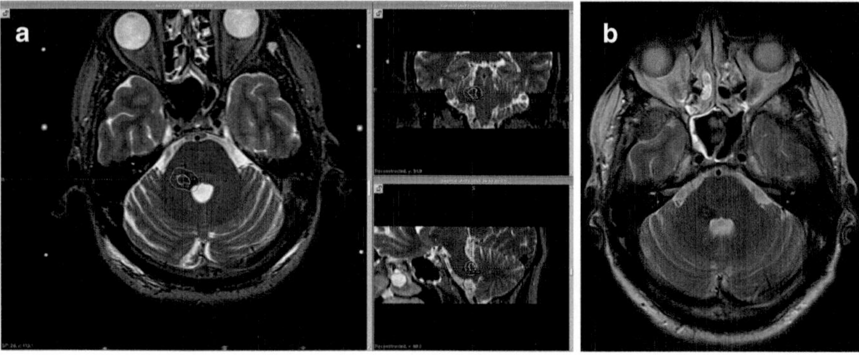

**Fig. 11.1** (**a**) Modern treatment planning of a right pontine CCM using T2-weighted high resolution MR images. (*Left:* axial, *right above:* coronal, and *right below:* sagittal slices.) (*Yellow:* 12 Gy 50% prescription isodose line, *green:* 4 Gy line.) (**b**) 1-year follow-up shows no significant change in the appearance (axial T2-weighted MRI)

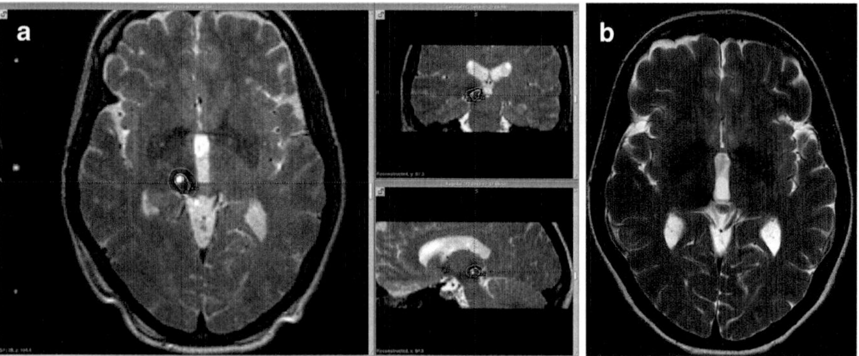

**Fig. 11.2** (**a**) Modern treatment planning of a right thalamic CCM using T2-weighted high resolution MR images. (*Left:* axial, *right above:* coronal, and *right below:* sagittal slices.) (*Yellow:* 12 Gy 50% prescription isodose line, *green:* 4 Gy line.) (**b**) 3-year follow-up shows a decrease in size the lesion, which is due to the resolution of intralesional hemorrhage (axial T2-weighted MRI)

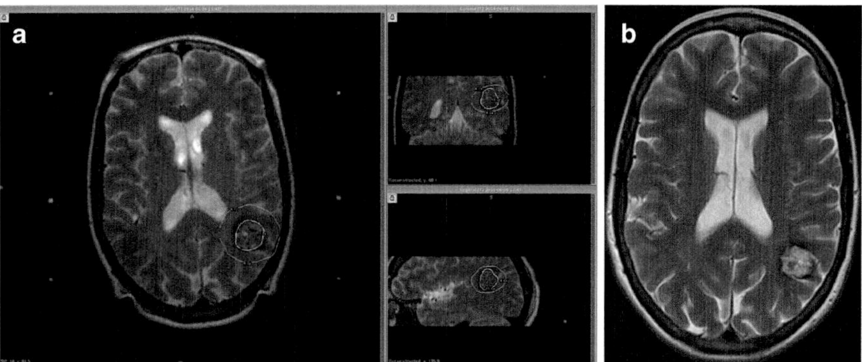

**Fig. 11.3** (**a**) Modern treatment planning of a left temporo-parieto-occipital (Wernicke's area) CCM using T2-weighted high resolution MR images. (*Left:* axial, *right above:* coronal, and *right below:* sagittal slices.) (*Yellow:* 13 Gy 50% prescription isodose line, *green:* 4 Gy line.) (**b**) 1-year follow-up shows no significant change in the appearance (axial T2-weighted MRI)

**Table 11.1** Principles of modern CCM SRS. After [6]

| Importance of patient selection and data analysis (proper interpretation of natural history) |
|---|
|     – Difference between hemispheric and deep eloquent location |
|     – Difference between first and rebleed |
| Modern treatment protocols |
|     – High conformity (gamma-radiation based SRS, MRI-based planning) |
|     – 12–15 Gy (<20 Gy) margin dose |
|     – Within the hemosiderin ring |
|     – Avoid DVA |
|     – At least 3 months after the last bleed (allow enough time for clot resolution) |

Regarding clinical outcome the first line of criticism addresses safety of SRS. Early studies, often cited by critics, reported high radiation-associated complication rates (adverse radiation effects, AREs). However, those studies were from an era with poor delineation of the target with CT or less conformal MRI, and with the use of higher dose protocols that came from a historic AVM-experience [84–87]. Clearly, these studies represent the early experimental phase of the collective learning curve of CCM SRS. On the other hand, modern studies applying the treatment protocol summarized in Tables 11.1 and 11.2 have reported low rates of AREs resulting in only mild persisting morbidity without mortality attributed to radiation. We experienced such a learning curve in Sheffield, from early attempts resulting high rate of AREs [86] until we adopted our contemporary treatment protocol leading to substantial decrease in the rate and severity of AREs [9]. Our contemporary technique uses a prescription dose less than 20Gy (typically 12–15 to the 50% isodose), highly conformal MRI-based treatment planning and treating only lesions without evidence of recent bleed (Type II or III [24], at least 3 months after last hemorrhage). We also learned that it was crucial the lesion to be defined strictly within the supposed radiosensitizer hemosiderin ring [88], and associated DVAs

**Table 11.2** Summary of CCM series using modern gamma-radiation based SRS (the latest report from each group)

| Study | Patients/ lesions (n) | Deep (n) | Superficial (n) | Marginal (prescription) dose (Gy) | Gross target volume (cm³) | Pre-trt first bleed (/year) | Pre-trt rebleed (/ year) | Post-trt bleed until 2 yr. (/ year) | Post-trt bleed after 2 yr. (/year) | Permanent ARE (%) | Post-trt bleed related morbidity (%) | Mortality related to treated CCM (%) | Treatment years |
|---|---|---|---|---|---|---|---|---|---|---|---|---|---|
| Kida and Hasegawa 2004† [71] | 152 | 87 | 65 | 14.9 | N/A | N/A | 31.8* | 8** | <5 | N/A | N/A | 2 | 1991–2001 |
| Liu et al. 2005‡ [72] | 125 | 63 | 49 | 12.1 | 3.12 | N/A | 29.2 | 10.3 | 3.3 | 2.5 | 9.6 | 0 | 1993–2002 |
| Kida 2009† [68] | 84 | 84 | 0 | 13.4 | N/A | N/A | N/A | 7.1 | 1.8 | N/A | N/A | 2.4 | N/A |
| Wang et al. 2010 [73] | 96 | 13 | 83 | 15.6 | N/A | N/A | N/A | 4.2 | <2.1 | 5.2 | N/A | 0 | 1995–2005 |
| Lunsford et al. 2010†† [14] | 103 | 93 | 10 | 16 | 1.31 | N/A | 32.5 | 10.8 | 1.06 | 1 | N/A | 1 | 1988–2005 |
| Lee et al. 2012‡ [74] | 49/50 | 50 | 0 | 11 | 3.2 | N/A | 31.3 | 3.3 | 1.74 | 4.1 | N/A | 0 | 1993–2010 |
| Jay et al. 2012 [75] | 16 | 16 | 0 | 13 | 0.42 | N/A | N/A | 3.72 | 3.59 | 0 | 0 | 6.25 | 1998–2009 |
| Park and Hwang 2013 [76] | 20 | 20 | 0 | 13 | 0.56 | N/A | 39.5 | 8.2 | 0 | 5 | 0 | 0 | 2005–2010 |
| Liscak et al. 2013 [69] | 112 | 50 | 62 | 16 | 0.9 | N/A | N/A | 3.2 | 0.5 | 0.9 | 3.6 | 2.7 | 1992–2000 |
| Frischer et al. 2014 [77] | 38 | 38 | 0 | 12 | 0.3 | N/A | 7.2 | 2.63 | 0.6 | 7.9 | N/A | N/A | 1987–2011 |

| | | | | | | | | | | | | | |
|---|---|---|---|---|---|---|---|---|---|---|---|---|---|
| Lee et al. 2014 [10] | 49 | 49 | 0 | 13.1 | 0.74 | N/A<br>N/A | 38.36 | 7.6***<br>9.84 | 2.3<br>1.5 | 2 | N/A | 0 | 1992–2011 |
| Kim et al. 2014 [78] | 39 | 39 | 0 | 13 | 1.1 | N/A | 33.6**** | 8.1 | 2.4 | 0 | N/A | 0 | 1997–2012 |
| Azimi et al. 2015 [79] | 100 | 74 | 26 | 13 | 1.5 | N/A | 34.3 | 4.1 | 1.9 | N/A | N/A | 0 | 2003–2011 |
| Fedorcsák et al. 2015 [49] | 45/51 | 14 | 37 | 14 | 1.38*****<br>1.53 | 2<br>0.3 | 21.7<br>0 | 7.1<br>0 | 0<br>0 | 7<br>0 | 7<br>0 | 0<br>0 | 2008–2012 |
| Kida et al. 2015 [80] | 298 | 178 | 118 | 14.6 | N/A | 3.9 | 21.4 | 7.4 | 2.8 | 3.7 | N/A | 2 | 1991–2012 |
| López-Serrano et al. 2017 [81] | 95 | 76 | 19 | 11.87 | 1.57 | N/A | N/A | 1.4 | 0.16 | 0 | 1.05 | 0 | 1994–2014 |
| Park et al. 2018 [82] | 45 | 45 | 0 | 13 | 1.82 | N/A | 40.06 | 3.33 | 2.13****** | 0 | N/A | 0 | 1998–2011 |
| Nagy et al. 2018a [16] | 210 | 210 | 0 | 12–13 | 0.24–0.54 | 2.4***<br>2.8 | 20.7 | 4.3<br>7.9 | 1.1<br>1.3 | 7.2 | 7.4 | 0.5–1 | 1995–2014 |
| Nagy et al. 2018b [17] | 96/109 | 0 | 109 | 15 | 0.6 | 2.5***<br>2.1 | 14.15 | 1.8<br>3.85 | 0.7<br>1.3 | 2 | 4.3 | 0.9–2.7 | 1995–2014 |
| Jacobs et al. 2018†† [83] | 76 | 76 | 0 | 15 | 0.66 | N/A | 31.3 | 9.58 | 1.83 | N/A | N/A******* | 2.9 | 1988–2016 |

*ARE* Adverse radiation effect, *N/A* Not applicable. *During 5 years prior to radiosurgery. **First year after treatment. ***First line one bleed, second line multiple bleeds prior to SRS. ****Only 5 of 39 patients had bled twice prior to SRS. *****First line deep-seated, second line superficial. ******1.48% in 2–5 years, 4.64% after 5 years. *******Symptom deterioration was reported in 23.7% of the patients either caused by rehemorrhage or ARE, but it is not clear whether these were temporary or persisting. †, ‡, ††: Data from the same groups analyzing either both deep-seated and superficial, or brainstem lesions only
All except one group used gamma knife®, the one exception used GammaART-6000™ [49]

should also be preserved, because irradiating them (as closing them with microsurgery [45]), was found to be associated with high rate of complications (Fig. 11.4) [89].

The other major concern addresses effectiveness of SRS. A reduction in rebleed rate of CCMs after a 2-year latency period has been reproduced by numerous groups and therefore widely accepted by now. It was first reliably demonstrated in 1995 by

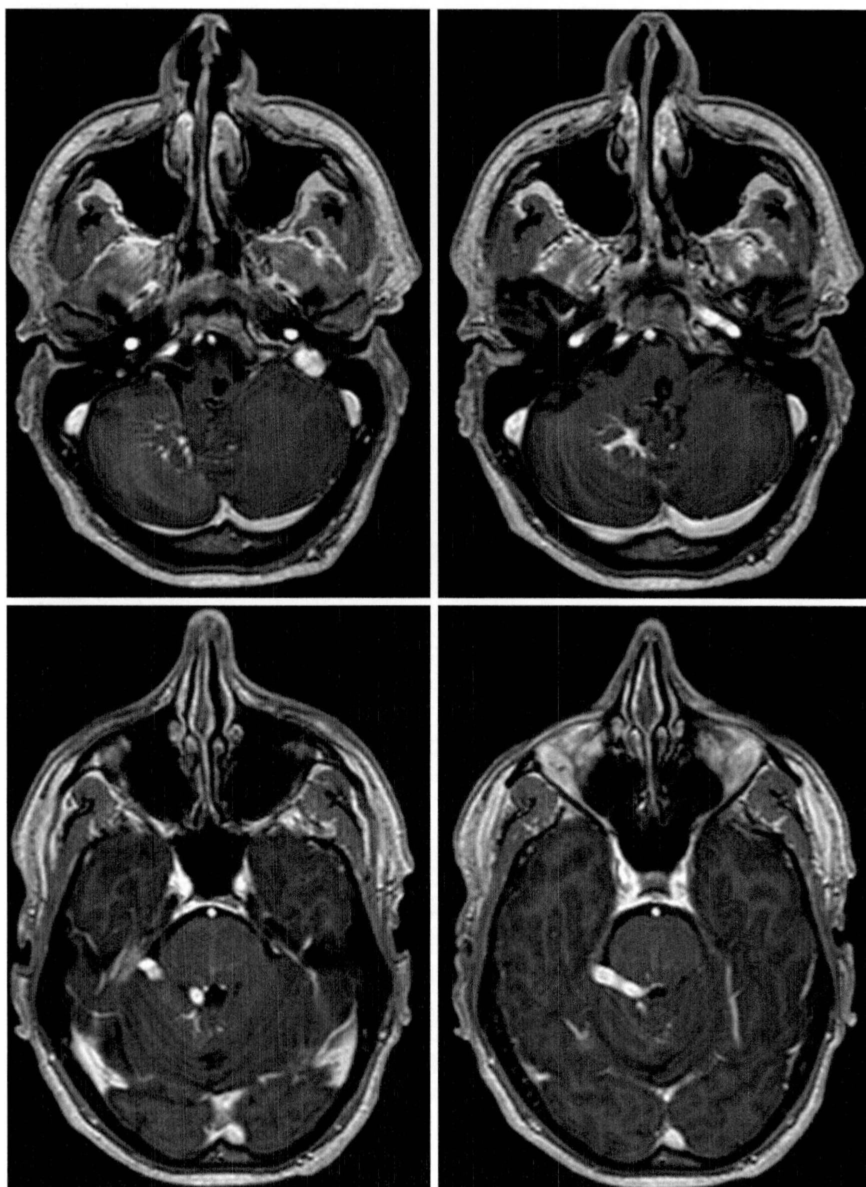

**Fig. 11.4** T1-weighted post-gadolinium axial MR images showing an extensive DVA involving the cerebellum and brainstem in association with a ponto-medullar CCM

the Pittsburgh group in a paper we consider the pioneer of modern CCM SRS not only in terms of data analysis but also in terms of definition of treatment protocol [4]. Admittedly, however, not all published studies demonstrated such a reduction. Temporary increase in rebleed rate [17, 69, 84], and reduction of rebleed rate only after a longer latency period [85] were reported, and more recently even the long-lasting protective effect of radiosurgery was also questioned [82]. We have mentioned the difficulties interpreting hemorrhagic events, particularly when attempts are made to account for pre-diagnosis clinical events: these exceptions may reflect the varied interpretation of what counts as a hemorrhage and may well be due to different patient selection and low number of patients resulting in unreliable statistical analysis. Natural history studies have also shown during the last decades that the key for proper interpretation of CCM SRS is the distinction between the risk of first and repeated hemorrhage. It is also the lesson from these studies that hemispheric lesions behave less aggressively than deep-seated CCMs.

The heterogeneous quality of literature on CCM SRS with distinct measures of natural history, post-treatment bleed rates and ill-definition of treatment standards provides ammunition for the critics who often cite early experimental and low quality contemporary studies that would support their negative view [7, 13]. This attitude is clear in surgical reviews that usually refer to early SRS reports [2, 90, 91]. The few systemic reviews dealing with CCM SRS typically pooled studies of heterogeneous quality. One applied criteria of modern evidence based medicine, and found only one study comparing SRS to surgery and one comparing SRS to observation [59]. However, both studies represented early attempts with poor definition of natural history, selection criteria and follow-up. A detailed extensive meta-analysis pooled all available SRS studies published until 2009 without distinction on natural history, anatomical location, and SRS technique [92]. As large modern SRS series have been published since then, this study unavoidably underestimates its effectiveness with overestimation of its morbidity. Another meta-analysis specifically focused on SRS of brainstem CCMs analyzing 5 series [93]. However, only 3 of these would meet the above strict methodical criteria [74, 76, 94]. A very detailed descriptive systemic review compared outcomes of surgical and radiosurgical interventions [53]. However, the ratio of hemispheric and deep eloquent, as well as hemorrhagic and non-hemorrhagic lesions was different between the two groups, reflecting on different patient populations. Comparing the effect of these two interventions on two distinct group of patients does not seem appropriate. We have recently tried another approach of reviewing the literature by critically weighting the published data based on the aforementioned standardized criteria (Table 11.1) [6]. Due to the lack of quality evidence we think that such a methodically critical analysis of the published data together with reanalysis of the results with increasing number of patients and longer follow up is the most realistic way to get a better view on safety and effectiveness until high level evidence becomes available. After a brief overview on our recent knowledge on the histopathological response to radiosurgery we present the results of our earlier critical review together with more recent data from Sheffield on outcome after CCM SRS in terms of morbidity, effect of bleeding and epilepsy in the following sections.

### 11.4.1 Histopathological Response to Radiosurgery

The idea to use SRS for AOVMs was initially based on the assumption that the majority of these lesions were partially thrombosed AVMs and therefore the vessels would be further obliterated by high dose focused radiation, as observed in the pathological vessels of true AVMs [95]. In AVMs it is well documented that radiation induces hyalinization and thickening of the wall of their endothelium-lined pathological vessels that leads to progressive thrombo-obliteration [96]. Although later histopathological studies found most AOVMs to be CCMs [23], numerous clinical studies demonstrated that these lesions respond in a similar timescale to true AVMs, with reduction of rebleed rate within a 2-year latency period after treatment. Moreover, histological studies of surgically resected previously irradiated CCMs showed to some degree similar radiation-induced vasculopathy as seen in AVMs: fibrinoid necrosis, endothelial destruction, hyalinization, marked fibrosis and scar tissue formation [85, 97–100]. Although complete obliteration was also found with signs of neovascularization [98], a comparative study demonstrated different histopathological effect of SRS on AVMs and CCMs with only about 20% luminal reduction in CCMs after SRS [99]. Of note, these specimens came from lesions that remained symptomatic after irradiation, and those rendered silent by the treatment may actually show complete response, were they removed for analysis. Alternatively, hyalinized vessel walls ("scaring") of such a low pressure lesion may sufficiently stabilize it to prevent a rebleed even without full obliteration.

### 11.4.2 Morbidity after Radiosurgery

Two types of morbidity should be considered after CCM SRS. First, as the beneficial effect of the treatment is expected only after a latency period and the risk of hemorrhage never reaches zero in a large patient population, post-treatment hemorrhage adds to persisting morbidity. In our critical review we found this to be 5.3% for deep-seated lesions [6], which is similar to our recent results of over 200 patients from Sheffield (7.7%) [16]. For hemispheric lesions we found slightly lower hemorrhage related morbidity, 4.3% [17]. It is also important to stress that not only the rate is low, but its severity is mild [16, 17]. Lesion specific mortality is below 1% (Table 11.2), and is exclusively caused by post-treatment hemorrhage, or is related to surgical removal after rebleed [6]. Once suffering from a bleed, the likelihood of permanent deficit seems to be the same with post-treatment hemorrhages as with pre-treatment hemorrhages, suggesting that the benefit of SRS is not to reduce the severity but the frequency of the bleed [9]. The second type of morbidity is related to radiation (adverse radiation effect, ARE). Perilesional edema, causing temporary neurological deficit in less than 10% of the cases [16, 17] or remaining clinically silent, is typically seen within 12 months after SRS. Persisting AREs typically present later than 1 year after treatment, their rates are low, 4.2%–7.2% in deep-seated lesions, resulting in only mild disability (an increase of 1 in modified Rankin Scale score), and the rate of persisting morbidity for hemispheric lesions is even lower, 0.8–1.95% [6, 16, 17].

## 11.4.3   Bleeding Rate After Radiosurgery

The most popular use of SRS is to reduce the risk of future hemorrhage and consequential neurological deterioration, especially for deep-seated lesions. The first report of large clinical series applying modern SRS technique with sufficient follow-up time found that rebleed rate fell from 32%/patient/year pre-treatment to 8.8 within the first 2 years after treatment and to 1.1 thereafter [4]. Moreover, it is also important to mention that this time course of decay of rebleed rates parallels histological changes after SRS found by a recent histopathological study [99]. Contemporary SRS studies focusing on deep eloquent CCMs that had bled at least twice prior to treatment (i.e. proven to behave more aggressively) consequently found a similar sharp drop in annual rebleed rates within a latency period of 2–3 years (Table 11.2). In our critical review we found that annual rebleed rate fell in this group from 32.3% pre-treatment to 8.3% within the first 2 years after SRS, and to 1.5% thereafter [6]. The rebleed rates are similar to the results from the original report from Pittsburgh in 1995 [4] and from our recent paper (20.7, 7.9 and 1.3% pre-treatment, within and after 2 years, respectively) [16]. When confining analysis exclusively to SRS for CCM that had bled only once prior to treatment, during the first 2 years after SRS a higher rate of hemorrhage (4.3–7.1%) [10, 16] was found when compared to first ever hemorrhage rate. Importantly, this is rebleed (the rate being still much lower than rebleed rate of untreated lesions) and therefore the increase is relative to first ever bleed rate. It is also important to note that the rate of further bleed after the 2-year latency period is minimal even in this population (1.1–2%). Hemispheric lesions with one or multiple prior hemorrhages treated with SRS follow a similar pattern with somewhat, but not significantly lower bleed rates [17].

## 11.4.4   Long Term Effects on Bleeding

The most pertinent question currently is whether the fall of rebleed rate within 2 years can really be attributed to the radiobiological effect of SRS or whether it simply reflects natural history, as hemorrhages may occur in clusters that was suggested by observational studies. In other words, does SRS bring any benefit over the natural history? Our understanding of natural history has significantly improved since 2010, when we and the Pittsburgh group published the results of the two largest cohorts of that time [9, 14]. Opponents at that time argued with a virtual patient model obtained by simulation based on available natural history data of heterogeneous quality [13], therefore that debate was merely speculative. As mentioned above, we have a better understanding on the natural history of CCMs as several good quality natural history studies analyzing large patient populations have been published since then.

Only two retrospective studies comparing treated and untreated populations address this question. Li et al. [42] did not find significant difference in terms of hemorrhage free survival between the conservative and SRS group. However, for the SRS group no treatment and patient selection parameters were provided, and such failure could also be explained with poor target definition (e.g. treating lesions prior to clot resolution). In contrast, Kida et al. [80] found statistically significant superiority of SRS over conservative management. Barker et al. [41] in their observational study of unselected population (50% of the lesions being deep-seated) found that 57% of the lesions bled after 5 years, which raised to 72% after 10 years. A recent multi-centric study estimated the 5 year hemorrhage risk to be 31% for brainstem CCMs that presented with bleed [15], and this was found about 50% in a single center study both for brainstem and thalamic lesions [42, 43]. In our recent study hemorrhage free survival of deep-seated CCMs with hemorrhagic presentation was 90% at 5 years after SRS, far superior to natural history [16]. Moreover, Barker et al. [41] found a fall of annual rebleed rate from 25 to 9.5% 2.5 year after initial bleed, a 2.4 fold decline, similar to what was found after 2 years in other papers [38]. In contrast, the decline was 3.9 to 6.1 fold 2 years after SRS in our study depending on the number of pre-treatment hemorrhages [16]. Comparing our results to the only long-term natural history results of brainstem CCMs with comparable size and follow-up time, the long-term benefit appears even more striking in favor of SRS [42]. While in the observation group of a mixed population of lesions with and without hemorrhagic presentation the hemorrhage free survival was 24% at 10, and only 10% at 15 years, we estimated it as 95–85% at 10 years, and 95–75% even 20 years after SRS, depending on hemorrhagic or non-hemorrhagic presentation. Moreover, comparing the more conservative 31% 5 year risk of first hemorrhage for brainstem CCMs with hemorrhagic presentation estimated in an unselected population [15] to the 8% risk we found 5 years after RS of lesions with single prior hemorrhages, we find a far better outcome in the RS group. Our results also suggest that lesions treated earlier have lower chance of rebleeding in the long term, although the difference between single and multiple bleed groups was not significant [16]. Moreover, the case-specific mortality was 6% at 15 years in the conservative group [42] and <1% during our follow-up period after SRS [16]. Taken together, recent data suggest that the reduction of bleed rate observed 2 years after SRS can hardly be accounted only for the "temporal clustering" seen in the natural history.

### 11.4.5   The Effect of CCM SRS on Epilepsy

The second, less popular goal of SRS is to treat epilepsy caused by CCMs as it may be a real treatment alternative for microsurgical resection in patients with intractable epilepsy in several conditions, such as eloquent location, the patient's medical condition, or the patient's preference. The role of SRS in the treatment of epilepsy caused by CCMs was first investigated in 2000 by a retrospective multicenter study analyzing 49 patients without any history of prior bleeding [101]. It was demonstrated that 53% of the patients suffering from epilepsy longer than 1 year refractory to medical therapy became seizure free ("modified "Engel Class IA and B), and 20% showed significant improvement (Class II) within a mean of 4 months after SRS, which is a 73% overall improvement rate. Patients with CCM located in the mesial temporal lobe had worse outcome. More recent studies found similar results, 39–54% of the patients became seizure free (Class I), and 14–20.5% improved significantly (Class II) [73, 102], and a meta-analysis found that 31% of the patients became seizure-free and 35% improved significantly after SRS [92]. On the first instance this seems inferior to surgical series, as Class I response was achieved in 69% of the surgical cases refractory to previous medical therapy [57]. However, considering pre-intervention seizure duration SRS appears to be as effective as surgery if applied early after seizure onset. Whilst 90% of the patients treated with SRS improved with short history of epilepsy ($\leq 3$ years) and only 38.5% with longer lasting epileptic disease [73], 81% improved with $\leq 1$-year history and 70% with longer duration of epilepsy in the surgical group, and good outcome could only be achieved with complete removal of both CCM and the surrounding hemosiderin ring even in the short history group (90.5% versus 60% with partial removal) [103]. In our recent study overall rate of improvement was 85%, 87% in the hemorrhagic and 78.6% in the non-hemorrhagic group, and favorable outcome was 81% for patients with seizures not controlled with antiepileptic medication prior to SRS [17]. However, favorable outcome in our material did not appear to depend on timing of the intervention. Nevertheless, our study is also in line with previous publications suggesting that SRS may be a good alternative for surgery in terms of seizure control.

## 11.5 The Role of Modern Radiosurgery on the Multimodality Management of CCMs

It is hard to recommend a universal optimal management algorithm of CCMs due to their heterogeneity [1]. Based on available data we have recently recommended a treatment algorithm (Fig. 11.5) [12]. As it was mentioned above, it is important to stress that despite the overlap between indications, the three management options are not competitive but complementing each other. It is also important to note that the final decision should be made on an individual basis taking into account not only CCM location and behavior, but age, and medical condition. Moreover, the final treatment decision is also influenced by neurosurgeon's experience and the preference of the fully informed patient.

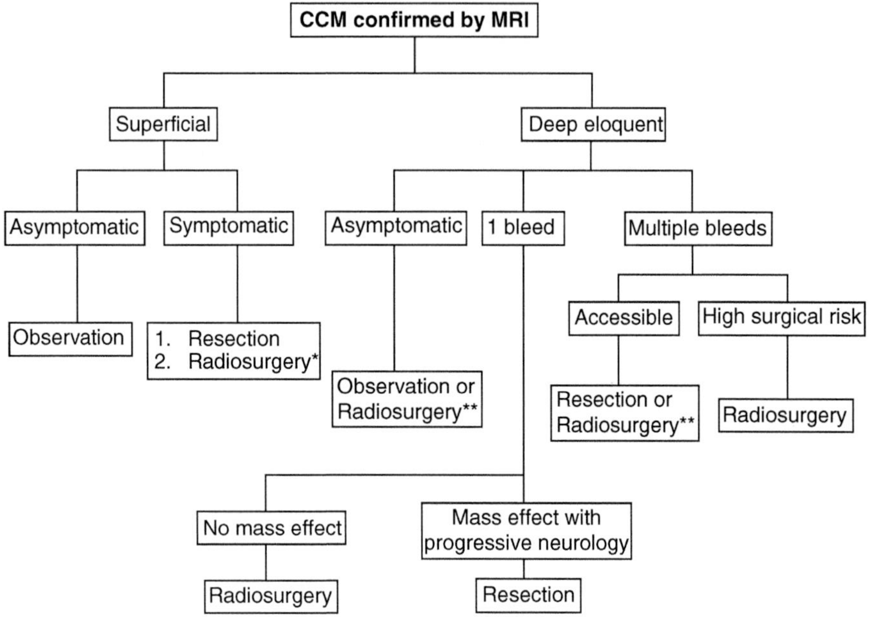



**Fig. 11.5** Proposed algorithm for the management of CCMs. *Surgery is first option in most cases, but radiosurgery is a valid alternative. **Both modalities may be an option, but currently there is no evidence to demonstrate superiority of either. After [12]

## 11.5.1  Deep Seated CCMs

There is currently no convincing data suggesting that intervention brings any benefit over natural history for incidental deep seated CCMs. SRS may be an option due to its low treatment specific morbidity and we do not decline to offer SRS for selected non-hemorrhagic cases. We have treated 26 such lesions until 2014 in Sheffield and preliminary results are promising with a long-term prospective annual hemorrhage risk of 1%. However, the statistical power is low to prove any benefit over the relatively benign natural history. Due to high surgical morbidity the question for lesions that have bled once prior to SRS and left the patients with no or only minimal neurological deficit is whether to observe or treat them with SRS, and surgery remains rather an option only for those lesions that become aggressive whilst still being resectable with acceptable morbidity. Repeated hemorrhages causing progressive neurological deficit or significant mass effect may strengthen the indication for a rapid surgical solution, reducing the risk of microsurgery. However, SRS may also be an alternative intervention when surgery is technically feasible but medically contraindicated or declined by the patient (Figs. 11.1 and 11.2).

## 11.5.2  Superficial CCMs

Surgery is safe and effective in most of the cases, therefore the question is whether SRS may be a treatment alternative for microsurgical resection in selected patients under some circumstances. As a general statement, there is no doubt that microsurgery is the treatment of choice for most of the hemispheric hemorrhagic CMs and we counsel our patients with this knowledge. Based on our recent paper on SRS of hemispheric CCMs published recently [17] we would strictly reserve SRS for a small group of selected patients harboring proven-aggressive CCMs in eloquent location preventing safe resection or in the case of the patient's poor medical condition. It should be also stressed, however, that even if the eligible patients are well informed, some would still be reluctant to undergo craniotomy. Moreover, our recent paper, together with few prior publications, demonstrated that SRS lead to good seizure control similar to microsurgery, and outcomes both after microsurgery and SRS appear to be superior to natural history or medical therapy alone. Therefore, it can be confidently recommended for selected patients as an alternative to open surgery (Fig. 11.3).

## 11.5.3  Failure of SRS and Retreatment

Failure of radiosurgical treatments is well known for all treated pathologies and therefore it is not unreasonable to suppose failure after SRS in the case of CCMs. We have recently tried to define failure of CCM SRS that is harder than in the case of other radiosurgical targets due to the lack of radiological measure to demonstrate the beneficial effect of SRS [104]. Thus, from a clinical point of view a strict definition of failure is hemorrhage following the first 2-year latency period that happens in approximately 5% of the cases, not far from failure rate found after SRS of other pathologies. In addition to true clinical hemorrhages, temporary neurological symptoms without evidence of concurrent hemorrhage or radiation induced perifocal edema may be recurrent requiring intervention due to their detrimental effect on the patients' quality of life. We found two reasons for treatment failure, inaccurate target definition and incomplete response to radiation.

When considering salvage treatment, we need to take into account the patient's clinical state and operability of the lesion. In the case of mass effect or progressive neurological decline, surgery is the treatment of choice. However, as most of the lesions treated with SRS had previously been deemed high risk for microsurgical resection, the risk of morbidity and mortality with microsurgery may be high and it also may happen that removal of the lesion is unsuccessful. We treated 2% of our CCM cases with repeat SRS as an alternative salvage treatment. Based on our initial experience reported in a pilot study, over a median follow-up time of 3 years none of the retreated lesions rebled or produced recurrent transient neurological events, and no transient or persistent AREs were observed. Admittedly, the small numbers and relatively short follow-up time make us cautious to make any strong statement about the effectiveness of repeat CCM SRS. However, the lack of adverse events encourages us to apply repeat SRS after treatment failure for cases not amenable for surgical resection. More cases and longer follow-up are certainly needed for validation.

## 11.6 Perspectives

All published contemporary radiosurgical studies are retrospective and with the lack of matched control group. Critics of this method advocate a prospective randomized controlled trial to clarify the conflicting issues surrounding different managements of CCMs [59]. Although data suggest the benefit of SRS over natural history in the case of deep seated CCMs, the weakest point is clearly the lack of quality evidence [1]. As we pointed out above, we consider SRS rather a complementary than a competing management modality, and we think that the ultimate question is whether to observe deep-seated lesions once becoming symptomatic or to treat them with SRS early after the first bleed. For hemispheric lesions treatment alternative for microsurgery is not as warranted when intervention comes into view. However, the few data on SRS demonstrate that its safety and effectiveness appears to be compatible with microsurgery both in terms of bleeding prevention and seizure control. For deep seated lesions without or with only minimal morbidity we consider SRS favorable to surgical resection, and a prospective randomized trial or a prospective case control study to compare conservative and early radiosurgical management after the first hemorrhage would be welcome. For symptomatic and eloquent superficial lesions, carrying higher surgical risk, it is reasonable to ask which treatment modality is better. As superficial CCMs are more common, this would be an optimal group for a prospective randomized trial or a prospective case control study in order to address these questions than in the rarer, and more aggressive deep seated group, as the chance of conducting such trials is low particularly due to the widely different immediate impact of the three management options that would limit enrolment [12]. Even if such trial came into reality in the near future, it would take years to collect reliable long-term results. Therefore, as a next step forward, a more realistic close goal would be to set up international prospective registries including all detected cases regardless of subsequent choice of management modalities, and to conduct a multi-centric retrospective case control study inviting investigators of published large series reporting either of three management modalities.

In order to get closer to the answer to the still existing open questions surrounding SRS and for any future collaboration, we previously suggested standard data collection (Table 11.3) [12]. It is important first to distinct clearly between hemorrhagic and non-hemorrhagic clinical events, by using standardized

**Table 11.3** Proposal for reporting standards for radiosurgery of CCMs. Modified after [NagyKemeny2013]

| Patient and lesion characteristics prior to treatment |
| --- |
| Age at presentation |
| Age at treatment |
| Sex |
| Family history |
| Presenting symptoms |
| Persisting deficits (modified Rankin scale – mRS) |
| Multiplicity |
| Rate of first bleed (/treated lesion/year) |
| Rate of rebleed (/treated lesion/year) |
| Bleeds 0, 1 or $\geq$ 2 (to be analyzed separately) |
| Location: Superficial/deep-seated (to be recorded separately) |
| Non-hemorrhagic clinical events |
| **Treatment parameters** |
| Gross target volume (GTV) |
| Prescription isodose volume (PIV) |
| Marginal (prescription) dose |
| **Post-treatment hemorrhage rates (/treated lesion/year)** |
| $\leq 2$ years |
| >2 years after treatment |
| Kaplan-Meier curve with estimated hemorrhage free survival |
| **Morbidity related to post-treatment hemorrhages (increase in mRS score)** |
| **Morbidity related to radiation (adverse radiation effects—ARE)** |
| Temporary (duration, requirement for medication) |
| Persisting (increase in mRS score) |
| **Mortality related to treated CCM** |
| **Radiology (if applicable)** |

definition of clinical hemorrhage [25]. We recommend to record retrospective annual first bleed rate for treated lesions (/lesion/year) separately to annual rebleed rate until treatment, and hemorrhage rates should also be calculated separately within 2 years post-treatment and thereafter. Due to their distinct natural history, it seems reasonable to analyze superficial and deep seated lesions separately, and lesions with 0, 1 or multiple bleeds. Although causal relationship with SRS is not proven for all cases, all lasting neurological deterioration unrelated to a post-treatment hemorrhage should be considered as adverse radiation effect, in order to determine the maximal potential morbidity of SRS. Due to delayed protection that is specific to this treatment modality, morbidity related to post-treatment hemorrhage should also be recorded accurately. For a contemporary treatment protocol we also consider a gamma-radiation based instrument the most precise SRS treatment due to its highest conformity achieved with multiple isocenters, owing to the lowest extralesional radiation dose and the largest experience accumulated worldwide.

## 11.7   Conclusion

Controversies of CCM SRS are yet to be resolved due to the lack of radiological proof of cure. However, over the last three decades we were able to confine treatment protocol to reduce the high initial morbidity of the experimental phase, which was the main basis of the early skepticism. Moreover, during the last decade accumulation of large population based data also led to a better understanding of the natural history of CCMs together with the publication of large SRS series moved the debate of the effect of SRS from a speculative to a data- and observation-based foundation. As a result it has been more often considered to complement microsurgery and a wait-and-see policy. Moreover, with the increasing positive experience with SRS and due to the cumulative morbidity of repeated hemorrhages our recommendation to use SRS for deep seated CCMs early after the first hemorrhage, once they become symptomatic, appears to gain broader acceptance. We acknowledge, however, that this debate remains ongoing until more data with more patients and longer follow-up time are available.

**Key Points**
1. SRS of CCMs remains controversial despite our better understanding of natural history and increasing number of radiological series using contemporary treatment protocol.
2. The natural history of deep eloquent CCMs—located in the brainstem, thalamus or basal ganglia—is more aggressive than of hemispheric lesions both in terms of bleed rate and morbidity. It is also likely that the chance for long-term hemorrhage free survival is low despite an initial reduction of the increased rebleed rate especially in deep eloquent lesions as rebleed rate remains higher than the rate of first bleed even 5 years after presentation.
3. Modern protocols are based on the proper understanding of natural history, and MRI-based accurate treatment planning with lower radiation dose as applied to AVMs and avoiding both hemosiderin ring and DVA.
4. SRS using current protocols is an effective treatment alternative for deep-seated CCMs with multiple hemorrhages reducing pre-treatment annual rebleed rates from about 30% to 1–2% within 2 years after treatment.
5. It appears also to stabilize lesions with only one prior hemorrhages after the two-year latency period with a slightly increased rebleed rate of 5%.
6. The rebleed rate after the treatment of hemispheric CCMs with SRS is similarly reduced.
7. SRS of CCMs causing seizures appears to be as effective as microsurgery in terms of seizure control.
8. In modern SRS series radiation only induces low rate of mild persisting morbidity (5–7%).
9. The rate of persisting morbidity caused by post-treatment hemorrhages is also low (5–7%) and the less than 1% mortality is also only caused by hemorrhages.

10. At present there is no high quality evidence to define the relative roles of microsurgery, SRS and wait-and-watch policy in the management of symptomatic CCMs. Although their indications are partly overlapping, their role in CCM management is rather complementary.

11. Recent data both on natural history and on long-term the outcomes of SRS reassure us to recommend early SRS soon after presentation in neurologically intact or minimally disabled patients, especially harboring deep-seated CCM. In our opinion, waiting for the cumulative morbidity of the natural history to justify an otherwise low-risk intervention does not serve the patient well.

# References


1. Akers A, Al-Shahi Salman R, Dahlem K, Flemming K, Hart B, et al. Synopsis of guidelines for the clinical management of cerebral cavernous malformations: consensus recommendations based on systematic literature review by the angioma alliance scientific advisory board clinical experts panel. Neurosurgery. 2017;80(5):665–80.
2. Gross BA, Batjer HH, Awad IA, Bendok BR. Cavernous malformations of the basal ganglia and thalamus. Neurosurgery. 2009;65(1):7–18. discussion −9.
3. Gross BA, Batjer HH, Awad IA, Bendok BR, Du R. Brainstem cavernous malformations: 1390 surgical cases from the literature. World Neurosurg. 2013;80(1–2):89–93.
4. Kondziolka D, Lunsford LD, Flickinger JC, Kestle JR. Reduction of hemorrhage risk after stereotactic radiosurgery for cavernous malformations. J Neurosurg. 1995;83(5):825–31.
5. Niranjan A, Bowden G, Flickinger JC, Lunsford LD. Radiosurgery for cavernous malformations and other vascular diseases. In: Chin LS, Regine WF, editors. Principles and practice of stereotactic radiosurgery. 2nd ed. New York: Springer; 2015. p. 623–36.
6. Nagy G, Kemeny AA. Radiosurgery for cerebral cavernomas. J Neurosurg Sci. 2015;59(3):295–306.
7. Bertalanffy H, Gerganov VM. Microsurgical or radiosurgical management of intracranial cavernomas. Acta Neurochir Suppl. 2013;116:103–6.
8. Brown RD Jr, Flemming KD, Meyer FB, Cloft HJ, Pollock BE, Link ML. Natural history, evaluation, and management of intracranial vascular malformations. Mayo Clin Proc. 2005;80(2):269–81.
9. Nagy G, Razak A, Rowe JG, Hodgson TJ, Coley SC, Radatz MW, et al. Stereotactic radiosurgery for deep-seated cavernous malformations: a move toward more active, early intervention. J Neurosurg. 2010;113(4):691–9.
10. Lee SH, Choi HJ, Shin HS, Choi SK, Oh IH, Lim YJ. Gamma knife radiosurgery for brainstem cavernous malformations: should a patient wait for the rebleed? Acta Neurochir. 2014;156(10):1937–46.
11. Niranjan A, Lunsford LD. Stereotactic radiosurgery guidelines for the management of patients with intracranial cavernous malformations. Prog Neurol Surg. 2013;27:166–75.
12. Nagy G, Kemeny AA. Stereotactic radiosurgery of intracranial cavernous malformations. Neurosurg Clin N Am. 2013;24(4):575–89.
13. Steiner L, Karlsson B, Yen CP, Torner JC, Lindquist C, Schlesinger D. Radiosurgery in cavernous malformations: anatomy of a controversy. J Neurosurg. 2010;113(1):16–21.
14. Lunsford LD, Khan AA, Niranjan A, Kano H, Flickinger JC, Kondziolka D. Stereotactic radiosurgery for symptomatic solitary cerebral cavernous malformations considered high risk for resection. J Neurosurg. 2010;113(1):23–9.

15. Horne MA, Flemming KD, Su IC, Stapf C, Jeon JP, Li D, et al. Clinical course of untreated cerebral cavernous malformations: a meta-analysis of individual patient data. Lancet Neurol. 2016;15(2):166–73.
16. Nagy G, Burkitt W, Stokes SS, Bhattacharyya D, Yianni J, Rowe JG, et al. Contemporary radiosurgery of cerebral cavernous malformations: Part 1. Treatment outcome for critically located hemorrhagic lesions. J Neurosurg. 2019;130(6):1817–25.
17. Nagy G, Stokes SS, Eross LG, Bhattacharyya D, Yianni J, Rowe JG, et al. Contemporary radiosurgery of cerebral cavernous malformations: Part 2. Treatment outcome for hemispheric lesions. J Neurosurg. 2019;130(6):1826–34.
18. Kalani MYS, Lawton MT, Spetzler RF. Letter to the Editor. Radiosurgery for cerebral cavernous malformations: a word of caution. J Neurosurg. 2019;130(6):2086–90.
19. Del Curling O Jr, Kelly DL Jr, Elster AD, Craven TE. An analysis of the natural history of cavernous angiomas. J Neurosurg. 1991;75(5):702–8.
20. Robinson JR, Awad IA, Little JR. Natural history of the cavernous angioma. J Neurosurg. 1991;75(5):709–14.
21. Sage MR, Brophy BP, Sweeney C, Phipps S, Perrett LV, Sandhu A, et al. Cavernous haemangiomas (angiomas) of the brain: clinically significant lesions. Australas Radiol. 1993;37(2):147–55.
22. Al-Holou WN, O'Lynnger TM, Pandey AS, Gemmete JJ, Thompson BG, Muraszko KM, et al. Natural history and imaging prevalence of cavernous malformations in children and young adults. J Neurosurg Pediatr. 2012;9(2):198–205.
23. Tomlinson FH, Houser OW, Scheithauer BW, Sundt TM Jr, Okazaki H, Parisi JE. Angiographically occult vascular malformations: a correlative study of features on magnetic resonance imaging and histological examination. Neurosurgery. 1994;34(5):792–9. discussion 9-800.
24. Zabramski JM, Wascher TM, Spetzler RF, Johnson B, Golfinos J, Drayer BP, et al. The natural history of familial cavernous malformations: results of an ongoing study. J Neurosurg. 1994;80(3):422–32.
25. Al-Shahi Salman R, Berg MJ, Morrison L, Awad IA. Hemorrhage from cavernous malformations of the brain: definition and reporting standards. Angioma Alliance Scientific Advisory Board. Stroke. 2008;39(12):3222–30.
26. Gross BA, Du R. Natural history of cerebral arteriovenous malformations: a meta-analysis. J Neurosurg. 2013;118(2):437–43.
27. Batra S, Lin D, Recinos PF, Zhang J, Rigamonti D. Cavernous malformations: natural history, diagnosis and treatment. Nat Rev Neurol. 2009;5(12):659–70.
28. Al-Shahi R, Bhattacharya JJ, Currie DG, Papanastassiou V, Ritchie V, Roberts RC, et al. Prospective, population-based detection of intracranial vascular malformations in adults: the Scottish intracranial vascular malformation study (SIVMS). Stroke. 2003;34(5):1163–9.
29. Porter PJ, Willinsky RA, Harper W, Wallace MC. Cerebral cavernous malformations: natural history and prognosis after clinical deterioration with or without hemorrhage. J Neurosurg. 1997;87(2):190–7.
30. Clatterbuck RE, Eberhart CG, Crain BJ, Rigamonti D. Ultrastructural and immunocytochemical evidence that an incompetent blood-brain barrier is related to the pathophysiology of cavernous malformations. J Neurol Neurosurg Psychiatry. 2001;71(2):188–92.
31. Tu J, Stoodley MA, Morgan MK, Storer KP. Ultrastructural characteristics of hemorrhagic, nonhemorrhagic, and recurrent cavernous malformations. J Neurosurg. 2005;103(5):903–9.
32. Pozzati E, Acciarri N, Tognetti F, Marliani F, Giangaspero F. Growth, subsequent bleeding, and de novo appearance of cerebral cavernous angiomas. Neurosurgery. 1996;38(4):662–9. discussion 9-70.
33. Fritschi JA, Reulen HJ, Spetzler RF, Zabramski JM. Cavernous malformations of the brain stem. A review of 139 cases. Acta Neurochir. 1994;130(1–4):35–46.
34. Kim DS, Park YG, Choi JU, Chung SS, Lee KC. An analysis of the natural history of cavernous malformations. Surg Neurol. 1997;48(1):9–17. discussion −8.

35. Moriarity JL, Wetzel M, Clatterbuck RE, Javedan S, Sheppard JM, Hoenig-Rigamonti K, et al. The natural history of cavernous malformations: a prospective study of 68 patients. Neurosurgery. 1999;44(6):1166–71. discussion 72-3.
36. Al-Shahi Salman R, Hall JM, Horne MA, Moultrie F, Josephson CB, Bhattacharya JJ, et al. Untreated clinical course of cerebral cavernous malformations: a prospective, population-based cohort study. Lancet Neurol. 2012;11(3):217–24.
37. Gross BA, Du R. Hemorrhage from cerebral cavernous malformations: a systematic pooled analysis. J Neurosurg. 2017;126(4):1079–87.
38. Taslimi S, Modabbernia A, Amin-Hanjani S, Barker FG 2nd, Macdonald RL. Natural history of cavernous malformation: systematic review and meta-analysis of 25 studies. Neurology. 2016;86(21):1984–91.
39. Kondziolka D, Lunsford LD, Kestle JR. The natural history of cerebral cavernous malformations. J Neurosurg. 1995;83(5):820–4.
40. Jeon JS, Kim JE, Chung YS, Oh S, Ahn JH, Cho WS, et al. A risk factor analysis of prospective symptomatic haemorrhage in adult patients with cerebral cavernous malformation. J Neurol Neurosurg Psychiatry. 2014;85(12):1366–70.
41. Barker FG 2nd, Amin-Hanjani S, Butler WE, Lyons S, Ojemann RG, Chapman PH, et al. Temporal clustering of hemorrhages from untreated cavernous malformations of the central nervous system. Neurosurgery. 2001;49(1):15–24. discussion −5.
42. Li D, Hao SY, Jia GJ, Wu Z, Zhang LW, Zhang JT. Hemorrhage risks and functional outcomes of untreated brainstem cavernous malformations. J Neurosurg. 2014;121(1):32–41.
43. Tian KB, Zheng JJ, Ma JP, Hao SY, Wang L, Zhang LW, et al. Clinical course of untreated thalamic cavernous malformations: hemorrhage risk and neurological outcomes. J Neurosurg. 2016;127:1–12.
44. Moultrie F, Horne MA, Josephson CB, Hall JM, Counsell CE, Bhattacharya JJ, et al. Outcome after surgical or conservative management of cerebral cavernous malformations. Neurology. 2014;83(7):582–9.
45. Porter RW, Detwiler PW, Spetzler RF, Lawton MT, Baskin JJ, Derksen PT, et al. Cavernous malformations of the brainstem: experience with 100 patients. J Neurosurg. 1999;90(1):50–8.
46. Tung H, Giannotta SL, Chandrasoma PT, Zee CS. Recurrent intraparenchymal hemorrhages from angiographically occult vascular malformations. J Neurosurg. 1990;73(2):174–80.
47. Li D, Hao SY, Tang J, Xiao XR, Jia GJ, Wu Z, et al. Clinical course of untreated pediatric brainstem cavernous malformations: hemorrhage risk and functional recovery. J Neurosurg Pediatr. 2014;13(5):471–83.
48. Robinson JR Jr, Awad IA, Magdinec M, Paranandi L. Factors predisposing to clinical disability in patients with cavernous malformations of the brain. Neurosurgery. 1993;32(5):730–5. discussion 5-6.
49. Fedorcsak I, Nagy G, Dobai JG, Mezey G, Bognar L. Radiosurgery of intracerebral cavernomas - Current Hungarian practice. Ideggyogy Sz. 2015;68(7–8):243–51. Az intracerebralis cavernomak sugarsebeszete--hol tart magyarorszag?
50. Jakimovski D, Schneider H, Frei K, Kennes LN, Bertalanffy H. Bleeding propensity of cavernous malformations: impact of tight junction alterations on the occurrence of overt hematoma. J Neurosurg. 2014;121(3):613–20.
51. Awad I, Jabbour P. Cerebral cavernous malformations and epilepsy. Neurosurg Focus. 2006;21(1):e7.
52. Josephson CB, Leach JP, Duncan R, Roberts RC, Counsell CE, Al-Shahi SR. Seizure risk from cavernous or arteriovenous malformations: prospective population-based study. Neurology. 2011;76(18):1548–54.
53. Poorthuis MH, Klijn CJ, Algra A, Rinkel GJ, Al-Shahi SR. Treatment of cerebral cavernous malformations: a systematic review and meta-regression analysis. J Neurol Neurosurg Psychiatry. 2014;85(12):1319–23.

54. Amin-Hanjani S, Ogilvy CS, Ojemann RG, Crowell RM. Risks of surgical management for cavernous malformations of the nervous system. Neurosurgery. 1998;42(6):1220–7. discussion 7-8.
55. Gross BA, Smith ER, Goumnerova L, Proctor MR, Madsen JR, Scott RM. Resection of supratentorial lobar cavernous malformations in children: clinical article. J Neurosurg Pediatr. 2013;12(4):367–73.
56. Pasqualin A, Meneghelli P, Giammarusti A, Turazzi S. Results of surgery for cavernomas in critical supratentorial areas. Acta Neurochir Suppl. 2014;119:117–23.
57. Englot DJ, Han SJ, Lawton MT, Chang EF. Predictors of seizure freedom in the surgical treatment of supratentorial cavernous malformations. J Neurosurg. 2011;115(6):1169–74.
58. Kivelev J, Niemela M, Hernesniemi J. Treatment strategies in cavernomas of the brain and spine. J Clin Neurosci. 2012;19(4):491–7.
59. Poorthuis M, Samarasekera N, Kontoh K, Stuart I, Cope B, Kitchen N, et al. Comparative studies of the diagnosis and treatment of cerebral cavernous malformations in adults: systematic review. Acta Neurochir. 2013;155(4):643–9.
60. Abla AA, Turner JD, Mitha AP, Lekovic G, Spetzler RF. Surgical approaches to brainstem cavernous malformations. Neurosurg Focus. 2010;29(3):E8.
61. Ulrich NH, Kockro RA, Bellut D, Amaxopoulou C, Bozinov O, Burkhardt JK, et al. Brainstem cavernoma surgery with the support of pre- and postoperative diffusion tensor imaging: initial experiences and clinical course of 23 patients. Neurosurg Rev. 2014;37(3):481–91. discussion 92.
62. Samii M, Eghbal R, Carvalho GA, Matthies C. Surgical management of brainstem cavernomas. J Neurosurg. 2001;95(5):825–32.
63. Bradac O, Majovsky M, de Lacy P, Benes V. Surgery of brainstem cavernous malformations. Acta Neurochir. 2013;155(11):2079–83.
64. Pollock BE, Link MJ, Stafford SL, Garces YI, Foote RL. Stereotactic radiosurgery for arteriovenous malformations: the effect of treatment period on patient outcomes. Neurosurgery. 2016;78(4):499–509.
65. McDermott MW, Sneed PK. Radiosurgery in metastatic brain cancer. Neurosurgery. 2005;57(5 Suppl):S45–53. discusssion S1–4.
66. Regis J, Carron R, Delsanti C, Porcheron D, Thomassin JM, Murracciole X, et al. Radiosurgery for vestibular schwannomas. Neurosurg Clin N Am. 2013;24(4):521–30.
67. Santacroce A, Walier M, Regis J, Liscak R, Motti E, Lindquist C, et al. Long-term tumor control of benign intracranial meningiomas after radiosurgery in a series of 4565 patients. Neurosurgery. 2012;70(1):32–9. discussion 9.
68. Kida Y. Radiosurgery for cavernous malformations in basal ganglia, thalamus and brainstem. Prog Neurol Surg. 2009;22:31–7.
69. Liscak R, Urgosik D, Simonova G, Vymazal J, Semnicka J. Gamma knife radiosurgery of brain cavernomas. Acta Neurochir Suppl. 2013;116:107–11.
70. Kim MS, Pyo SY, Jeong YG, Lee SI, Jung YT, Sim JH. Gamma knife surgery for intracranial cavernous hemangioma. J Neurosurg. 2005;102(Suppl):102–6.
71. Kida Y, Hasegawa T. Radiosurgery for cavernous malformations: results of long-term follow-up. In: Kondziolka D, editor. Radiosurgery. Basel: Karger; 2004. p. 153–60.
72. Liscak R, Vladyka V, Simonova G, Vymazal J, Novotny J Jr. Gamma knife surgery of brain cavernous hemangiomas. J Neurosurg. 2005;102(Suppl):207–13.
73. Wang P, Zhang F, Zhang H, Zhao H. Gamma knife radiosurgery for intracranial cavernous malformations. Clin Neurol Neurosurg. 2010;112(6):474–7.
74. Lee CC, Pan DH, Chung WY, Liu KD, Yang HC, Wu HM, et al. Brainstem cavernous malformations: the role of gamma knife surgery. J Neurosurg. 2012;117(Suppl):164–9.
75. Jay SM, Chandran H, Blackburn TP. Gamma knife stereotactic radiosurgery for thalamic and brainstem cavernous angiomas. Br J Neurosurg. 2012;26(3):367–70.
76. Park SH, Hwang SK. Gamma knife radiosurgery for symptomatic brainstem intra-axial cavernous malformations. World Neurosurg. 2013;80(6):e261–6.

77. Frischer JM, Gatterbauer B, Holzer S, Stavrou I, Gruber A, Novak K, et al. Microsurgery and radiosurgery for brainstem cavernomas: effective and complementary treatment options. World Neurosurg. 2014;81(3–4):520–8.
78. Kim BS, Yeon JY, Kim JS, Hong SC, Lee JI. Gamma knife radiosurgery of the symptomatic brain stem cavernous angioma with low marginal dose. Clin Neurol Neurosurg. 2014;126:110–4.
79. Azimi P, Shahzadi S, Bitaraf MA, Azar M, Alikhani M, Zali A, et al. Cavernomas: outcomes after gamma-knife radiosurgery in Iran. Asian J Neurosurg. 2015;10(1):49–50.
80. Kida Y, Hasegawa T, Iwai Y, Shuto T, Satoh M, Kondoh T, et al. Radiosurgery for symptomatic cavernous malformations: a multi-institutional retrospective study in Japan. Surg Neurol Int. 2015;6(Suppl 5):S249–57.
81. Lopez-Serrano R, Martinez NE, Kusak ME, Quiros A, Martinez R. Significant hemorrhage rate reduction after gamma knife radiosurgery in symptomatic cavernous malformations: long-term outcome in 95 case series and literature review. Stereotact Funct Neurosurg. 2017;95(6):369–78.
82. Park K, Kim JW, Chung HT, Paek SH, Kim DG. Long-term outcome of gamma knife radiosurgery for symptomatic brainstem cavernous malformation. World Neurosurg. 2018;116:e1054–e9.
83. Jacobs R, Kano H, Gross BA, Niranjan A, Monaco EA 3rd, Lunsford LD. Defining long-term clinical outcomes and risks of stereotactic radiosurgery for brainstem cavernous malformations. World Neurosurg. 2018;. Epub 2018/12/12
84. Amin-Hanjani S, Ogilvy CS, Candia GJ, Lyons S, Chapman PH. Stereotactic radiosurgery for cavernous malformations: Kjellberg's experience with proton beam therapy in 98 cases at the Harvard cyclotron. Neurosurgery. 1998;42(6):1229–36. discussion 36-8.
85. Karlsson B, Kihlstrom L, Lindquist C, Ericson K, Steiner L. Radiosurgery for cavernous malformations. J Neurosurg. 1998;88(2):293–7.
86. Mitchell P, Hodgson TJ, Seaman S, Kemeny AA, Forster DM. Stereotactic radiosurgery and the risk of haemorrhage from cavernous malformations. Br J Neurosurg. 2000;14(2):96–100.
87. Pollock BE, Garces YI, Stafford SL, Foote RL, Schomberg PJ, Link MJ. Stereotactic radiosurgery for cavernous malformations. J Neurosurg. 2000;93(6):987–91.
88. St George EJ, Perks J, Plowman PN. Stereotactic radiosurgery XIV: the role of the haemosiderin 'ring' in the development of adverse reactions following radiosurgery for intracranial cavernous malformations: a sustainable hypothesis. Br J Neurosurg. 2002;16(4):385–91.
89. Lindquist C, Guo WY, Karlsson B, Steiner L. Radiosurgery for venous angiomas. J Neurosurg. 1993;78(4):531–6. Epub 1993/04/01.
90. Bertalanffy H, Benes L, Miyazawa T, Alberti O, Siegel AM, Sure U. Cerebral cavernomas in the adult. Review of the literature and analysis of 72 surgically treated patients. Neurosurg Rev. 2002;25(1–2):1–53. discussion 4-5.
91. Gross BA, Batjer HH, Awad IA, Bendok BR. Brainstem cavernous malformations. Neurosurgery. 2009;64(5):E805–18. discussion E18.
92. Pham M, Gross BA, Bendok BR, Awad IA, Batjer HH. Radiosurgery for angiographically occult vascular malformations. Neurosurg Focus. 2009;26(5):E16.
93. Lu XY, Sun H, Xu JG, Li QY. Stereotactic radiosurgery of brainstem cavernous malformations: a systematic review and meta-analysis. J Neurosurg. 2014;120(4):982–7.
94. Monaco EA, Khan AA, Niranjan A, Kano H, Grandhi R, Kondziolka D, et al. Stereotactic radiosurgery for the treatment of symptomatic brainstem cavernous malformations. Neurosurg Focus. 2010;29(3):E11.
95. Kondziolka D, Lunsford LD, Coffey RJ, Bissonette DJ, Flickinger JC. Stereotactic radiosurgery of angiographically occult vascular malformations: indications and preliminary experience. Neurosurgery. 1990;27(6):892–900.
96. Szeifert GT, Levivier M, Lorenzoni J, Nyary I, Major O, Kemeny AA. Morphological observations in brain arteriovenous malformations after gamma knife radiosurgery. Prog Neurol Surg. 2013;27:119–29.

97. Gewirtz RJ, Steinberg GK, Crowley R, Levy RP. Pathological changes in surgically resected angiographically occult vascular malformations after radiation. Neurosurgery. 1998;42(4):738–42. discussion 42-3.

98. Nyáry I, Major O, Hanzély Z, Szeifert GT. Histopathological findings in a surgically resected thalamic cavernous hemangioma 1 year after 40-Gy irradiation. J Neurosurg. 2005;102(Suppl):56–8.

99. Tu J, Stoodley MA, Morgan MK, Storer KP, Smee R. Different responses of cavernous malformations and arteriovenous malformations to radiosurgery. J Clin Neurosci. 2009;16(7):945–9.

100. Shin SS, Murdoch G, Hamilton RL, Faraji AH, Kano H, Zwagerman NT, et al. Pathological response of cavernous malformations following radiosurgery. J Neurosurg. 2015;123(4):938–44.

101. Régis J, Bartolomei F, Kida Y, Kobayashi T, Vladyka V, Liscak R, et al. Radiosurgery for epilepsy associated with cavernous malformation: retrospective study in 49 patients. Neurosurgery. 2000;47(5):1091–7.

102. Liu KD, Chung WY, Wu HM, Shiau CY, Wang LW, Guo WY, et al. Gamma knife surgery for cavernous hemangiomas: an analysis of 125 patients. J Neurosurg. 2005;102(Suppl):81–6.

103. Jin Y, Zhao C, Zhang S, Zhang X, Qiu Y, Jiang J. Seizure outcome after surgical resection of supratentorial cavernous malformations plus hemosiderin rim in patients with short duration of epilepsy. Clin Neurol Neurosurg. 2014;119:59–63.

104. Nagy G, Yianni J, Bhattacharyya D, Rowe JG, Kemeny AA, Radatz MWR. Repeat radiosurgery treatment after cavernous malformation radiosurgery. World Neurosurg. 2018;118:e296–303.

# Chapter 12
# Cavernomas in Children


Nejat Akalan


## 12.1   Introduction

In spite of intensive research, pathogenesis of cerebral cavernomas has not yet been elucidated. Cavernomas are originally believed to be primarily congenital in origin and loss–of-function mutations in at least three genes has been demonstrated in familial forms that are responsible for almost one third of the diagnosed cases. On the other hand, documented cases of de novo formation after radiation therapy, at stereotactic biopsy trajectory and association with developmental venous anomaly (DVA) brought controversy against the congenital hypothesis. Similar to the true arteriovenous malformations (AVM), where several theories have been proposed against congenital origin including inflammation, angiogenic and hormonal factors induced by hypoxia due to the presence of DVA. Nevertheless, cavernomas detected at pediatric age including fetal period suggest a congenital origin cannot be underestimated [1]. Diverse clinical course of the disease in both familial and isolated cases has been explained by the existence of powerful genetic and/or environmental disease modifiers [2]. Currently, there is no unifying hypothesis that would explain the occurrence of symptomatic cavernomas in a wide age spectrum beginning from fetal period. Ongoing debate on the origin and pathogenesis of cerebral cavernomas raises the question whether pediatric cavernomas should be regarded as a different disease entity or as a result of different germ-line mutations owing their diverse presentation compared to adults [3].


N. Akalan (✉)
Department of Neurosurgery, Medipol University School of Medicine, Istanbul, Turkey
e-mail: nejata@tr.net



© Springer Nature Switzerland AG 2020

O. Bradáč, V. Beneš (eds.), *Cavernomas of the CNS*,
https://doi.org/10.1007/978-3-030-49406-3_12

## 12.2 Epidemiology

Exact incidence of cavernomas remains unknown due to asymptomatic cases, revealed in autopsy. Prevalence estimations depend mostly on either autopsy or radiological series and the incidence has been reported to be 0.15–0.56 per 100,000 persons per year, with a prevalence of 0.17–0.9% while 70–95% of lesions remain life-time asymptomatic [4–9]. Previous estimates are largely based on adult series very few children have been included in those. Recent data argues they are not uncommon and its prevalence ranges from 0.37 to 0.53%, being second most common cause of spontaneous intracerebral hemorrhage in children, after AVMs [10–13].

## 12.3 Clinical Presentation

Seizure, hemorrhage or focal neurological deficits which are cardinal presentations of cerebral AVM are also valid for cavernomas. Cerebral cavernomas are typically presented with seizures and focal neurological deficits due to mass effect and hemorrhage [5, 14–17]. Hemorrhage is the most feared complication for a true AVM responsible for serious morbidity and mortality which all modes of treatment aim to avoid. Although hemorrhage has also been presented as a major complication in cavernomas, the magnitude and consequences of bleeding are incomparable to AVM's. Owing to their morphology, hemorrhage is episodic, confined within the lesion; initially asymptomatic detected by radiology. While sudden bleeding from a high-flow AVM can result with acute symptoms secondary to direct parenchymal injury, cavernomas become symptomatic only after smaller, silent intralesional hemorrhages reach a critical mass to disturb surrounding parenchyma [14, 18]. Discrepancy between AVM and cavernoma bleeding is believed to cause confusion and misconception effecting especially natural history studies reporting a wide range of frequencies, partly due to differences in definition of hemorrhage [19, 20]. Several associations such as American Heart Association and Angioma Alliance have recommended standards to define cavernoma hemorrhage only with acute or subacute onset symptoms concordant with radiological location, surgical findings or pathological examination (Fig. 12.1). Presence of hemosiderin or enlarged diameter of the CM is not considered hemorrhage [19, 21]. Nevertheless, symptoms related to cavernoma hemorrhage following asymptomatic repeated episodes are closely related to size and location. Those who have reached enough size at the supratentorial area produce neurological deficits secondary to local mass effect usually preceded by sudden headache, impaired consciousness or seizure. Mixed series with adult predominance report hemorrhage in 8–37% cases as the initial presenting feature [22]. Among pediatric population, cavernomas represent 20–25% of

| Presentation | Clinical Evidence |
|---|---|
| Acute or subacute onset symptoms of headache, seizure, impaired consciousness, new/worsened focal neurological deficit referable to the anatomic location of the cavernoma | Radiological, pathological, surgical or cerebrospinal fluid evidence of recent extra- or intralesional hemorrhage |

A mere existence of hemosiderin halo, or solely an increase in cavernoma diameter without other evidence of recent hemorrhage, are not considered as to represent a hemorrhage associated symptomatology

**Fig. 12.1** Criteria advised by Angioma Alliance Scientific Advisory Board for accurate definition of cavernoma hemorrhage with matching symptoms with radiological, pathological or surgical findings (Figure adapted from Salman RA-S et al. [21])

spontaneous ICH in children. Hemorrhage was observed in 33–64% of the pediatric cases at the time of initial diagnosis [23–25]. Significant fatal hemorrhage is a rare phenomenon compared to AVM's, with a reported annual risk of 0.25–6% in cavernomas [5, 16, 26–29]. Although cavernomas are identified by repeated microhemorrhages, extralesional/parenchymal, subarachnoid and intraventricular hemorrhages have also been described [30, 31]. Several clinical series report a higher propensity for overt hemorrhage in women and children [30, 32–34] (Fig. 12.2). Cavernomas situated in the vicinity of the ventricular system can cause blood oozing through the disrupted ependyma during episodes of hemorrhage. Shirvani and Hajimirzabeigi [35] have reviewed 136 intraventricular cavernoma cases in the literature where 23% of patients were in the pediatric and adolescent group and 19%, infants. They have concluded that lack of perilesional brain tissue inside the ventricles promotes the rapid growth and increases the probability of bleeding. These figures indicate that the ratio of intraventricular location is higher in the pediatric age among symptomatic cases (Fig. 12.3). It is not clear whether paraventricular location and relatively large size is an evidence indicating pediatric cavernoma to be a different disease entity compared to adults or simply early detection due to localization. Similar concern is valid for infratentorial localization, published large series report a higher incidence of infratentorial cavernomas in children over 30%, compared to adult series [25, 36–38]. Contrarily, reported high incidence has been attributed to the tendency to report such a less common location in the medical literature, rather than reflecting the actual incidence [37]. Nevertheless, brainstem cavernomas, both in adults and children, are presented with focal neurological signs almost always accompanied by cranial nerve involvement along with motor deficits, ataxia and even neuropathic pain [25, 36, 39] (Fig. 12.4). Neurological deficits are secondary

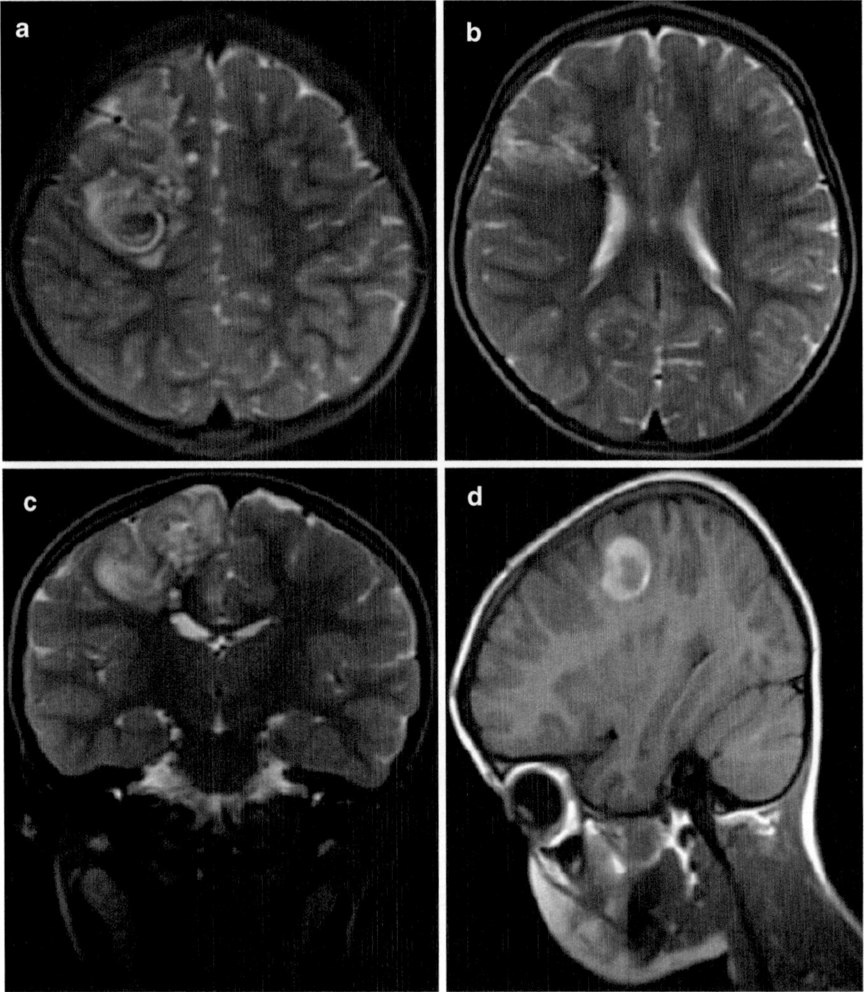

**Fig. 12.2** Cavernoma with extra-lesional, parenchymal hemorrhage presented with right sided hemiparesis following focal seizure in a 3 year old boy; T2 weighed axial (**a, b**), coronal (**c**) sections revealing a paraventricular lesion with mixed signal intensity surrounded by a rim of hypointensity consistent with cavernoma and hyperintense extralesional signal at the neighbouring cortex at the T1 weighed sagittal image (**d**), representing recent hemorrhage

to local mass effect rather than direct parenchymal injury although they invariably exhibit varying degrees of micro hemorrhage in the brainstem.

An exclusive characteristic of cavernoma hemorrhage is that; even when they are too small to be symptomatic, they may contribute to seizure development. Progressive deposition of hemosiderin in the cerebral parenchyma surrounding the cavernous malformation is a potent epileptogenic agent with the iron content [40, 41].

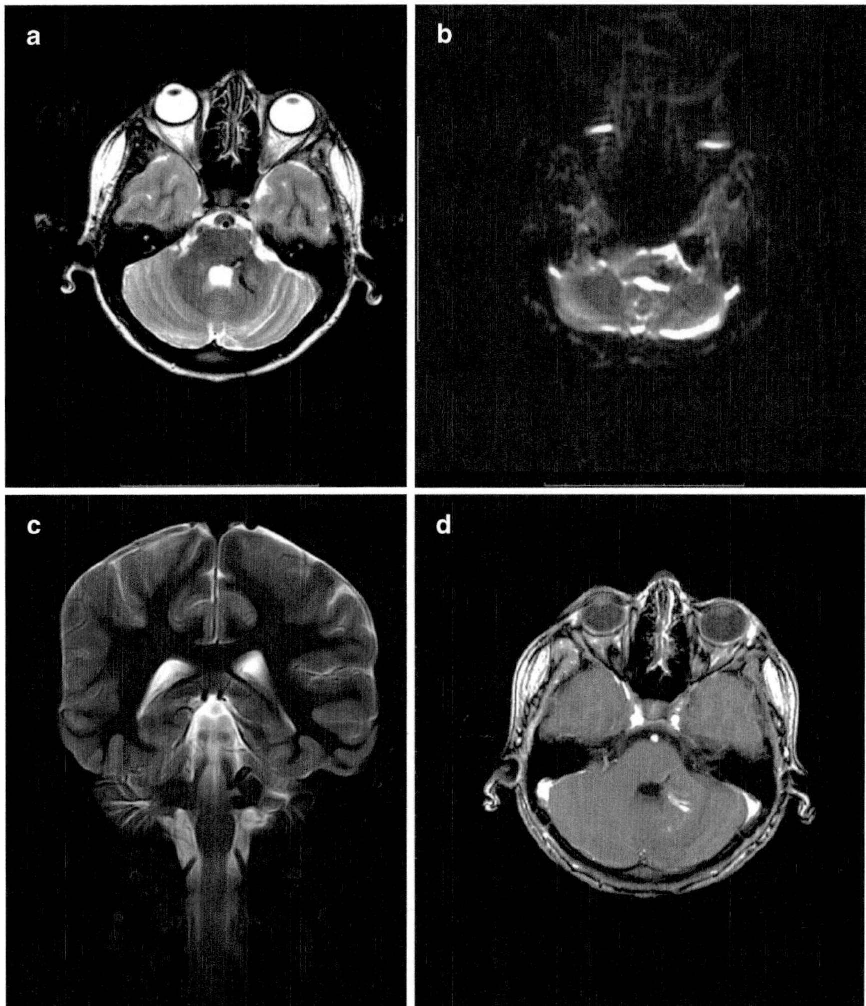

**Fig. 12.3** MR study of a 23 month old boy due to sudden irritability and nuchal rigidity revealing subependymal lesion at the wall of the IV. Ventricle at medullar level, homogenous and hypointense in axial T2 (**a**) and coronal (**c**), and diffusion weighed (**b**) images; with adjacent DVA in T1 axial image with contrast (**d**), suggestive for a cavernoma apparent by oozing into the ventricle

Whether preceded by a recent hemorrhagic event or not, seizure is the most frequent single presenting symptom in most of the published series [23, 42–48]. Bilginer et al. [23], in their review of 36 operated pediatric cavernoma cases found that seizure was the most common single presenting symptom in 38.9%, added those with additional symptoms and signs, 61.1%of the patients had had at least one seizure on admission (Fig. 12.5).

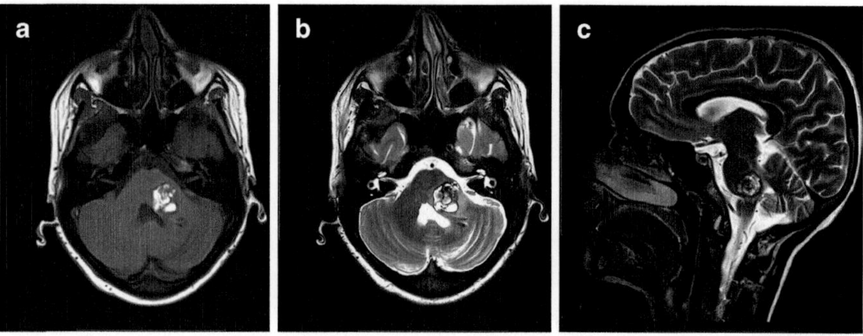

**Fig. 12.4** 12 year old girl admitted with the complaint of facial weakness on the right, with MR request to rule-out a tumor revealing a non-homogenous lesion with hiper- and hypointense patchy appearance on axial T1 (**a**) and T2 (**b**) and sagittal (**c**) weighed images, at the pontomedullary junction at the level of facial nucleus, consistent with a cavernoma

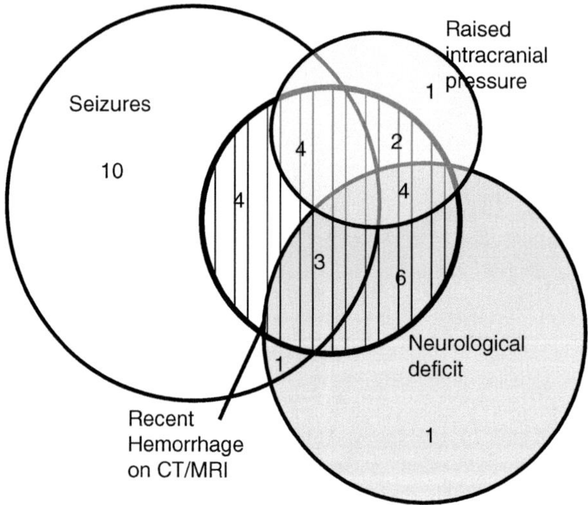


**Fig. 12.5** Association of symptoms on admission in 36 pediatric cavernomas, demonstrating recent hemorrhage is imaging corresponds closely to the presentation except that only seizures where no recent hemorrhage was detected at the majority (Figure adapted from Bilginer et al. [23])

## 12.4 Natural History

"Understanding the natural history of a disease is an important prerequisite for designing studies that assess the impact of interventions, both chemotherapeutic and environmental.… may provide important indicators for drug targets and surrogate outcomes for clinical trials. However, collecting and visualizing data on natural history is challenging in part because disease processes are complex and evolve in different chronological periods for different subjects." [49]. This concept is valid for central nervous system diseases with congenital background, including cavernomas. Cerebral AVM's and pediatric aneurysms to some extent are vascular pathologies with congenital origin and may stay asymptomatic during life-time. Apart from those which become symptomatic by hemorrhage, intention to treat is to avoid hemorrhage, once detected. Consequence of hemorrhagic insult is well established as well as the life-time risks of bleeding with epidemiological natural history studies. Accumulated data on their natural history enables to make straightforward decisions for treatment in asymptomatic cases. Cavernomas, as a member of central nervous system vascular malformations have disadvantages in evaluating their natural history due to their diverse morphology and different flow dynamics. This can be appreciated from the diversity of the estimations for prevalence and hemorrhage rates reported so far.

Inconsistency among figures have several reasons; depending on the methodology of the study and composition of the target population. Above all, hemorrhage risk, as the main variable to be calculated has been appreciated differently in the studies. Unlike AVM's, the hemorrhage referred is almost always intralesional recurrent oozing, not necessarily symptomatic. Symptoms usually depend on the size and location of the cavernomas rather than the parenchymal disruption due to hematoma. Adding cases with image based diagnosis to symptomatic cases may result with under- or overestimation of the bleeding rate. Moreover, existence of the familial vs. sporadic, congenital and de-novo, single or multiple, adult and pediatric forms all together have a potential selection bias. Like all other vascular malformations, estimate of the natural history of cavernomas is important to compare the untreated clinical course and outcome in terms of morbidity and mortality to risks and complications of potential treatment.

Pediatric cavernomas detected even in infants may be regarded on the congenital origin but estimates based on this assumption may result in an artificially low figures because annual rate of bleeds before surgery overall may be underestimated as it is impossible to quantify the length of time that a patient has had the lesion [19, 24]. On the other hand, calculations based on children who present with hemorrhage may result in artificially high hemorrhage risk estimates. In adult series, while the annual risk of hemorrhage in incidentally detected cases was found as 0.33%, while the risk rebleeding after the first hemorrhage increases up to 60% [7, 16, 28, 50–55]. Nevertheless, Al-Shahi Salman et al. [7], in their population based cohort study of 139 adult cases, concluded that the risk of a first-ever intracranial hemorrhage is low; functional impairment from hemorrhage is mild at initial presentation and although the risk of recurrence is higher than the risk of a first event, it seems to decline over time.

In limited number of recent publications in pediatric cavernoma series, hemorrhage rate was 0.2–1.6% in incidental cases and 7.4–18.2% after the first incident, which are apparently lower than the average values in adult series [14, 24]. On the other hand, brain stem location is brainstem was associated with a higher rate of symptomatic hemorrhage [38, 56, 57].

## 12.5  Treatment

For any cerebral vascular malformation whether symptomatic or has the potential of initiating morbidity or mortality, definitive treatment modality is surgical excision. This is also valid for cavernomas as a member of cerebral vascular malformations. From surgical point of view, cavernomas, adult or pediatric, more likely resemble cerebral benign tumors rather than vascular malformations. In fact, cavernomas do not demonstrate the adverse properties of intra-axial tumors and AVM's that hamper resection. They are well circumscribed and can be differentiated from the surrounding brain parenchyma without any invasion as seen in most of the intra-axial tumors no high flow, arterial bleeding is expected within the lesion, unlike AVM's. These properties offer a rather safe and easy excision of a cavernoma compared to most of the intra-axial lesions. On the other hand, as a presumably congenital anomaly, diverse natural history along with the variable size, multiplicity and eloquent location of cavernomas complicates the decision-making process. Pediatric patients with cavernomas have additional disadvantages such as having a higher probability of having hemorrhage with a longer life span, facing detrimental effects of neurological impairments and seizures to neurocognitive and psychosocial development. Moreover, although not universally confirmed, pediatric cavernomas are reported to be larger, more aggressive at eloquent locations [22, 58, 59]. Epidemiologic studies based on autopsy findings assume that as high as 95% of cavernomas may remain asymptomatic [60, 61]. This probability supports the decision of observation in incidentally detected cavernomas especially when they are single, located supratentorially at a deep or non-eloquent area. Although several studies have reported younger age as a risk factor for hemorrhage and worse natural history, exclusively pediatric case series stated comparable hemorrhage rates with adults indicating age at time of diagnosis did not correlate with hemorrhage risk [24, 38, 51, 62]. There is enough evidence for managing conservatively an asymptomatic incidental cavernoma in a child, both for presumably low risk of hemorrhage as well as minor consequences when become symptomatic, due to non-eloquent location. Once detected, there is no clear-cut policy on how frequently and for which criteria should an asymptomatic cavernoma be followed. Annual magnetic resonance imaging is a logical option although a life-time screening for a child seems to be irrational. There are conflicting conclusions on how to manage silent growth based on radiology alone; whether location or size is predictive for further hemorrhage and symptoms. While deep hemispheric and brainstem locations are regarded as a risk factor by some, most studies have failed to confirm this in adults [38, 63–69]. Size, as well as location in terms of predicting hemorrhage is not regarded as a major risk factor in most of the studies [28, 38, 42, 66, 67]. On the other hand, cavernomas associated with developmental venous anomaly (DVA) have a higher risk of hemorrhage [22, 47, 63, 70–74]. Nevertheless, incidentally detected pediatric cavernomas with eloquent cortex or brainstem location, especially when accompanied by a DVA require a close monitoring (Fig. 12.6).

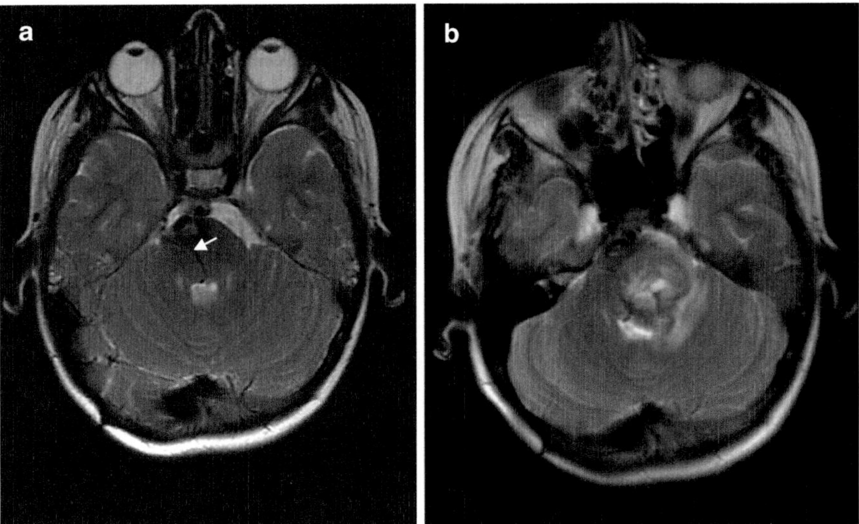

**Fig. 12.6** Six year old boy, MR imaging after temporary conjugate gaze palsy following headache revealed a pontine heterogenous lesion consistent with cavernoma supplemented by hipointense rim and adjacent linear hypointensity (arrow), representing DVA (**a**). He was decided to be followed until a second insult 4 years later at an age of 10, due to a new lesion posterior to the regressed cavernoma (**b**)

Surgery is the single best treatment option for symptomatic as well as growing asymptomatic cavernomas. Anticipated long life span of children weighed against the natural history of cavernomas early aggressive treatment is advocated [75–78]. Mode of presentation related to the location of the lesion is the most important variable dictating the timing and extent of surgical intervention. In most locations, larger the size of the lesion provides easier access through the intervening parenchyma concerning the architecture of cavernomas have detectable demarcation and less chance to bleed compared to most tumors and AVM's. On the contrary, small and deep seated cavernomas should not be recommended for surgery. Multiple lesions, especially in familial forms whether asymptomatic or with symptoms that cannot clearly be attributed to a single lesion, eloquent cortex and brainstem cavernomas, recently expanded lesions with perilesional reaction are difficult to decide to treat.

## 12.5.1  Supratentorial Cavernomas

Seizure by far is the most frequent symptom for newly diagnosed supratentorial cavernomas in adults except for those with extralesional bleeding. In children, neurological impairment due to mass effect is more frequent than adults, either alone or accompanied by seizures. Larger lesions tend to be more common as the age approaches to infancy. Lobar cavernomas with symptoms due to their size and remote to eloquent cortex can be removed without morbidity through the shortest trajectory from the non-eloquent cortex. Similarly, single lesions found incidentally with a considerable mass in children are advised to be resected as the probability of morbidity due to hemorrhage risk and further lesion growth during long life-span outweighs surgical morbidity [79]. Regardless their size, periventricular cavernomas incidentally with an exophytic component extending into the ventricle are candidates for surgery to avoid rupture into the ventricle [80–83]. Ventricular location provides safe approach without interrupting normal cortex and relatively direct access to the lesion through ventricular surface (Fig. 12.7).

Decision for surgery is complicated for lesions at the eloquent cortex and those presenting with seizures. Eloquent area cavernomas already symptomatic in children should be considered for early surgery as progressive morbidity is inevitable if left alone. Size and proximity to cortex may permit to reach the lesion through the already compromised cortex without adding further morbidity. As cavernomas have no intervening neural tissue or vasculature contributing to the surrounding, excision is less likely to increase the morbidity (Fig. 12.8). Contrarily, eliminating the mass effect is expected to counterbalance the injury of the limited cortical incision in amelioration of the symptoms. Frameless stereotaxy or intraoperative ultrasound is very helpful in determining the closest and less dangerous incision point and trajectory to reach the lesion. One exception is a deep and small lesion where reaching to the lesion requires considerable retraction. Observing for repeat hemorrhages until the size reaches to a resectable size or progressive neurological decline seems to be a more logical option.

Cavernomas manifested with seizures may be problematic for the surgical decision in children. For a cavernoma apparent with a single seizure along with mass effect surgical treatment is straightforward. In those with drug resistant epilepsy or seizure semiology that does not correspond the location of the cavernoma surgical decision and the extent of resection is not easily justified (Fig. 12.9). With

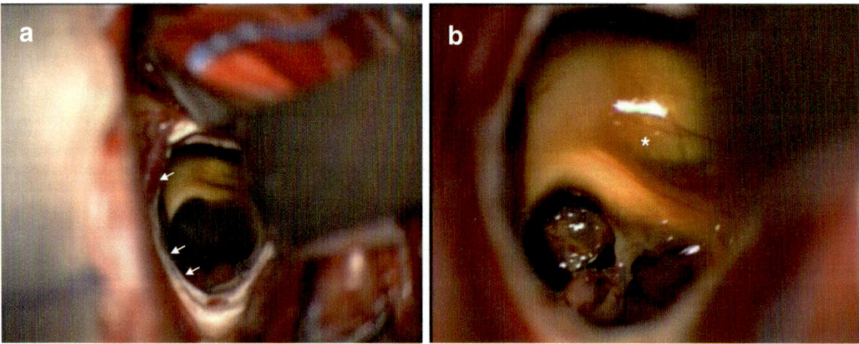

**Fig. 12.7** Intraventricular cavernoma situated in the III. ventricle; operated through anterior interhemispheric transcallosal approach where encapsulated hematoma was observed at the foramen of Monroe (**a**), excised without any neural tissue interruption except for a half centimeters of corpus callosum (**b**). Yellow hemosiderin deposits over the ependyma (asterix), incision in corpus callosum (arrows)

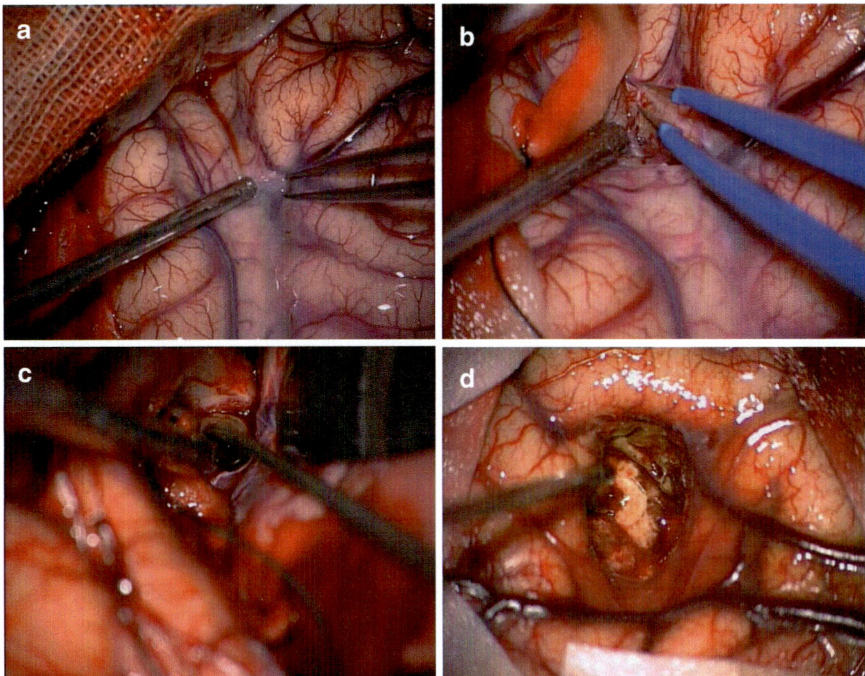

**Fig. 12.8** Right insular cavernoma in a left handed 5 year old boy disclosed due a temporary, sudden speech arrest and right hemiparesis, surgery through Sylvian dissection with the aid of navigation (**a**, **b**) cavernoma easily identified within the cortex (**c**) and excision without interrupting the neighbouring cortex hemosiderin ring (**d**)

| Cavernoma & epilepsy association | Definition |
| --- | --- |
| Definititive association | Seizure with at least 1 CM and evidence of a seizure onset zone in the immediate vicinity |
| Probable association | Seizure with at least 1 CM and with evidence that the it is focal and arises from same hemisphere as the CM |
| Unrelated | Seizure with at least 1 CM with evidence that they are not causally related |

**Fig. 12.9** Definitions for the association of epilepsy to the cavernoma proposed by Surgical Task Force of the ILAE Commission on Therapeutic Strategies (*CM: Cavernoma) (Figure adapted from Aker et al. [20] and Rosenow et al. [41])

a single seizure in the pediatric age, which is the most common most common neurological symptom at the pediatric age, it may be challenging to prove cause and effect relationship. It might be more appropriate to observe the child if electrophysiology is uninformative and the cavernoma is rather silent in terms of size and location. Those with recurrent focal seizures and seizure semiology concordant with cavernoma location, excision provides the best chance for seizure freedom. When the pathophysiological background of seizure related to cavernoma is considered, excision of the hemosiderin deposition within normal parenchyma around the lesion is argued for a better seizure control [44, 84, 85]. Particularly for lesions that are located non-eloquently and in which the usually relatively small perilesional deposits can be resected safely [44].

One other focus discussion is the resection extent in temporal lobe epilepsy related cavernomas. As far as the surgery is aimed to eliminate the seizures rather than the mass effect of the cavernoma, question is whether lesionectomy is enough to achieve seizure control. For any given lesion at the mesial temporal lobe that has been found responsible for seizures, extended mesial resections including hippocampus has been proven to be superior to lesion excision [86]. Likewise, there is enough evidence that better postoperative seizure outcome is achieved with extended resections over lesionectomy and hemosiderin rim alone in temporal lobe epilepsy [44, 87–89]. In childhood temporal lobe epilepsy syndromes, extended cortical resections including amygdala and hippocampus is argued to be superior to lesionectomy for better seizure control even if the lesion including cavernomas is located in temporal neocortex [90] (Fig. 12.10). This requires a thorough preoperative evaluation and testing to identify the epileptogenic zone in specialized epilepsy centers.

## 12.5.2 *Brainstem*

Unlike their supratentorial counterparts, significant morbidity exists with the surgical treatment of brainstem cavernomas. On the other hand, Both subsequent amount of data is present in the literature that brainstem cavernomas have a higher rate of symptomatic hemorrhage than cavernous malformations at other locations (brainstem [38, 56, 57]). Children with incidentally detected brainstem cavernomas with lesions deep to the surface or prior hemorrhagic episode and acceptable neurologic deficits should be followed conservatively. Nevertheless, once bled and become symptomatic, progressive natural history of brainstem cavernomas ultimately require surgical resection. Pediatric cavernomas are found to be larger than the adult population and become symptomatic differently from their adult counterparts with their relatively reduced intracranial volume indicating a potential for a greater mass effect [37, 38]. Therefore, it is reasonable to accept that surgery may offer a high probability of altering the natural history of the disease by preventing future hemorrhages and avoiding neurologic decline, as demonstrated on published surgical series. Experience gained from brainstem surgery from low grade lesions of the brainstem in children promotes surgical intervention whose longer life expectancy increases the driving force to seek definitive treatment. As in the supratentorial locations, larger the cavernoma, less eloquent brainstem tissue is need to traversing to reach the lesion. In respect to the location of the cavernoma within the brainstem; mesencephalic, pontine or intramedullary, one of the standard

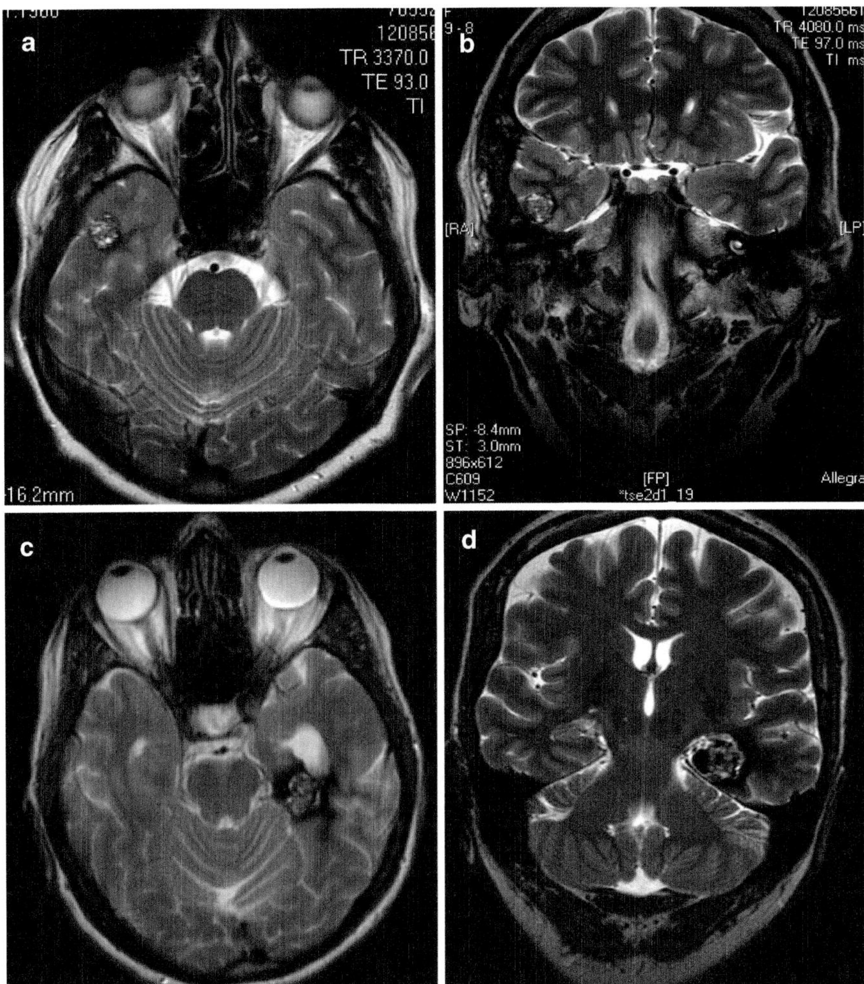

**Fig. 12.10** Drug resistant temporal lobe epilepsy cases, 8-year-old boy with cavernoma at the right inferior temporal gyrus (**a** and **b**); 12-year-old girl, cavernoma detected on the left posterior parahippocampus (**c** and **d**). Temporal lobectomy and amigdalohippocampectomy where both cavernomas are situated within the limits of standard lobectomy borders were performed in both cases

posterior fossa approaches such as midline suboccipital, retrosigmoid, supracerebellar-infratentorial can be utilized. Lesions that are exophytic or apparent by a hemosiderin-stained area at the surface can be approached through a direct route (Fig. 12.11). Those imbedded within the neural tissue require careful preoperative planning to estimate the displaced tracts and find the safest entry point with minimal destruction. Displacement by the lesion may result with unexpected morbidity when previously defined safe entry zones are used. Again, once the lesion

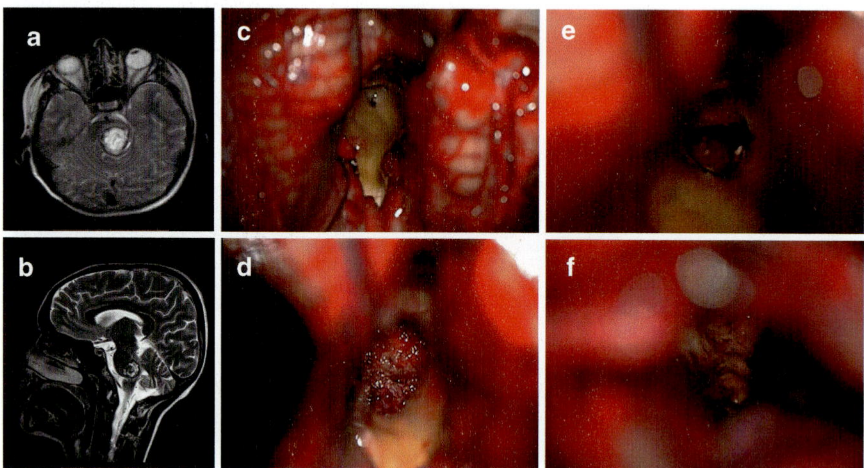

Fig. 12.11 Brain stem (medullary) cavernoma in a 11 year old boy with swallowing difficulty and conjugate gaze disturbance (**a, b**) operated through a midline posterior fossa telavolar approach; hematoma detected at the floor of the ventricle within hemosiderin staining (**c**), exposing the mass after enlarging the ruptured area of the hematoma (**d**), leaving the hemosiderin stained tissue, intact (**e** and **f**)

is reached, the morphology of the cavernoma allows safe excision with better appreciation of the normal tissue interface compared to tumors and without the risk of unexpected bleeding as in AVM's. One important point to remember in both supra- and infratentorial cavernomas is to preserve the DVA, accompanying to subsequent number cavernomas. Reader is advised to refer to the related chapters in this book for further information about microsurgical techniques as there is no difference to mention separately for pediatric cavernomas.

## 12.6  Radiosurgery for Pediatric Cavernomas

Stereotactic radiosurgery (SRS) has been used as an alternative treatment for symptomatic cavernomas in elequent areas although it is not clear whether cavernomas respond to high dose irradiation the same way as AVM's [20, 91–93]. While studies report that hemorrhage rates is expected to decrease after 2–4 years, there appears to be a temporary increase in the hemorrhage rate up to 22.4% per patient per year with temporary morbidity rates varying from 10.5 to 59% and from 1.7 to 22.7%, permanently, in adult series (pri&pre). There is ongoing debate as to whether the effects of SRS in fact merely reflect the cavernomas' natural history [20] As far as radiation exposure enhancing the genesis of new cavernoma formation in pediatric cases along with no clear information existing for SRS optimal dose to reduce hemorrhage and unknown late effects of focused radiation in children, it seems irrational to propose SRS for pediatric cavernomas.

# References


1. Leung KY, Tang MH, Lam TP, Fan YW, Shek TW, Wong KY, Ngai CS. Prenatal diagnosis of a cavernous angioma associated with intracranial hemorrhage: report of one case and review of the literature. Ultrasound Obstet Gynecol. 2004;24(7):800–3.
2. Tang AT, Choi JP, Kotzin JJ, Yang Y, Hong CC, Hobson N, Girard R, Zeineddine HA, Lightle R, Moore T, Cao Y, Shenkar R, Chen M, Mericko P, Yang J, Li L, Tanes C, Kobuley D, Võsa U, Whitehead KJ, Li DY, Franke L, Hart B, Schwaninger M, Henao-Mejia J, Morrison L, Kim H, Awad IA, Zheng X, Kahn ML. Endothelial TLR4 and the microbiome drive cerebral cavernous malformations. Nature. 2017;545(7654):305–10.
3. Tirakotai W, Fremann S, Soerensen N, Roggendorf W, Siegel AM, Mennel HD, Zhu Y, Bertalanffy H, Sure U. Biological activity of paediatric cerebral cavernomas: an immunohistochemical study of 28 patients. Childs Nerv Syst. 2006;22(7):685–91.
4. Morris Z, Whiteley WN, Longstreth WT Jr, Weber F, Lee YC, Tsushima Y, Alphs H, Ladd SC, Warlow C, Wardlaw JM, Al-Shahi Salman R. Incidental findings on brain magnetic resonance imaging: systematic review and meta-analysis. BMJ. 2009;339:b3016.
5. Kim DS, Park YG, Choi JU, Chung SS, Lee KC. An analysis of the natural history of cavernous malformations. Surg Neurol. 1997;48:9–17.
6. Moriarity J, Clatterbuck R, Rigamonti D. The natural history of cavernous malformations. Neurosurg Clin N Am. 1999;10:411–7.
7. Al-Shahi Salman R, Hall JM, Horne MA, Moultrie F, Josephson CB, Bhattacharya JJ, Counsell CE, Murray GD, Papanastassiou V, Ritchie V, Roberts RC, Sellar RJ, Warlow CP. Scottish audit of intracranial vascular malformations (SAIVMs) collaborators. Untreated clinical course of cerebral cavernous malformations: a prospective, population-based cohort study. Lancet Neurol. 2012;11:217–24.
8. Berry R, Alpers B, White J. The site, structure and frequency of intracranial aneurysms, angiomas and arteriovenous abnormalities. In: Millikan CH, editor. Research publications: Association for Research in nervous and mental disease. Baltimore: Williams and Wilkins; 1966. p. 4–72.
9. Otten P, Pizzolato G, Rilliet B, et al. 131 cases of cavernous angioma (cavernomas) of the CNS, discovered by retrospective analysis of 24,535 autopsies. Neurochirurgie. 1989;35:128–31.
10. Robinson JR, Awad IA, Neurosurg LJRJ. Natural history of the cavernous angioma. J Neurosurg. 1991;75(5):709–14.
11. Alexiou GA, Mpairamidis E, Sfakianos G, Prodromou N. Surgical management of brain cavernomas in children. Pediatr Neurosurg. 2009;45(5):375–8.
12. Rigamonti D, Hadley M, Drayer B, et al. Cerebral cavernous malformations. Incidence and familial occurrence. N Engl J Med. 1988;319:343–7.
13. Bergeson PS, Rekate HL, Tack ED. Cerebral cavernous angiomas in the newborn. Clin Pediatr (Phila). 1992;31(7):435–7.
14. Gross BA, Du R, Orbach DB, Scott RM, Smith ER. The natural history of cerebral cavernous malformations in children. J Neurosurg Pediatr. 2016;17(2):123–8.
15. Fortuna A, Ferrante L, Mastronardi L, Acqui M, d'Addetta R. Cerebral cavernous angioma in children. Childs Nerv Syst. 1989;5:201–7.
16. Aiba T, Tanaka R, Koike T, Kameyama S, Takeda N, Komata T. Natural history of intracranial cavernous malformations. J Neurosurg. 1995;83:56–9.
17. Frim DM, Scott RM. Management of cavernous malformations in the pediatric population. Neurosurg Clin N Am. 1999;10:513–8.
18. Zabramski J, Wascher T, Spetzler R, Johnson B, Golfinos J, Drayer BP, Brown B, Rigamonti D, Brown G. The natural history of familial cavernous malformations: results of an ongoing study. J Neurosurg. 1994;80:422–32.
19. Flemming KD, Brown RD Jr. Epidemiology and natural history of intracranial vascular malformations. In: Winn HR, editor. Youmans & Winn neurological surgery. 7th ed. Amsterdam: Elsevier; 2017. p. 3446–3463e7.

20. Akers A, Al-Shahi Salman RA, Awad I, et al. Synopsis of guidelines for the clinical management of cerebral cavernous malformations: consensus recommendations based on systematic literature review by the Angioma Alliance Scientific Advisory Board Clinical Experts Panel. Neurosurgery. 2017;80(5):665–80.
21. Salman RA-S, Berg M, Morrison L, et al. Hemorrhage from cavernous malformations of the brain: definition and reporting standards. Angioma Alliance Scientific Advisory Board. Stroke. 2008;39:3129–30.
22. Maraire J, Awad I. Intracranial cavernous malformations: lesion behavior and management strategies. Neurosurgery. 1995;37:591–605.
23. Bilginer B, Narin F, Hanalioglu S, Oguz KK, Soylemezoglu F, Akalan N. Cavernous malformations of the central nervous system (CNS) in children: clinico-radiological features and management outcomes of 36 cases. Childs Nerv Syst. 2014;30(8):1355–66.
24. Al-Holou WN, O'Lynnger TM, Pandey AS, Gemmete JJ, Thompson BG, Muraszko KM, Garton HJ, Maher CO. Natural history and imaging prevalence of cavernous malformations in children and young adults. J Neurosurg Pediatr. 2012;9(2):198–205.
25. Ghali MG, Srinivasan VM, Mohan AC, Jones JY, Kan PT, Lam S. Pediatric cerebral cavernous malformations: genetics, pathogenesis, and management. Surg Neurol Int. 2016;7(Suppl 44):S1127–34.
26. Raychaudhuri R, Batjer HH, Awad IA. Intracranial cavernous angioma: a practical review of clinical and biological aspects. Surg Neurol. 2005;63(4):319–28.
27. Pollock BE, Garces YI, Stafford SL, Foote RL, Schomberg PJ, Link MJ. Stereotactic radiosurgery for cavernous malformations. J Neurosurg. 2000;93:987–91.
28. Porter PJ, Willinsky RA, Harper W, Wallace MC. Cerebral cavernous malformations: natural history and prognosis after clinical deterioration with or without hemorrhage. J Neurosurg. 1997;87:190–7.
29. Del Curling O Jr, Kelly DL Jr, Elster AD, Craven TE. Ananalysis of the natural history of cavernous angiomas. J Neurosurg. 1991;75:702–8.
30. Barrow D, Krisht A. Cavernous malformations and hemorrhage. In: Awad I, Barrow D, editors. Cavernous malformations. Park Ridge: AANS; 1993. p. 65–80.
31. Ueda S, Saito A, Inomori S, et al. Cavernous angioma of the cauda equina producing subarachnoid hemorrhage. Case report. J Neurosurg. 1987;66:134–6.
32. Hubert P, Choux M, Houtteville J. Cerebral cavernomas in infants and children. Neurochirurgie. 1989;35:104–5.
33. Mazza C, Scienza R, Bernardin BD, et al. Cerebral cavernous malformations (cavernomas) in children. Neurochirurgie. 1989;35:106–8.
34. Scott R, Barnes P, Kupsky W, et al. Cavernous angiomas of the central nervous system in children. J Neurosurg. 1992;76:38–46.
35. Shirvani M, Hajimirzabeigi A. Intraventricular cavernous malformation: review of the literature and report of three cases with neuroendoscopic resection. J Neurol Surg A Cent Eur Neurosurg. 2017;78(3):269–80.
36. Li D, Hao SY, Tang J, Xiao XR, Jia GJ, Wu Z, Zhang LW, Zhang JT. Clinical course of untreated pediatric brainstem cavernous malformations: hemorrhage risk and functional recovery. J Neurosurg Pediatr. 2014;13(5):471–83.
37. Di Rocco C, Tamburrini G, Rollo M. Cerebral arteriovenous malformations in children. Acta Neurochir. 2000;142:145–56.
38. Abla AA, Lekovic GP, Garrett M, Wilson DA, Nakaji P, Bristol R, Spetzler RF. Cavernous malformations of the brainstem presenting in childhood: surgical experience in 40 patients. Neurosurgery. 2010;67(6):1589–98. discussion 1598–9.
39. Smit LM, Halbertsma FJ. Cerebral cavernous hemangiomas in childhood. Clinical presentation and therapeutic considerations. Childs Nerv Syst. 1997 Oct;13(10):522–5.
40. McCormick W. The pathology of vascular malformations. J Neurosurg. 1966;24:807–16.

41. Rosenow F, Alonso-Vanegas MA, Baumgartner C, et al. Cavernoma-related epilepsy: review and recommendations for management. Report of the Surgical Task Force of the ILAE Commission on therapeutic strategies. Epilepsia. 2013;54:2025–35.
42. Robinson J, Awad I, Little J. Natural history of the cavernous angioma. J Neurosurg. 1991;75:709–14.
43. Buckingham MJ, Crone KR, Ball WS, Berger TS. Management of cerebral cavernous angiomas in children presenting with seizures. Childs Nerv Syst. 1989;5(6):347–9.
44. Dammann P, Schaller C, Sure U. Should we resect peri-lesional hemosiderin deposits when performing lesionectomy in patients with cavernoma-related epilepsy (CRE)? Neurosurg Rev. 2017;40(1):39–43.
45. Del Curling O Jr, Kelly DL Jr, Elster AD, et al. An analysis of the natural history of cavernous angiomas. J Neurosurg. 1991;75:702–8.
46. Awad I, Jabbour P. Cerebral cavernous malformations and epilepsy. Neurosurg Focus. 2006;21(1):e7.
47. Gross BA, Lin N, Du R, et al. The natural history of intracranial cavernous malformations. Neurosurg Focus. 2011;30(6):E24.
48. Giombini S, Morello G. Cavernous angiomas of the brain. Account of fourteen personal cases and review of the literature. Acta Neurochir. 1978;40:61–82.
49. Jewell NP. Natural history of diseases: statistical designs and issues. Clin Pharmacol Ther. 2016;100(4):353–61.
50. Flemming KD. Predicting the clinical behaviour of cavernous malformations. Lancet Neurol. 2012;11:202–3.
51. Barker F, Amin-Hanjani S, Butler W, Lyons S, Ojemann RG, Chapman PH, et al. Temporal clustering of hemorrhages from untreated cavernous malformations of the central nervous system. Neurosurgery. 2001;49:15–25.
52. Mathiesen T, Edner G, Kihlstrom L. Deep and brainstem cavernomas: a consecutive 8-year series. J Neurosurg. 2003;99:31–7.
53. Wang W, Liu A, Zhang J, et al. Surgical management of brainstem cavernous malformations: report of 137 cases. Surg Neurol. 2003;59:444–4542.
54. Fritschi J, Reulen H, Spetzler R, et al. Cavernous malformations of the brain stem. A review of 139 cases. Acta Neurochir. 1994;130:35–46.
55. Kondziolka D, Monaco EA 3rd, Lunsford LD. Cavernous malformations and hemorrhage risk. Prog Neurol Surg. 2013;27:141–6.
56. Abla AA, Lekovic GP, Turner JD, de Oliveira JG, Porter R, Spetzler RF. Advances in the treatment and outcome of brainstem cavernous malformation surgery: a single-center case series of 300 surgically treated patients. Neurosurgery. 2011;68(2):403–14. discussion 414–5.
57. Garrett M, Spetzler RF. Surgical treatment of brainstem cavernous malformations. Surg Neurol. 2009;72(Suppl 2):S3–9. discussion S9–10.
58. Mottolese C, Hermier M, Stan H, Jouvet A, Saint-Pierre G, Froment JC, Bret P, Lapras C. Central nervous system cavernomas in the pediatric age group. Neurosurg Rev. 2001;24(2–3):55–71. discussion 72–3.
59. Van Lindert EJ, Tan TC, Grotenhuis JA, Wesseling P. Giant cavernous hemangiomas: report of three cases. Neurosurg Rev. 2007;30:83–92.
60. Jellinger K. Vascular malformations of the central nervous system: a morphological overview. Neurosurg Rev. 1986;9:177–216.
61. McCormick W. Pathology of vascular malformations of the brain. In: Wilson C, Stein B, editors. Intracranial arteriovenous malformations. Baltimore: Williams and Wilkins; 1984. p. 44–63.
62. Kupersmith MJ, Kalish H, Epstein F, Yu G, Berenstein A, Woo H, et al. Natural history of brainstem cavernous malformations. Neurosurgery. 2001;48:47–54.
63. Porter RW, Detwiler PW, Spetzler RF, Lawton MT, Baskin JJ, Derksen PT, et al. Cavernous malformations of the brainstem: experience with 100 patients. J Neurosurg. 1999;90:50–8.

64. Labauge P, Brunereau L, Lévy C, Laberge S, Houtteville JP. The natural history of familial cerebral cavernomas: a retrospective MRI study of 40 patients. Neuroradiology. 2000;42:327–32.

65. Cantu C, Murillo-Bonilla L, Arauz A, Higuera J, Padilla J, Barinagarrementeria F. Predictive factors for intracerebral hemorrhage in patients with cavernous angiomas. Neurol Res. 2005;27:314–8.

66. Kondziolka D, Lunsford LD, Kestle JR. The natural history of cerebral cavernous malformations. J Neurosurg. 1995;83:820–4.

67. Moriarity JL, Wetzel M, Clatterbuck RE, Javedan S, Sheppard JM, Hoenig-Rigamonti K, et al. The natural history of cavernous malformations: a prospective study of 68 patients. Neurosurgery. 1999;44:1166–73.

68. Sarwar M, McCormick WF. Intracerebral venous angioma. Case report and review. Arch Neurol. 1978;35:323–5.

69. McCormick WF. Intracerebral venous angioma. Case report and review. Arch Neurol. 1978;35:323–5.

70. Abdulrauf SI, Kaynar MY, Awad IA. A comparison of the clinical profile of cavernous malformations with and without associated venous malformations. Neurosurgery. 1999;44:41–7.

71. Cakirer S. De novo formation of a cavernous malformation of the brain in the presence of a developmental venous anomaly. Clin Radiol. 2003;58:251–6.

72. Campeau NG, Lane JI. De novo development of a lesion with the appearance of a cavernous malformation adjacent to an existing developmental venous anomaly. AJNR Am J Neuroradiol. 2005;26:156–9.

73. Detwiler PW, Porter RW, Zabramski JM, Spetzler RF. De novo formation of a central nervous system cavernous malformation: implications for predicting risk of hemorrhage. Case report and review of the literature. J Neurosurg. 1997;87:629–32.

74. Pozzati E, Acciarri N, Tognetti F, Marliani F, Giangaspero F. Growth, subsequent bleeding, and de novo appearance of cerebral cavernous angiomas. Neurosurgery. 1996;38:662–70.

75. Olivecrona H, Riives J. Arteriovenous aneurysms of the brain, their diagnosis and treatment. Arch Neurol Psychiatr. 1948;59:567–602.

76. Humphreys RP, Hoffman HJ, Drake JM, Rutka JT. Choices in the 1990s for the management of pediatric cerebral arteriovenous malformations. Pediatr Neurosurg. 1996;25:277–85.

77. LeBlanc R, Ethier R, Little JR. Computerized tomography findings in arteriovenous malformations of the brain. J Neurosurg. 1979;51:765–72.

78. Takahashi S, Sonobe M, Shirane R, Kubota Y, Kawakami H. Computer tomography of ruptured intracranial arteriovenous malformations in the acute stage. Acta Neurochir. 1982;66:87–94.

79. Ozgen B, Senocak E, Oguz KK, Soylemezoglu F, Akalan N. Radiological features of childhood giant cavernous malformations. Neuroradiology. 2011;53(4):283–9.

80. Nieto J, Hinojosa J, Muñoz MJ, Esparza J, Ricoy R. Intraventricular cavernoma in pediatric age. Childs Nerv Syst. 2003;19(1):60–2.

81. Katayama Y, Tsubokawa T, Maeda T, Yamamoto T. Surgical management of cavernous malformation of the third ventricle. J Neurosurg. 1994;80:64–72.

82. Reyns N, Assaker R, Louis E, Lejeune JP. Intraventricular cavernomas: three cases and review of the literature. Neurosurgery. 1999;44:648–53.

83. Tatagiba M, Schönmayr R, Samii M. Intraventricular cavernous angioma. A survey. Acta Neurochir. 1991;110:140–5.

84. Chusid JG, Kopeloff LM. Epileptogenic effects of pure metals implanted in motor cortex of monkeys. J Appl Physiol. 1962;17:697–700.

85. Kwon CS, Sheth SA, Walcott BP, Neal J, Eskandar EN, Ogilvy CS. Long-term seizure outcomes following resection of supratentorial cavernous malformations. Clin Neurol Neurosurg. 2013;115:2377–81.

86. Schramm J, Aliashkevich AF. Surgery for temporal mediobasal tumors: experience based on a series of 235 patients. Neurosurgery. 2008;62(6 Suppl 3):1272–82.

87. Shan YZ, Fan XT, Meng L, An Y, Xu JK, Zhao GG. Treatment and outcome of epileptogenic temporal cavernous malformations. Chin Med J. 2015;128:909–13.
88. Van Gompel JJ, Rubio J, Cascino GD, Worrell GA, Meyer FB. Electrocorticography-guided resection of temporal cavernoma: is electrocorticography warranted and does it alter the surgical approach? J Neurosurg. 2009;110:1179–85.
89. Yeon JY, Kim JS, Choi SJ, Seo DW, Hong SB, Hong SC. Supratentorial cavernous angiomas presenting with seizures: surgical outcomes in 60 consecutive patients. Seizure. 2009;18:14–20.
90. Ormond DR, Clusmann H, Sassen R, Hoppe C, Helmstaedter C, Schramm J, Grote A. Pediatric temporal lobe epilepsy surgery in Bonn and review of the literature. Neurosurgery. 2019;84(4):844–56.
91. Smith ER, Scott RM. Cavernous and venous malformations. In: Albright AL, Pollack IF, Adelson PD, editors. Principles and practice of pediatric neurosurgery. Third ed. New York: Thieme Medical Publishers; 2015. p. 858–65.
92. Gross BA, Batjer HH, Awad IA, Bendok BR, Du R. Brainstem cavernous malformations: 1390 surgical cases from the literature. World Neurosurg. 2013;80(1–2):89–93.
93. Sager O, Beyzadeoglu M, Dincoglan F, et al. Evaluation of linear accelerator (LINAC)-based stereotactic radiosurgery (SRS) for cerebral cavernous malformations: a 15-year single-center experience. Ann Saudi Med. 2014;34(1):54–8.

# Chapter 13
# Cavernomas During Pregnancy


**Nejat Akalan**


Pregnancy can cause exacerbation of an existing neurological disorder and sometimes may even be detected for the first-time during pregnancy in which it might be an incidental finding [1]. Although infrequent, cerebrovascular insult can be manifested during pregnancy and the puerperium with an incidence from 0.3 to 9 per 100,000 deliveries and 12–80% of maternal deaths are caused by cerebrovascular disorders [2–7]. The most common pathology responsible for cerebrovascular insult in pregnant women is aneurysmal subarachnoid hemorrhage followed by arteriovenous malformations (AVM) and hypertensive intracerebral hemorrhage [8]. Almost all aneurysmal hemorrhages during pregnancy are detected as the first incident while some of the AVM cases have already been diagnosed previously. Nevertheless, it is not so easy to document whether pregnancy actually exacerbates hemorrhage from the previously diagnosed or unknown pathology. Actual rarity of aneurysms and AVM's raise the question of coincidental bleeding rather than the pregnancy induction. Only available information comes from case reports and small case series and the data is controversial on whether pregnancy increases the risk for aneurysm or AVM rupture [9–14].

As a member of congenital vascular malformations, cavernomas are also to have similar increased risk for hemorrhage and aggressive behavior in pregnant woman. They have been reported to increase in size and become symptomatic during pregnancy [15–24].

Mechanism inducing hemorrhage of aneurysms and AVM's are usually attributed to physiologic changes during certain periods of pregnancy, especially at the second and third trimesters which are associated with the increase in cardiac output. This may not be case for cavernomas, as they have no high-flow characteristics within the tissue, Endocrinological mechanisms in women and during pregancy to


N. Akalan (✉)
Department of Neurosurgery, Medipol University School of Medicine, Istanbul, Turkey
e-mail: nejata@tr.net



© Springer Nature Switzerland AG 2020
O. Bradáč, V. Beneš (eds.), *Cavernomas of the CNS*,
https://doi.org/10.1007/978-3-030-49406-3_13

explain the tendency to bleed have not been elucidated although menstrual and reproductive characteristics of the patient are believed to play a role in the risk for aneurysmal rupture [25–27]. Hormonal stimulation has also been proposed for the pathogenesis of increased risk of hemorrhage in cavernomas [16, 28, 29]. Hormonal mechanisms and angiogenic factors inducing pregnancy-related vasculogenesis have been also suspected to promote growth, thrombosis, and hemorrhage of vascular lesions [30]. This has raised the discussion whether female gender may be associated with an increased risk for hemorrhage. Several studies found a female preponderance in patients with symptomatic hemorrhage, particularly in those with brainstem and spinal cord lesions, with female-to-male ratios as high as 1.6: 1 and 2.3: 1, respectively [31]. Nevertheless, there are also series where male predominance is suggested, however, the ratios are reversed and males predominate by similar ratios [32, 33]. In more recent series the risk for clinical symptoms and hemorrhage for cavernomas are no different in pregnancy than the nonpregnant state [34–36]. Flemming et al. [34] out of 117 pregnant women harboring cavernomas, none had symptoms during pregnancy.

In the review of University of Toronto Vascular Malformation Study Group on 186 women with cerebral cavernous malformations with 349 pregnancies and 283 live births, there were 49 hemorrhages during childbearing years, only 3 of which were during pregnancy. When the number of clinically significant hemorrhages divided by the time in the pregnant state with the number of hemorrhages during the nonpregnant state between the ages of 15 and 44 years, hemorrhage rate for pregnant women was 1.15% per person-year compared with 1.01% per person-year for nonpregnant women [36].

At the prospective study on female patients at the Barrow Neurological Institute 28 sporadic and 36 familial cases with 168 pregnancies were identified. Out of 64 cases, 5 cases had symptomatic hemorrhage. Most common symptom was seizure, identified in 4 cases. The overall risk of symptomatic hemorrhage for pregnant women in the sporadic group was 2% per person-year and 4% per person-year in the familial group, which is within the range for the general cavernoma population [35].

Currently, there is no quantitative data for counselling cavernoma bearing pregnancies nor an individualized treatment protocol in case of symptomatic hemorrhage during pregnancy. Management of symptomatic hemorrhage from cavernous malformations during pregnancy should be the same with any cavernoma case with similar symptomatology and imaging characteristics unless maternal and fetal life is endangered. If hemorrhage and associated symptoms otherwise suitable for observation in an usual case have a threat to mothers' life surgery should be undertaken.

# References


1. Haider B, Oertzen JV. Neurological disorders. Best Pract Res Clin Obstet Gynaecol. 2003;27:867–75.
2. Sachs BP, Brown DA, Driscoll SG, et al. Maternal mortality in Massachusetts. Trends and prevention. N Engl J Med. 1987;316:667–72.

3. Sharshar T, Lamy C, Mas JL. Incidence and causes of strokes associated with pregnancy and puerperium. A study in public hospitals of Ile de France. Stroke in pregnancy study group. Stroke. 1995;26:930–6.
4. Guyer B, Strobino DM, Ventura SJ, et al. Annual summary of vital statistics—1994. Pediatrics. 1995;96:1029–39.
5. Wiebers DO, Whisnant JP. The incidence of stroke among pregnant women in Rochester, Minn, 1955 through 1979. JAMA. 1985;254:3055–7.
6. Gibbs CE. Maternal death due to stroke. Am J Obstet Gynecol. 1974;119:69–75.
7. Sawin P. Spontaneous subarachnoid hemorrhage in pregnancy and the puerperium. Neurosurg Aspects Pregnancy. 1996:85–99.
8. Roark CD, Thompson BG Jr. Pregnancy and the vascular lesion. In: Richard Winn H, editor. Youmans & Winn neurological surgery. 7th ed. Amsterdam: Elsevier; 2017. p. 3607–3610 e2.
9. Fox MW, Harms RW, Davis DH. Selected neurologic complications of pregnancy. Mayo Clin Proc. 1990;65:1595–618.
10. Del Zotto E, Giossi A, Volonghi I, et al. Ischemic stroke during pregnancy and puerperium. Stroke Res Treat. 2011;2011:606–780.
11. Tiel Groenestege AT, Rinkel GJE, van der Bom JG, et al. The risk of aneurysmal subarachnoid hemorrhage during pregnancy, delivery, and the puerperium in the Utrecht population: case-crossover study and standardized incidence ratio estimation. Stroke. 2009;40:1148–51.
12. Mas JL, Lamy C. Stroke in pregnancy and the puerperium. J Neurol. 1998;245:305–13.
13. Kim YW, Neal D, Hoh BL. Cerebral aneurysms in pregnancy and delivery: pregnancy and delivery do not increase the risk of aneurysm rupture. Neurosurgery. 2013;72:143–9.
14. Robinson JL, Hall CJ, Sedzimir CB. Subarachnoid hemorrhage in pregnancy. J Neurosurg. 1972;36:27–33.
15. Zabramski JM, Kalani YS. Natural history of cavernous malformations. In: Richard Winn H, editor. Youmans & Winn neurological surgery. 7th ed. Amsterdam: Elsevier; 2017. p. 3537–3546 e2.
16. Robinson JR, Awad IA, Little JR. Natural history of the cavernous angioma. J Neurosurg. 1991;75:709–14.
17. Porter RW, Detwiler PW, Spetzler RF, et al. Cavernous malformations of the brainstem: experience with 100 patients. J Neurosurg. 1999;90:50–8.
18. Pozzati E, Acciarri N, Tognetti F, et al. Growth, subsequent bleeding, and de novo appearance of cerebral cavernous angiomas. Neurosurgery. 1996;38:662–669, discussion 669–670.
19. Katayama Y, Tsubokawa T, Maeda T, et al. Surgical management of cavernous malformations of the third ventricle. J Neurosurg. 1994;80:64–72.
20. Yamasaki T, Handa H, Yamashita J, et al. Intracranial and orbital cavernous angiomas. A review of 30 cases. J Neurosurg. 1986;64:197–208.
21. Awada A, Watson T, Obeid T. Cavernous angioma presenting as pregnancy-related seizures. Epilepsia. 1997;38:844–6.
22. Lopate G, Black JT, Grubb RL Jr. Cavernous hemangioma of the spinal cord: report of 2 unusual cases. Neurology. 1990;40:1791–3.
23. Aiba T, Tanaka R, Koike T, Kameyama S, Takeda N, Komat T. Natural history of intracranial cavernous malformations. J Neurosurg. 1995;83:56–9.
24. Yamasaki T, Handa H, Yamashita J, Paine JT, Tashiro Y, Uno A, Ishikawa M, Asato R. Intracranial and orbital cavernous angiomas. A review of 30 cases. J Neurosurg. 1986;64:197–208.
25. Mosiewicz A, Jakiel G, Janusz W, et al. Treatment of intracranial aneurysms during pregnancy. Ginekol Pol. 2001;72:86–92.
26. Robinson JL, Hall CS, Sedzimir CB. Arteriovenous malformations, aneurysms, and pregnancy. J Neurosurg. 1974;41:63–70.
27. Okamoto K, Horisawa R, Kawamura T, et al. Menstrual and repro¬ductive factors for subarachnoid hemorrhage risk in women: a case-control study in Nagoya, Japan. Stroke. 2001;32:2841–4.
28. Porter RW, Detwiler PW, Spetzler RF, Lawton MT, Baskin JJ, Derksen PT, et al. Cavernous malformations of the brainstem: experience with 100 patients. J Neurosurg. 1999;90:50–8.
29. Pozzati E, Acciarri N, Tognetti F, Marliani F, Giangaspero F. Growth, subsequent bleeding, and de novo appearance of cerebral cavernous angiomas. Neurosurgery. 1996;38:662–70.

30. Safavi-Abbasi S, Feiz-Erfan I, Spetzler RF, Kim L, Dogan S, Porter RW, Sonntag VK. Hemorrhage of cavernous malformations during pregnancy and in the peripartum period: causal or coincidence? Case report and review of the literature. Neurosurg Focus. 2006;21(1):e12.
31. Al-Shahi R, Bhattacharya JJ, Currie DG, et al. Prospective, population-based detection of intracranial vascular malformations in adults: the Scottish intracranial vascular malformation study (SIVMS). Stroke. 2003;34:1163–9.
32. Kondziolka D, Nixon B, Lasjaunias P, et al. Cerebral arteriovenous malformations and associated arterial aneuryms: hemodynamic and therapeutic considerations. Can J Neurol Sci. 1988;15:130–4.
33. Troupp H, Marttila I, Halonen V. Arteriovenous malformations of the brain. Prognosis without operation. Acta Neurochir. 1970;22:125–8.
34. Flemming K, Link M, Christianson T, et al. The prospective hemorrhage risk of intracerebral cavernous malformations. Neurology. 2012;78:632–6.
35. Kalani MY, Zabramski JM. Risk for symptomatic hemorrhage of cerebral cavernous malformations during pregnancy. J Neurosurg. 2013;118:50–5.
36. Witiw CD, Abou-Hamden A, Kulkarni AV, et al. Cerebral cavernous malformations and pregnancy: hemorrhage risk and influence on obstetrical management. Neurosurgery. 2012;71:626–630, discussion 631.

# Chapter 14
# Spinal Cavernous Malformations


Norbert Svoboda, Vladimír Beneš, and Ondřej Bradáč


## 14.1  Intramedullary Spinal Cavernous Malformation

### 14.1.1  Introduction

Historically, the first account of intramedullary cavernoma (IC) was published in 1903 by Hadlich [1] as an autopsy finding, and 9 years later Schultze [2] performed the first gross total resection of IC. ICs were thought to be extremely rare because, until the introduction of magnetic resonance (MR) in 1985, only 19 cases had been reported. Nowadays the incidence is reported to be higher. However, ICs are still far less frequent than brain cavernomas (BCs). ICs account for 3–5% [3] of all CNS lesions and 5–12% of all spinal vascular tumors [4–6]. Although ICs have identical histological features to BCs, the natural history and surgical approach is different. As ICs are specifically located in highly eloquent tissue of the spinal cord, they pose a great threat to the proper function of the cord. Even a small change in diameter of the lesion in the spinal cord can lead to severe impairment of neurologic functions. This resembles the character of brainstem cavernomas, however, the risk of rebleeding of ICs is significantly lower. Patients with ICs have generally worse clinical outcomes than those with brainstem cavernomas [7, 8]. Surgical resection remains the only curative treatment option, and issues surrouding the correct timing of surgery are still a matter of discussion, particularly in patients presenting only with pain.


N. Svoboda · V. Beneš · O. Bradáč (✉)

Department of Neurosurgery and Neurooncology, First Medical Faculty, Military University Hospital and Charles University, Prague, Czech Republic

e-mail: ondrej.bradac@uvn.cz



© Springer Nature Switzerland AG 2020

O. Bradáč, V. Beneš (eds.), *Cavernomas of the CNS*,

https://doi.org/10.1007/978-3-030-49406-3_14

### 14.1.2 Epidemiology, Histology, and Localization

ICs are found in 1.86 per 100,000 population [9]. The average age at presentation is around 40 years [4, 10], ranging from 2 to 80 years [3, 4, 6, 10–22]. Previously suggested female predominance [23, 24] has not been confirmed in later publications. The proposed male to female ratio is currently counted as 1.1/1 [10]. Patients with IC have an increased risk for multiple cavernous malformations [25–27]. Coexistent brain cavernoma is found in up to 40% [28, 29] and 10–15% have a positive family history of IC [4, 9, 10, 27, 30–32]. Nevertheless, the proportion of familial occurrence of ICs is likely to be higher than this, as these studies based their results on the presence of diagnosed ICs in the family. This means they may have overlooked asymptomatic undiagnosed lesions. As many as 40% of patients with multiple neuraxis cavernoma have a sporadic non-familiar form of multifocal IC [29]. Inheritance of the familiar form follows an autosomal-dominant pattern. Rarely, IC may be diagnosed in patients with systemic cavernous malformations such as Klippel-Trenaunay-Weber syndrome [33] or Cobb syndrome [34].

The gross appearance of IC does not differ from that of brain cavernoma. IC is a well-demarcated, lobulated, soft, and bluish or reddish-brown mulberry-shaped vascular lesion without intervening spinal tissue [35]. From the hemodynamic point of view, ICs are low blood flow and low-pressure lesions. The surrounding glial tissue stained by hemosiderin deposits have a yellowish discoloration and rubbery character, which is used as guidance during surgical dissection. The size of ICs range from millimeters to centimeters, on average reaching 9.2 mm [10]. Most frequently ICs are located superficially and posteriorly. In such cases, the location of ICs can be identified due to a typical blueish discoloration seen macroscopically on the cord surface. The change of color is not present in the case of deep-seated or small ICs. Calcification or focal ossification is rare [36]. Naim-Ur-Rahman et al. [37] reported an atypical IC with a heavily ossified shell, and bone formations invading surrounding tissue that made safe total resection impossible. Intramedullary cavernous malformations are most commonly located in thoracic (57%), less in the cervical (38%), and most infrequently in the lumbar (5%) spinal cord [10].

### 14.1.3 Clinical Presentation

The manifestation of ICs is highly variable and non-specific. In some cases, the clinical course may be misleading, and the correct diagnosis is clarified when the MRI is done. On account of the non-specific symptomatology, the median duration of symptoms is relatively long-lasting, typically for 29 months [10] preceding the final diagnosis. Most patients suffer from sensory and motor deficits. These deficits affect about two-thirds of individuals with IC. ICs may manifest by variable sensory deficits such as radicular and central pain [40], hyperaesthesia or dysesthesia [41], paresthesia [41] (even episodic [42]), thermosensory deficit [37], allodynia [43], central neuropathic itch [35] and rarely by hypothermia of extremities [44]. Motor deficit usually develops below the level of IC, nevertheless, curious ascending flaccid paraplegia over several weeks has been also reported [45]. Autonomic disorders are seen less frequently, occurring in approximately one-third of patients [10]. Interestingly, Liang et al. [17] diagnosed sphincter dysfunction in 68 patients (71%) out of their 96 patients with IC. A relatively large retrospective meta-analysis of 632 patients by Badhiwala et al. [10] showed that only the minority of patients have no symptoms (1%) or present with respiratory distress (0.5%) [10].

The variable clinical course follows three different patterns—acute, stepwise, and slow progressive neurological deterioration. It is supposed that acute neurological decline is caused by bleeding into the cord parenchyma or into the wall of the cavernoma itself. Patients with acute intramedullary hemorrhage present with sudden onset with a rapid decline over hours even days. The annual rate of hemorrhage broadly varies from 1.4 to 6.8% [3, 6, 8, 14, 16, 18, 24, 41, 42, 46, 47]. This wide range is on account of a different definition of bleeding in published studies. Some defined bleeding as acute neurological deterioration, others characterized the hemorrhage on radiological evidence. According to a recent study [42], symptomatic patients and those having experienced acute hemorrhage have a higher annual hemorrhage rate (9.5% and 9.7% respectively). On the other hand, asymptomatic patients have a considerably lower annual hemorrhage rate (0.8%). Even though there is similar eloquence to brain stem cavernomas, where only a subtle hemorrhage may lead to significant neurological decline, the annual rate is noticeably lower (brain stem cavernoma rebleeding reaches 5–75% per patient-year) [48–51]. The exact pathophysiological mechanism responsible for the difference in annual hemorrhage rate among supratentorial, infratentorial, and spinal cavernomas is unknown. As ICs lack association with developmental venous anomalies, the structural or venous drainage variations are supposed to prevent re-hemorrhage in ICs [43]. The next possible pathophysiological mechanism of acute neurological worsening is thrombosis of hyalinized vascular channels [36]. Rarely, IC is associated with subarachnoid hemorrhage presenting with prominent lower or upper back pain [52, 53].

Relatively frequently, patients present with discrete episodes of neurologic deterioration with varying degrees of recovery between episodes [36]. Based on histological findings, it has been suggested that repetitive hemorrhage or thrombosis within ICs are responsible for gradual enlargement leading to stepwise deterioration. These episodes repeat over months or even years. Alarmingly, such a clinical course may resemble that of multiple sclerosis or transverse myelitis.

At last, there is the course of slow progressive neurological decline without improvement. This is supposed to be due to the hyalinization and thickening of vascular walls, or gradual thrombosis [36]. McCormick et al. [5] proposed that neurotoxicity of hemosiderin deposits and compromised surrounding microcirculation may be another pathophysiological mechanism responsible for this course. Importantly, slow progressive neurological deterioration caused by IC may be mistaken for chronic progressive radiculomyelopathy or Foix-Alajouanine syndrome [54].

**Table 14.1** Modified from McCormick et al. [76]

| I | Intact neurologically, normal ambulation, minimal dysesthesia |
|---|---|
| II | Mild motor or sensory deficit, functional independence |
| III | Moderate deficit, limitation of function, independent with external aid |
| IV | Severe motor or sensory deficit, limited function, dependent |
| V | Paraplegia or quadriplegia, eve with flickering movement |

Acute and stepwise neurological decline was tracked in 45%, and slow progressive in 55% of patients [10]. It has been reported that the onset of symptoms may be associated with minor trauma, strenuous activity or pregnancy [5]. A modified McCormick scale is usually used for objective pre- and post-operative scoring of patient's clinical status (Table 14.1, [55]).

### 14.1.4 Imaging Techniques

Hemorrhage, widening of the spine and rarely calcification can be nonspecifically appreciated on computed tomography (CT) scans. Due to its low blood flow feature, ICs are usually occult with digital subtraction angiography. MRI remains the gold standard imaging modality. ICs have mixed signal intensity on T1- and T2-weighted images. T1-weighted images usually demonstrate a isointense to hyperintense lobulated lesion a hypointense rim. On T2-weighted images, a pathognomonic appearance of "popcorn ball" with complete hypointense hemosiderin rim may often be appreciated [56, 57] (Fig. 14.1). Rarely, ICs may present with a homogenous hyper or hypointense appearance [57]. When compared to brain cavernomas, calcification is less frequent in ICs [4]. The differential diagnosis contains the full range of intramedullary tumors, and in peculiar cases, distinguishing it from the demyelinating lesions of multiple sclerosis may be challenging. MR has an irreplaceable position in preoperative planning. As there is a high risk of multiplicity, some authors recommend completing MR imaging of the whole neuraxis. Others believe that there is no need for diagnosing asymptomatic ICs as there is, after all, no justification for any intervention of such a lesion [58].

### 14.1.5 Surgery

Currently, surgical removal of IC remains the only curative treatment option. Meticulous presurgical planning is essential to achieve the best possible result. As there are multiple surgical approaches available, the spinal cord surgeon should pick out the most appropriate one in advance of the surgery. ICs may be located superficially or deep-seated; anteriorly, laterally, or posteriorly. Notwithstanding the variety of approaches to the spinal cord, the posterior approach (PA) is the most frequently elected. It is of great advantage that the posterior approach provides

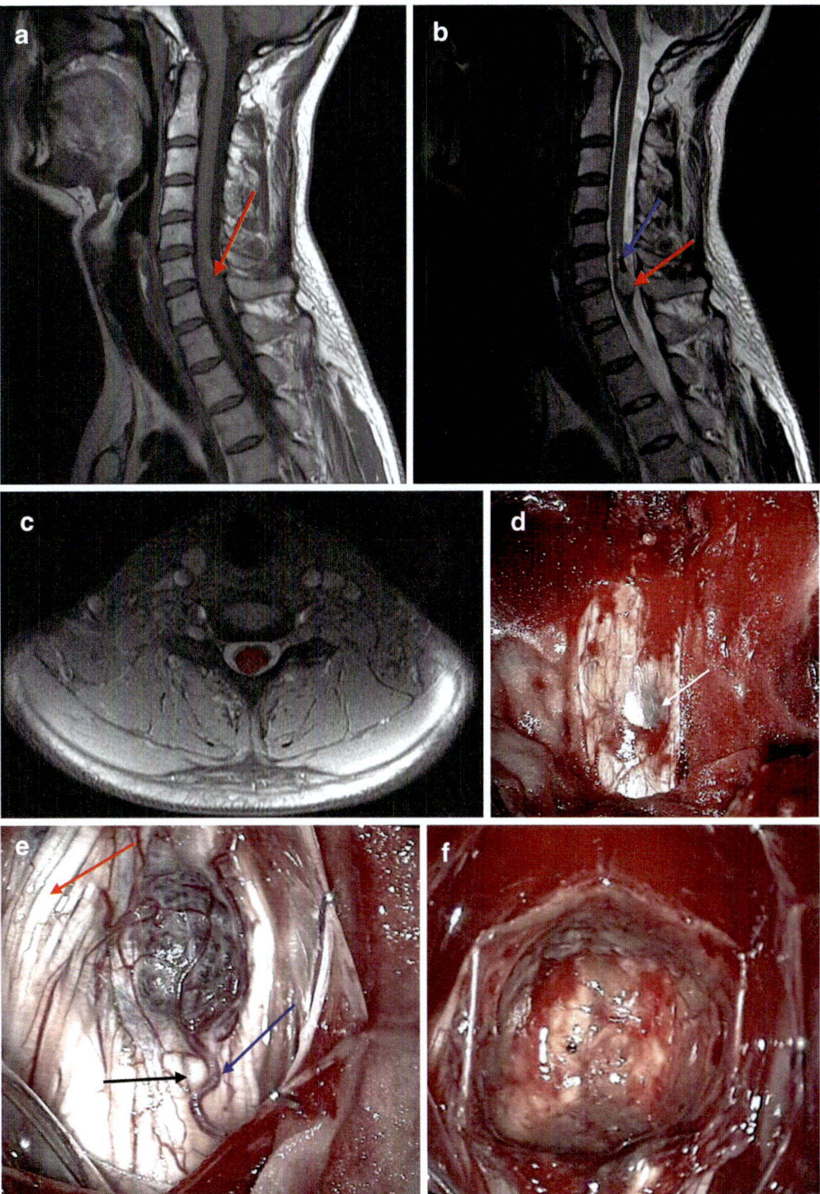

**Fig. 14.1** Cervical intramedullary cavernoma: (**a**) T1-weighted sagittal, (**b**) T2-weighted sagittal, and (**c**) Multiple Echo Recombined Gradient Echo (MERGE) axial images show intramedullary cavernoma (red arrows, reddish area). On T2-weighted image is visible hemosiderin cap sign (blue arrow). (**d, e, f**) Surgical images. (**d**) Bluish discoloration and bulging of the dura (white arrow). (**e**) Spinal Cord with Intramedullary Cavernoma: posterior spinal vein (blue arrows), posterior median sulcus (black arrow), C6 posterior nerve root (red arrow). (**f**) The cavity after total IC removal. (**g**) T1-weighted sagittal, (**h**) T2-weighted sagittal, (**i**) T2 Fast Relaxation Fast Spin Echo (FRFSE) axial postoperative image without remnant of the tumor. (**j**) Micrograph showing hyalinized blood vessels lined with single layer of endothelium (hematoxylin and eosin stain, magnification × 100)

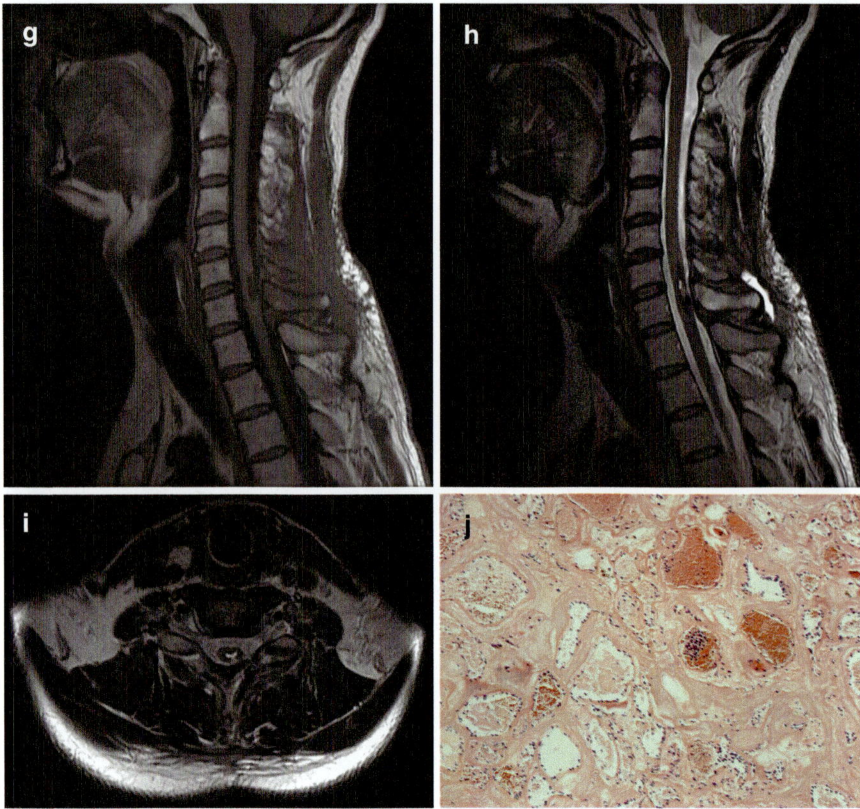

**Fig. 14.1** (continued)

extensive exposure of the spinal cord, it is relatively safe, and furthermore, it is an approach which all neurosurgeons are familiar with. Nevertheless, PA cannot be used for every IC. Especially in the case of ventrally or ventrolaterally located IC, the posterior approach would lead to extensive myelotomy or stretch of the spinal cord while rotated. In such cases, other surgical routes should be also considered: An anterior [59–61], anterolateral [62], transthoracic [63, 64], or posterolateral approach [65, 66]. These approaches are technically advanced, providing a decreased exposure of the operating field which is limiting during all stages of the procedure including watertight suture of the dura.

As mentioned above, the spinal cord is highly eloquent tissue similar to that of the brain stem. Based on this anatomical fact the use of a two-point method [67] is advocated to find the safest entry point. The two-point method is using a line drawn on an axial MRI scan connecting the center of IC with the most superficial part of the IC in regard to the pial surface or the non-eloquent entry zone. There are three recommended non-eloquent entry zones in the spinal cord—dorsal root entry zone (DREZ), dorsal median sulcus, and lateral. The lateral entry zone is located between the ventral and dorsal nerve roots [68]. Since there is a ballooning effect due to hemosiderin deposits, T2 weighted images tend to overstate the real lesion, and therefore the T1 weighted sequence is more appropriate for estimation of the relation between ICs and pial surface.

For the majority of ICs a posterior approach the most suitable [69]. There are three possibilities for bone removal—laminectomy, laminoplasty, and hemilaminectomy. Several authors have reported progressive spinal deformity following laminectomy and laminoplasty [10, 70, 71]. Nonetheless, it is our belief that thoroughly fixed laminoplasty is well functioning over a long period provided there is desired wide exposure. Dura is incised using the dural hook with scalpel No 11 and micro-scissors in a linear fashion. Dural leaflets are retracted and attached by several 4-0 stitches to surrounding soft tissue. Similarly, the arachnoid is incised by fixing the leaflets to the dura by Wecks clips. In the next step, the pial surface is inspected using high magnification on the microscope to find the typical reddish-brown or bluish discoloration that identifies a superficially located IC. Such ICs should be accessed directly by cutting overlaying pia. If IC is deep-seated, a midline myelotomy should be performed. In that case, the surgeon must identify the posterior median sulcus (PMS). As anatomical circumstances inside the spinal canal can be changed due to the growth of IC, PMS is often moved aside. There are three useful hints which may help to identify PMS. At first, the posterior spinal vein (PSV) is running over the PMS. PSV should be mobilized and moved away from the midline preserving its trunk. Small incoming branches can be sacrificed if necessary to gain sufficient mobilization. Secondly, if PSV is not visible, the PSV can be localized by a mesothelial septum (MS). MS is a thin fibrous vertical layer in the PMS in which converge small pial vessels from both sides. Finally, the PMS is located in between both posterior spinal arteries. Still, identifying the PMS is in many cases challenging, as pial veins and PSAs are displaced and curved due to the underlying IC. When PMS identified, it is entered using bipolar forceps or the micro-bayonets until the surface of the IC is noticed. The surgeon should be extremely careful when entering PMS as inappropriate movements and cauterization may harm posterior sulcal branches supplying dorsal columns. Electrophysiological monitoring should be routinely available while manipulating the spinal cord. IC should be removed en bloc. The dissection plane between IC and spinal cord is followed leaving periphery gliotic tissue left in place. Debulking and using CUSA is generally not recommended unless handling a large cavernoma which needs to be reduced for safe removal. After resection and meticulous cauterization, the cord is approximated with 6-0 running pial suture. Watertight suture of dura is done as a matter of course.

Still, there are cases when the posterior approach is insufficient. In the case of laterally and anterolaterally located ICs, the surgeon may require adjustment of exposure. This can be gained by the removal of lateral bony structures by means of drilling pedicle and facet joins (posterolateral approach). Additionally, the exposure to the ventral surface could be achieved by gentle traction from 6-0 sutures on dentate ligaments, providing dorsal rotation of the spinal cord. Based on our experience the posterior and posterolateral approaches were sufficient for gross total resection of patients with ICs treated in our department from the year 1998. It should be emphasized that the posterolateral approach is notably more challenging and should be performed by experienced hands.

### *14.1.6 Outcome*

According to current knowledge, the final postoperative outcome is dependent on pre-hospital symptoms and preoperative clinical status, MR findings, and the chosen therapeutic option. It is claimed that the length of symptoms is an important factor predicting postsurgical recovery. Patients having symptoms of less than 3 months were found to have better postsurgical outcomes [10, 12, 24, 42]. Zevgaridis et al. [24] reported improvement in 76% of patients with symptom duration less than 3 years and only in 52% of patients with longer-lasting symptomatology. Similarly, patients with acute or stepwise clinical course are prone to benefit more significantly from surgery when compared to those with progressive neurological decline [10]. It is general agreement that patients with motor deficits have the highest possibility of postsurgical improvement reaching up to 86% [4, 10, 15, 41–43, 72]. Interestingly, several studies pointed out that sensory deficit, pain (radicular or central), and bladder dysfunction often do not favor a full recovery following the surgery. It has been repeatedly claimed that those presenting with a purely sensory deficit are associated with a slower and less complete recovery [4, 10, 41, 45, 48]. Park et al. [41] performed total removal of IC in 14 patients, and reported that only 7% of patients with preoperative sensory deficit recovered completely by the final post-operative follow up (compared to a 46% rate of complete recovery in a group of patients with the preoperative motor deficit). Currently, there are ambiguous data regarding relief of pain following the surgery. Kharkar et al. [16] operated on four patients with both pain and weakness. They detected complete pain resolution in one patient only, the others had limited or no improvement. In a series of 23 patients presenting with pain by Kim et al., 78% had improvement of pain immediately following the surgery, but only 52% reported pain relief lasting over a year. On the contrary, Deutsch et al. [13] surgically treated five patients with predominant complaints about pain. According to their results, all patients had some degree of pain resolution. Kivelev et al. [43] reported a 90% rate of radicular pain relief after surgical removal. Only one patient (10%) developed permanent painful allodynia in her hand. Data about the recovery of bladder function are scarce and heterogeneous. Several studies have reported improvement of sphincter function following surgery [10, 38, 39, 49–51, 73]. On the other hand, Kivelev et al. [43] reported no significant improvement of bladder dysfunction in any of five patients undergoing IC resection. As previously mentioned, asymptomatic patients are diagnosed rarely (1%), and data about their natural course are limited. Goyal et al. [42] treated 22 asymptomatic patients, and calculated the annual risk for haemorrhage to be 0.8%. Nowadays, watchful follow-up is the standard proposed course of action for asymptomatic patients [3, 10, 17, 20, 42, 74, 75], and some authors recommend operating on asymptomatic patients with proven growth in time [20].

The importance of two MRI quantities is discussed—depth and size. Deep-seated ICs have been thought to have a worse outcome [31]. However this finding was not confirmed in a pooled analysis by Badhiwala et al. [10], in which there was no correlation between the favorable outcome of patients with superficial versus deep-seated ICs. Goyal et al. reported a worse outcome in patients with IC >1 cm.

They supposed that this phenomenon is due to the disequilibrium between the extension of spinal cord dissection in order to resect small lesions. Interestingly, no significant difference between resection of IC smaller and bigger than 1 cm was not found in a recent meta-analysis [4, 10].

Surgery is generally accepted as the primary treatment option [3–5, 10, 18, 28, 29, 47, 66, 69, 75–78] and still the only curative treatment. Gross-total resection is the most important factor in eliminating the risk of a new haemorrhage in the future, Table 14.2. It is achieved in 94% [10]. The transient worsening of patients immediately following the surgery is seen in 24–50% [4, 10, 15, 22, 55] and the majority resolves during the first 3 months. Long-term clinical worsening is seen in about 12% of patients after IC removal [4, 10, 15, 22, 55]. Only a minority of published studies have reported results of patients with IC treated conservatively [16, 17, 24, 31, 42, 43, 57, 72, 77, 79], and their conclusions are biased by the selectivity of patients. Kharkar et al. presented the results of 10 symptomatic patients approached conservatively. They did not notice any deterioration during the mean follow-up of 80 months. Goyal et al. observed 64 patients with IC. They reported that 48 patients (75%) did not experience a new hemorrhage during follow-up (total 336.6 person-years). It is important to emphasize that 19 patients (36%) were asymptomatic.

**Table 14.2** Outcomes of patients with ICs according to results of the meta-analysis by Badhiwala et al

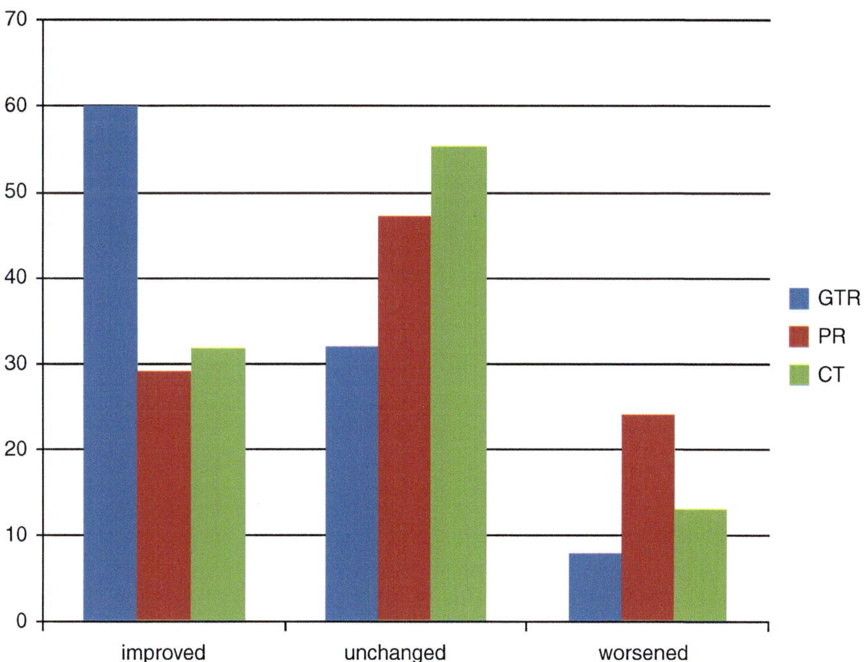


*CT* conservative treatment, *GTR* gross total resection, *PR* partial resection

### 14.1.7 Our Results and Policy

#### 14.1.7.1 Methods

The data of patients undergoing resection of ICs from 1998 to 2019 were analyzed retrospectively. A total of 26 consecutive patients were included. The localization and the volume of ICs were evaluated on MRI scans. The clinical deficits were categorized as sensory, motor and bladder/bowel dysfunction. The clinical course was divided into three patterns: acute, stepwise and slow progressive. Hemorrhage was defined as acute clinical deterioration. Patients were scored using a modified McCormick scale. The patient's status was evaluated preoperatively and 2 years postoperatively, or at the last follow-up in patients who had undergone surgery after the year 2017.

#### 14.1.7.2 Results

65 surgical removals of intramedullary tumors have been performed from 1998 to 2019 in our department. 26 (16%) of these were ICs. The male-female ratio was 18:8 with the median age of 45 years. The majority of ICs were located in the thoracic region (62%), followed by cervical (38%) spinal cord. The mean volume of IC accounted for 0.7 ml (0.1–6 ml). Coexistent cavernoma of the central nervous system was diagnosed in 35% and hereditary mutation of gene CCM1 was detected in one patient (4%) with positive familiar history. The most common neurological deficits were sensory (73%), followed by a motor (69%) and less commonly bladder/bowel dysfunction (35%). Most frequently patients presented with acute (46%), fewer with slow progressive (35%), and least frequently with stepwise neurological decline (19%). One patient with the stepwise neurological decline was misdiagnosed for multiple sclerosis (MS). He was treated for MS for long as 20 years until a diagnostic MRI scan of the thoracic spine was done. The calculated annual risk of hemorrhage reached 2.5%. Gross total resection was achieved in all patients. Although CSF wound leakage occurred in six patients, good wound healing was restored following surgical reoperation in all cases. In long-term follow-up 42% improved (11 patients), 46% remained stable (12 patients), and 12% (3 patients) deteriorated compared to their presurgical neurological status. However, only one patient suffered from progression of motor weakness.

#### 14.1.7.3 Our Recommendation

We feel there is a need for active surgical treatment in patients who suffer from IC. The resection of IC is a relatively safe procedure in skilled hands, as shown not only by our results. This is especially in force for patients with symptomatic

ICs when the removal may lead to clinical improvement. It is important to mention that only one of the deteriorated patients in our group experienced a motor decline. This patient was admitted in poor condition of grade III on McCormick scale. Two others worsened in sensory functions by one grade. Both developed new abnormal dermal sensation, which was treated with pregabalin. We believe that the benefit of eliminating the potential risk of severe disability of symptomatic ICs significantly overweights the potential risk of the surgery. It is important to note that none of the patients who presented only with pain worsened in long-term follow-up. In our eyes, the surgical approach is justified as it is a curative option, eliminating the risk of a new hemorrhage. Regarding asymptomatic patients, we believe that the decision of the surgeon should be based on the patient's age, clinical status, and MR finding. Surgery should be considered primarily in young patients in whom the risk of future haemorrhage is more probable. We would consider surgical removal of asymptomatic IC with proven growth, or if its size exceeds 1 cm. We assume it is very likely that such an IC has already repeatedly bled, increasing the risk of a new haemorrhage. A new haemorrhage of an IC larger than 1 cm would very likely lead to severe impairment of neurological function due to compression of the spinal cord. Nevertheless, good general condition is a cornerstone for surgery on asymptomatic IC. Otherwise, in older patients with incidental IC smaller than 1 cm we recommend to watch-and-wait as long as symptoms occur.

## 14.2  Extradural Spinal Cavernoma

### 14.2.1  *Epidemiology, Histology, and Localization*

In 1867 Virchow described the first vertebral hemangiomas (VHs) and later in 1926 Perman published the first radiological description of VH [80]. Currently, VHs are the most common spine bone tumors with incidence 10–12% determined by autopsy and radiography [81]. Solitary occurrence accounts for 70%. When multiple, VHs may affect up to five vertebrae. Usually VHs are located in the thoracic and lumbar spine, rarely in cervical and sacral [82]. They may affect only vertebral body 25%, posterior spinal arch 25% or both in 50%. VHs are usually located limited to the vertebra, however they can spread into epidural space even into the intervertebral foramen with a dumb-bell shape expansion [83]. Pure epidural cavernomas (ECs) are extremely rare [83–91]. Only 100 cases have been published so far [85]. VHs are vasoformative lesions growing in normal marrow that ends up with hypertrophic sclerotic trabeculation in the craniocaudal direction. Despite the fact that VHs are benign, and malignant transformation does not exist, they may have an aggressive growth pattern causing neurological decline.

### 14.2.2  Clinical Presentation

VHs are symptomatic only in 1% [92, 93]. These are called aggressive. Out of all aggressive VHs, 55% are associated with pain and the remaining 45% cause neurological deficits [94]. The pathophysiological background for the neurological decline is underlying spinal stenosis, pathological fracture, or disc herniation. The stenosis may be caused by bony hypertrophy of the posterior cortex of the vertebral body and/or hypertrophy of the laminae and facets. Similarly, the spinal canal may be narrowed by extravertebral epidural growth of VHs. In a series by Fox et al. [81] two thirds had symptoms caused by an enlargement of bony structures and by epidural soft tissue extension in one third. Progressive symptoms typically take a form of thoracic myelopathy. This may be caused by epidural growth of the tumor, expansion of bone, compression by vessels feeding or draining the lesion, compression fracture of the involved vertebra, spontaneous hemorrhage with epidural hematoma [95], and spinal cord ischemia due to steal syndrome.

### 14.2.3  Imaging Technique

There are several characteristic findings on different imaging modalities. On plain film or sagittal CT scan, one can appreciate the prominent vertical trabeculation (corduroy pattern or honeycomb appearance). On an axial CT scan a characteristically visible polka-dot sign is seen [96]. MRI demonstrates small hemangiomas as round and hyperintense on T1- and T2-weighted images. Larger VHs tend to be hypointensive on both T1- and T2-weighted images. A characteristic finding is a 'salt and pepper appearance' of the vertebral body. VHs are highly enhancing lesions due to their significant vascularity. Nevertheless, Cross et al. in their review of 109 cases showed that these characteristic findings were missing in 35% of plain films, 20% of CT scans, and 48% of MRI scans of aggressive VHs. DSA is helpful to distinguish nonaggressive from aggressive lesions (due to a higher vascularity).

Interestingly, ECs lack many MR features characteristic for cavernomas. ECs have no hypointense rim in T1- nor T2-weighted images. They may enhance homogenously or slightly heterogeneously. Additionally, as mentioned earlier, they may have a dumb-bell shape. Such an appearance resembles that of other extradural tumors such as schwannoma or neurofibroma (Fig. 14.2).

### 14.2.4  Treatment

Aggressive VHs cases should be considered for [97, 98] therapeutic intervention. There are several options such as surgery, vertebroplasty/kyphoplasty, direct ethanol injection, radiotherapy, embolization of the feeding arteries, or a combination of

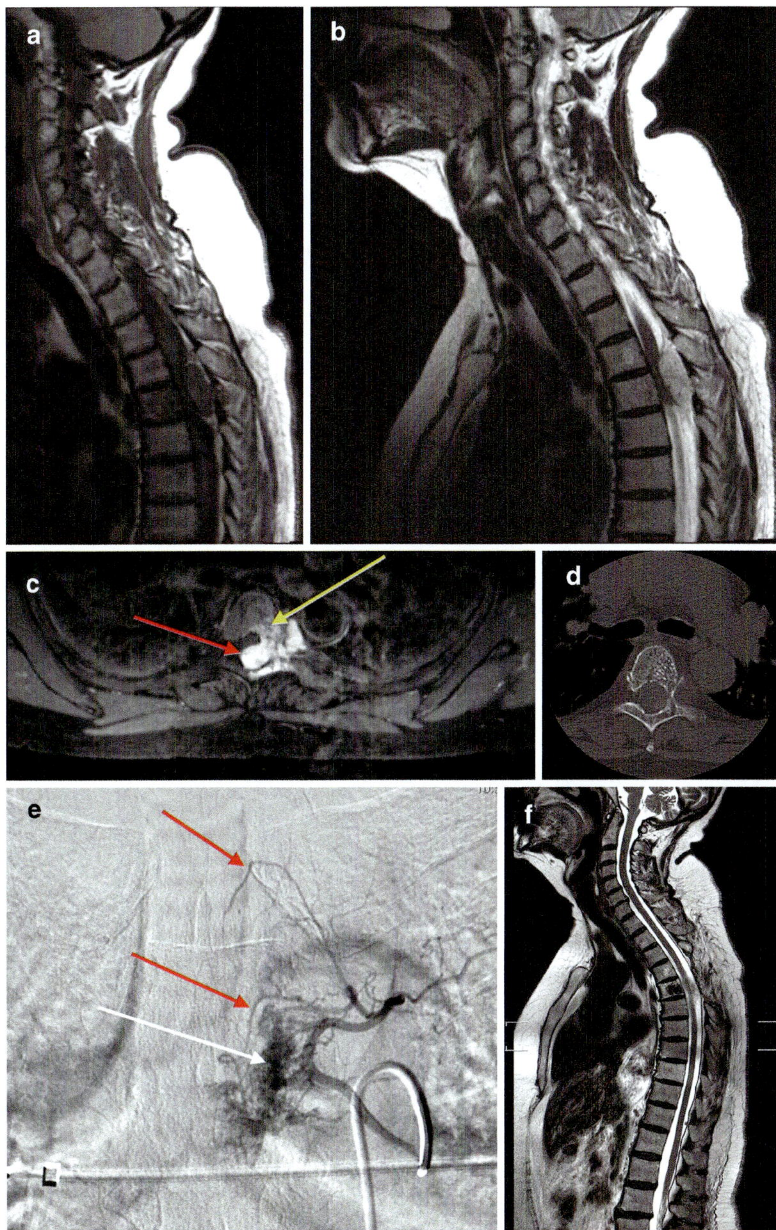

**Fig. 14.2** Vertebral hemangioma of fifth thoracic vertebra: (**a**) T1-weighted sagittal, (**b**) T2-weighted sagittal, and (**c**) T1-weighted axial with enhancement pre-surgical images. Epidural component of the tumor (red arrow) with its extra-foraminal extension and connection to the vertebra (yellow arrow). (**d**) Pre-operative CT scan showing polka-dot sign. (**e**) Angiographic image showing the rich vascular supply of the tumor (white arrow) and supply of the anterior spinal artery as a branch of intercostal artery (red arrows). (**f**) T2-weighted postoperative image demonstrates complete removal of the epidural component of the tumor. (**g**) CT postoperative scan with high density of bone cement within the vertebra after CT navigated vertebroplasty. (**h**) Micrograph showing typical features of cavernous malformation (hematoxylin and eosin stain, magnification × 100)

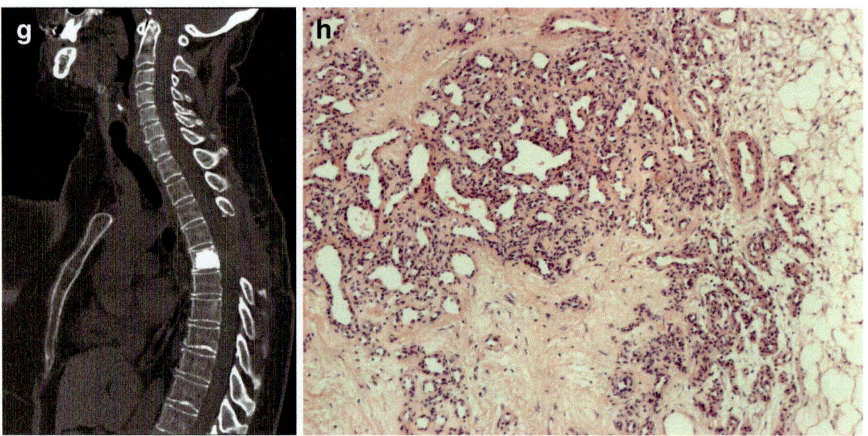

**Fig. 14.2** (continued)

these methods. Every method has been proved to be effective when properly indicated, nevertheless, complication rate, economical impact, learning curve, and technical requirement vary significantly [80].

There are two surgical approaches: Decompression, and vertebrectomy or en bloc resection. Decompression is a well-tolerated procedure with less risk of life-threatening bleeding [94] and it is also less technically demanding. It may be combined with vertebroplasty or radiotherapy to lower the risk of recurrence. Verterectomy is technically demanding, and threatens high blood loss (an estimated 2.5 liters). It is claimed that vertebrectomy or en bloc resection is associated with a lower risk of recurrence [80]. Vertebroplasty or injection of ethanol leads to shrinkage of VHs. Additionally, vertebroplasty prevents a collapse of the largely destroyed vertebra. Both procedures may be complicated by leakage of the agent into the spinal cord. VHs are radiosensitive, and radiotherapy can obliterate VHs and reduce pain. Jiang et al. [80] recommend radiotherapy for patients with pain or mild neurological decline. It may be also used preoperatively as a surgical adjunct, or postoperatively for residual VHs in case of incomplete removal. The recommended total dosage is 40 Gy fractionated within approximately 1 month. DSA provides faster pain improvement than radiotherapy, and may be used preoperatively to diminish procedural blood loss.

### 14.2.5 Conclusion

Asymptomatic VHs are very common and do not deserve any medical intervention or follow-up. A biopsy may be indicated in unclear findings from imaging methods. In contrast, aggressive VHs are rare entities that frequently need treatment. There is a wide range of effective therapeutic options to choose from. The choice should be based on the patient's condition and clinical course, age, imaging findings, and experience of the therapist.

## 14.3 Intradural Extramedullary Cavernoma

### 14.3.1 Epidemiology, Histology, and Localization

Intradural extramedullary cavernomas (IECs) are extremely rare lesions. The first note about IEC resection was published by Roger et al. in 1951 [99]. Since this, about 50 cases have been reported in international journals [100]. IECs occur in adults from age 18 to 79. IECs can be found in patients with familial multiple cavernous syndromes. They occur most often (80%) in the thoracic region. The histological structure is similar to that of cavernomas of other locations, usually having well-defined borders. They may arise from nerve roots (in the majority of cases), the inner surface of the dura and the pial surface of the spinal cord [101].

### 14.3.2 Clinical Presentation

Patients experienced variable complaints and variable courses of presentation. Patients with IECs develop symptoms similar to the symptoms of other intradural extramedullary tumors. Sensory dysfunction is the most common symptom, found in 40% of cases, followed by motor disturbances and pain, both found in 35% of cases [100]. Additionally, IECs may present with several types of often-repeated bleeding—subdural, subarachnoid (most frequent), and in one case an intramedullary clot in the close proximity to IEC was evacuated [102]. A minority of patients suffered from sphincter dysfunction [102, 103], headache, hydrocephalus [104], and Brown-Sequard syndrome [102]. The course of presentation can be acute, repeating or progressive [70, 74, 77, 99–102, 104–108].

### 14.3.3 Imaging Technique

MR scans are the most sensitive and specific type of radiologic imaging. IECs have mixed signals due to recurrent bleeding in both T1- and T2-weighted images sometimes with a characteristic hypointensive edge surrounding the lesion (due to macrophage uptake of hemosiderin). Generally, hemosiderin is less abundant compared to ICs [67, 107]. They are homogeneously enhancing and may have a dural tail mimicking other intradural extramedullary tumors [70, 100] (Fig. 14.3).

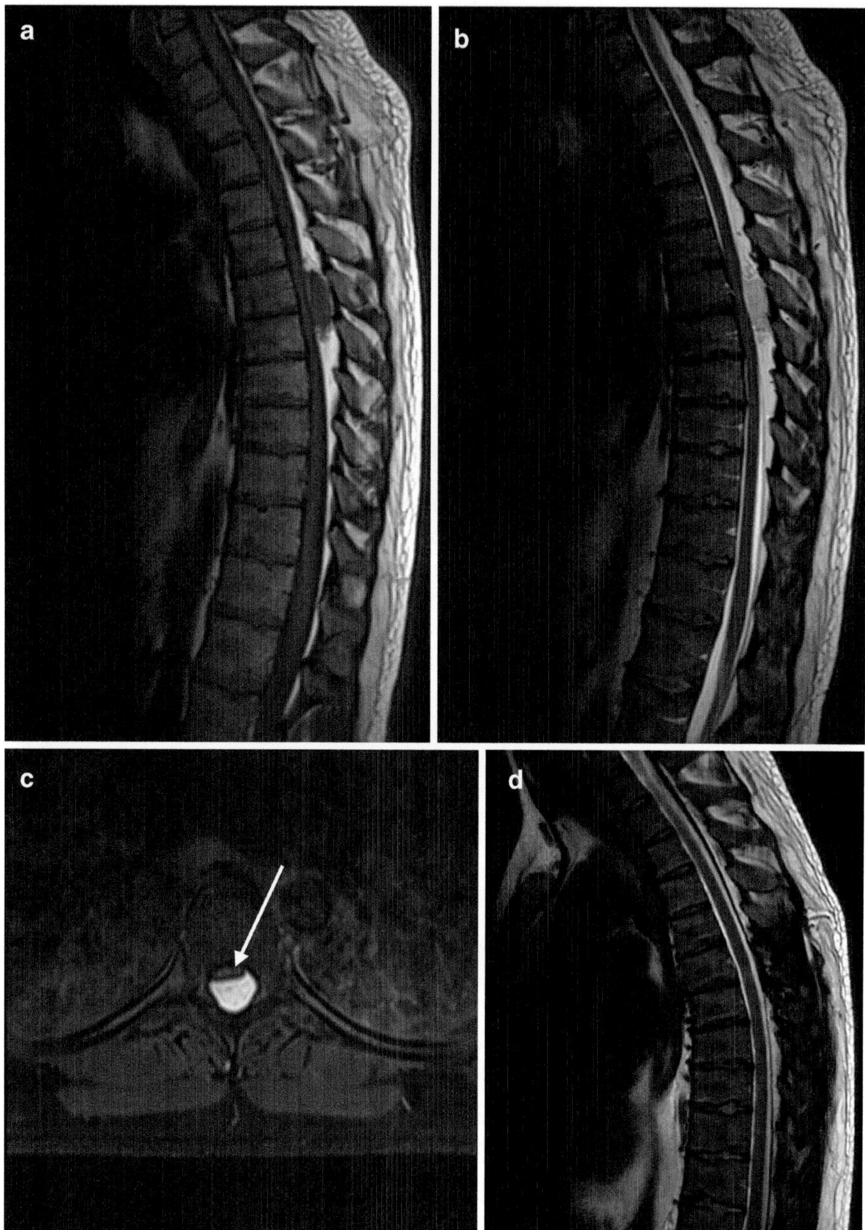

**Fig. 14.3** Extradural Cavernoma: (**a**) T1-weighted sagittal, (**b**) T2-weighted sagittal, and (**c**) T1-weighted enhanced axial pre-operative images depict purely extramedullary lesion compressing spinal cord (white arrow). (**d**) T2-weighted sagittal, (**e**) T1-weighted enhanced axial postoperative images show total resection of the tumor. (**f**) Micrograph showing caverns with thin-walled epithelial-lined spaces (hematoxylin and eosin stain, magnification × 100)

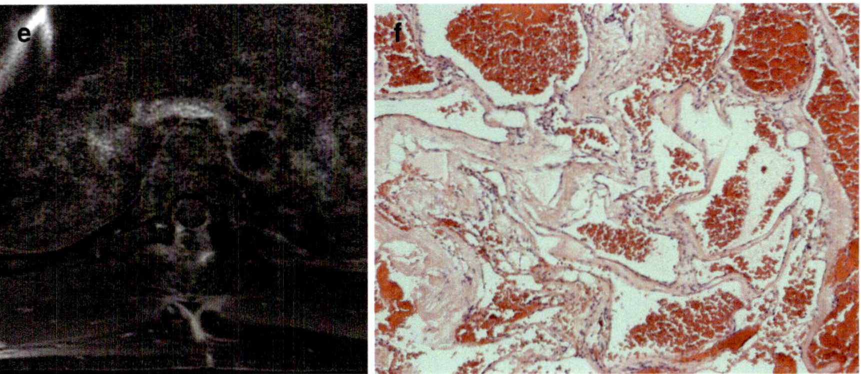

**Fig. 14.3** (continued)

### 14.3.4 Treatment Approach

The IECs were removed from each case reported here. Surgery provided excellent outcomes with a complete recovery of 70%. Patients with a lesion adhering to the spinal cord or with symptoms that lasted a long time preceding the surgery had worse outcomes. Although IECs are rare, they should be considered while setting a broad differential diagnosis.

## 14.4  Conclusion

It is worth noting that the problem of SCM is diverse, and comprises many different aspects. From the neurosurgical point of view, the most important aspect is that of IC. Despite the fact that ICs are relatively rare, neurosurgeons should provide adequate treatment. Eliciting a proper approach may be extremely challenging as long as the patient has no symptoms or presents only with pain. Intradural extramedullary and pure epidural cavernomas are extremely rare, and one should keep them in mind as they can mimic different tumors such as meningioma, schwannoma, and neurofibroma. VHs are the most common. Asymptomatic VHs are very frequent and do not deserve any medical intervention or follow-up. A biopsy may be indicated in unclear in unclear cases. Aggressive VHs are rare and often need treatment. One has a wide range of choices for effective therapy. The choice of therapy should be based on the patient's condition and clinical course, age, imaging findings, and therapist experiences.

**Key Points**

**IC**

- ICs are found in 1.86 per 100,000 population. The average age at presentation is around 40 years, ranging from 2 to 80 years.
- Coexistent brain cavernoma is found in up to 40% and 10–15% have a positive family history of IC.
- Most patients suffer from sensory and motor deficits. These deficits affect about two-thirds of individuals with IC.
- The annual rate of hemorrhage broadly varies from 1.4 to 6.8%.
- Surgical removal of IC remains the only curative treatment option. Meticulous presurgical planning is essential to achieve the best possible result.
- The final postoperative outcome is dependent on pre-hospital symptoms and pre-operative clinical status, MR findings, and the chosen therapeutic option. The length of symptoms is an important factor predicting postsurgical recovery. Patients having symptoms of less than 3 months were found to have better post-surgical outcomes.

**VH**

- VHs are symptomatic only in 1%. These are called aggressive. Out of all agressive VHs, 55% are associated with pain and the remaining 45% cause neurological deficits.
- Aggressive VHs cases should be considered for therapeutic intervention. There are several options such as surgery, vertebroplasty/kyphoplasty, direct ethanol injection, radiotherapy, embolization of the feeding arteries, or a combination of these methods.

**IEC**

- Intradural extramedullary cavernomas are extremely rare lesions.
- Patients experienced variable complaints and variable courses of presentation. Patients with IECs develop symptoms similar to the symptoms of other intradural extramedullary tumors.
- Surgery provide excellent outcomes with a complete recovery of 70%. Patients with a lesion adhering to the spinal cord or with symptoms that lasted a long time preceding the surgery have worse outcomes.

# References


1. Hadlich R. Ein Fall von tumor cavernosus de Rückenmarks mit besonderer Berücksichtigung der neuren Theorienüber die gene des Cavernomas. Virchows Arch. 1903;172:429–41.
2. Schultze F. Weiterer Beitrag zur diagnose und operativen Behandlung von Geschwülsten der Rüeckenmarkshäute und des Rüeckenmarks: Erfolgreiche operation eines intramedullaeren tumors. Dtsch Med Wochenschr. 1912;38:1676–9.
3. Bian LG, et al. Intramedullary cavernous malformations: clinical features and surgical technique via hemilaminectomy. Clin Neurol Neurosurg. 2009;111(6):511–7.

4. Gross BA, et al. Intramedullary spinal cord cavernous malformations. Neurosurg Focus. 2010;29(3):E14.
5. McCormick PC, et al. Cavernous malformations of the spinal cord. Neurosurgery. 1988;23(4):459–63.
6. Sandalcioglu IE, et al. Intramedullary spinal cord cavernous malformations: clinical features and risk of hemorrhage. Neurosurg Rev. 2003;26(4):253–6.
7. Cantu C, et al. Predictive factors for intracerebral hemorrhage in patients with cavernous angiomas. Neurol Res. 2005;27(3):314–8.
8. Kivelev J, et al. A proposed grading system of brain and spinal cavernomas. Neurosurgery. 2011;69(4):807–13, discussion 813–4.
9. El-Koussy M, et al. Incidence, clinical presentation and imaging findings of cavernous malformations of the CNS. A twenty-year experience. Swiss Med Wkly. 2011;141:w13172.
10. Badhiwala JH, et al. Surgical outcomes and natural history of intramedullary spinal cord cavernous malformations: a single-center series and meta-analysis of individual patient data: clinic article. J Neurosurg Spine. 2014;21(4):662–76.
11. Ardeshiri A, et al. A retrospective and consecutive analysis of the epidemiology and management of spinal cavernomas over the last 20 years in a single center. Neurosurg Rev. 2016;39(2):269–76. discussion 276.
12. Cantore G, et al. Intramedullary cavernous angiomas of the spinal cord: report of six cases. Surg Neurol. 1995;43(5):448–51. discussion 451–2.
13. Deutsch H, et al. Spinal intramedullary cavernoma: clinical presentation and surgical outcome. J Neurosurg. 2000;93(1 Suppl):65–70.
14. Choi GH, et al. The clinical features and surgical outcomes of patients with intramedullary spinal cord cavernous malformations. Acta Neurochir. 2011;153(8):1677–84. discussion 1685.
15. Jallo GI, et al. Clinical presentation and optimal management for intramedullary cavernous malformations. Neurosurg Focus. 2006;21(1):e10.
16. Kharkar S, et al. The natural history of conservatively managed symptomatic intramedullary spinal cord cavernomas. Neurosurgery. 2007;60(5):865–72. discussion 865–72.
17. Liang JT, et al. Management and prognosis of symptomatic patients with intramedullary spinal cord cavernoma: clinical article. J Neurosurg Spine. 2011;15(4):447–56.
18. Lu DC, Lawton MT. Clinical presentation and surgical management of intramedullary spinal cord cavernous malformations. Neurosurg Focus. 2010;29(3):E12.
19. Padovani R, et al. Cavernous angiomas of the spinal district: surgical treatment of 11 patients. Eur Spine J. 1997;6(5):298–303.
20. Santoro A, et al. Intramedullary spinal cord cavernous malformations: report of ten new cases. Neurosurg Rev. 2004;27(2):93–8.
21. Spetzger U, Gilsbach JM, Bertalanffy H. Cavernous angiomas of the spinal cord clinical presentation, surgical strategy, and postoperative results. Acta Neurochir. 1995;134(3–4):200–6.
22. Vishteh AG, et al. Surgical resection of intramedullary spinal cord cavernous malformations: delayed complications, long-term outcomes, and association with cryptic venous malformations. Neurosurgery. 1997;41(5):1094–100. discussion 1100–1.
23. Canavero S, et al. Spinal intramedullary cavernous angiomas: a literature meta-analysis. Surg Neurol. 1994;41(5):381–8.
24. Zevgaridis D, et al. Cavernous haemangiomas of the spinal cord. A review of 117 cases. Acta Neurochir. 1999;141(3):237–45.
25. Abid R, et al. Brain and spinal cord cavernoma. Value of MRI and review of the literature. Apropos of a case. J Radiol. 1993;74(11):563–7.
26. Bourgouin PM, et al. Multiple occult vascular malformations of the brain and spinal cord: MRI diagnosis. Neuroradiology. 1992;34(2):110–1.
27. Vishteh AG, Zabramski JM, Spetzler RF. Patients with spinal cord cavernous malformations are at an increased risk for multiple neuraxis cavernous malformations. Neurosurgery. 1999;45(1):30–2. discussion 33.

28. Mitha AP, et al. Outcomes following resection of intramedullary spinal cord cavernous malformations: a 25-year experience. J Neurosurg Spine. 2011;14(5):605–11.
29. Cohen-Gadol AA, et al. Coexistence of intracranial and spinal cavernous malformations: a study of prevalence and natural history. J Neurosurg. 2006;104(3):376–81.
30. Bicknell JM. Familial cavernous angioma of the brain stem dominantly inherited in Hispanics. Neurosurgery. 1989;24(1):102–5.
31. Labauge P, et al. Outcome in 53 patients with spinal cord cavernomas. Surg Neurol. 2008;70(2):176–81. discussion 181.
32. Zabramski JM, et al. The natural history of familial cavernous malformations: results of an ongoing study. J Neurosurg. 1994;80(3):422–32.
33. Yoshinaga T, et al. Cerebral and spinal cavernomas associated with Klippel-Trenaunay syndrome: case report and literature review. Acta Neurochir. 2018;160(2):287–90.
34. Matsui Y, et al. Coexistence of multiple cavernous angiomas in the spinal cord and skin: a unique case of Cobb syndrome. J Neurosurg Spine. 2014;20(2):142–7.
35. Dey DD, Landrum O, Oaklander AL. Central neuropathic itch from spinal-cord cavernous hemangioma: a human case, a possible animal model, and hypotheses about pathogenesis. Pain. 2005;113(1–2):233–7.
36. Ogilvy CS, Louis DN, Ojemann RG. Intramedullary cavernous angiomas of the spinal cord: clinical presentation, pathological features, and surgical management. Neurosurgery. 1992;31(2):219–29. discussion 229–30.
37. Gomez-Soriano J, et al. Sensory function after cavernous haemangioma: a case report of thermal hypersensitivity at and below an incomplete spinal cord injury. Spinal Cord. 2012;50(9):711–5.
38. Zhang L, et al. Comparison of outcome between surgical and conservative management of symptomatic spinal cord cavernous malformations. Neurosurgery. 2016;78(4):552–61.
39. Goyal A, et al. Clinical presentation, natural history and outcomes of intramedullary spinal cord cavernous malformations. J Neurol Neurosurg Psychiatry. 2019;90:695–703.
40. Kim LJ, et al. Analysis of pain resolution after surgical resection of intramedullary spinal cord cavernous malformations. Neurosurgery. 2006;58(1):106–11. discussion 106–11.
41. Park SB, Jahng TA, Chung CK. The clinical outcomes after complete surgical resection of intramedullary cavernous angiomas: changes in motor and sensory symptoms. Spinal Cord. 2009;47(2):128–33.
42. Yuce I, et al. A rare cause of episodic paresthesia: spinal cavernoma. Spine J. 2015;15(9):2092–3.
43. Chabert E, et al. Intramedullary cavernous malformations. J Neuroradiol. 1999;26(4):262–8.
44. Varoglu AO, et al. Intramedullary angioma with bilateral arm hypothermia. Br J Neurosurg. 2008;22(5):687–9.
45. Huntley GD, et al. Ascending spinal cord infarction secondary to recurrent spinal cord cavernous malformation hemorrhage. J Stroke Cerebrovasc Dis. 2017;26(4):e72–3.
46. Aoyama T, Hida K, Houkin K. Intramedullary cavernous angiomas of the spinal cord: clinical characteristics of 13 lesions. Neurol Med Chir (Tokyo). 2011;51(8):561–6.
47. Svoboda N, Bradac O, Benes V. Long-term postoperative clinical outcomes after intramedullary Cavernoma resection. Cesk Slov Neurol N. 2017;80(113(5)):564–8.
48. Aiba T, et al. Natural history of intracranial cavernous malformations. J Neurosurg. 1995;83(1):56–9.
49. Fritschi JA, et al. Cavernous malformations of the brain stem. A review of 139 cases. Acta Neurochir. 1994;130(1–4):35–46.
50. Kondziolka D, Lunsford LD, Kestle JR. The natural history of cerebral cavernous malformations. J Neurosurg. 1995;83(5):820–4.
51. Porter RW, et al. Cavernous malformations of the brainstem: experience with 100 patients. J Neurosurg. 1999;90(1):50–8.
52. Marconi F, et al. Spinal cavernous angioma producing subarachnoid hemorrhage. Case report. J Neurosurg Sci. 1995;39(1):75–80.

53. Mori K, et al. Intradural-extramedullary spinal cavernous angioma--case report. Neurol Med Chir (Tokyo). 1991;31(9):593–6.
54. Cosgrove GR, et al. Cavernous angiomas of the spinal cord. J Neurosurg. 1988;68(1):31–6.
55. Matsuyama Y, et al. Surgical results of intramedullary spinal cord tumor with spinal cord monitoring to guide extent of resection. J Neurosurg Spine. 2009;10(5):404–13.
56. Fontaine S, et al. Cavernous hemangiomas of the spinal cord: MR imaging. Radiology. 1988;166(3):839–41.
57. Turjman F, et al. MRI of intramedullary cavernous haemangiomas. Neuroradiology. 1995;37(4):297–302.
58. Otten M, McCormick P. Natural history of spinal cavernous malformations. Handb Clin Neurol. 2017;143:233–9.
59. Bucci MN, et al. Management of anteriorly located C1-C2 neurofibromata. Surg Neurol. 1990;33(1):15–8.
60. Hakuba A, et al. Transuncodiscal approach to dumbbell tumors of the cervical spinal canal. J Neurosurg. 1984;61(6):1100–6.
61. Weil AG, Bhatia S. Resection of a ventral intramedullary cervical spinal cord cavernous malformation through an anterior approach. Neurosurg Focus. 2014;37(Suppl 2):Video 18.
62. Nishikawa M, et al. The anterolateral partial vertebrectomy approach for ventrally located cervical intramedullary cavernous angiomas. Neurosurgery. 2006;59(1 Suppl 1):ONS58–63. discussion ONS58–63.
63. Raynor RB, Weiner R. Transthoracic approach to an intramedullary vascular malformation of the thoracic spinal cord. Neurosurgery. 1982;10(5):631–4.
64. Santoro A, et al. Total removal of an intramedullary cavernous angioma by transthoracic approach. Ital J Neurol Sci. 1998;19(3):176–9.
65. Martin NA, Khanna RK, Batzdorf U. Posterolateral cervical or thoracic approach with spinal cord rotation for vascular malformations or tumors of the ventrolateral spinal cord. J Neurosurg. 1995;83(2):254–61.
66. Spetzler RF, Zabramski JM, Flom RA. Management of juvenile spinal AVM's by embolization and operative excision. Case report. J Neurosurg. 1989;70(4):628–32.
67. Crispino M, et al. Spinal intradural extramedullary haemangioma: MRI and neurosurgical findings. Acta Neurochir. 2005;147(11):1195–8. discussion 1198.
68. Mitha AP, Turner JD, Spetzler RF. Surgical approaches to intramedullary cavernous malformations of the spinal cord. Neurosurgery. 68(2 Suppl Operative):2011, 317–24. discussion 324.
69. Brotchi J. Intrinsic spinal cord tumor resection. Neurosurgery. 2002;50(5):1059–63.
70. Alobaid A, et al. Mixed capillary-cavernous extramedullary intradural hemangioma of the spinal cord mimicking meningioma: case report. Br J Neurosurg. 2015;29(3):438–9.
71. Ziechmann R, et al. Intradural extramedullary thoracic cavernoma in a man with familial multiple cavernomas. Cureus. 2018;10(8):e3115.
72. Hegde A, et al. Spinal cavernous malformations: magnetic resonance imaging and associated findings. Singap Med J. 2012;53(9):582–6.
73. Deutsch H. Pain outcomes after surgery in patients with intramedullary spinal cord cavernous malformations. Neurosurg Focus. 2010;29(3):E15.
74. Nozaki K, et al. Spinal intradural extramedullary cavernous angioma. Case report. J Neurosurg. 2003;99(3 Suppl):316–9.
75. Reitz M, et al. Intramedullary spinal cavernoma: clinical presentation, microsurgical approach, and long-term outcome in a cohort of 48 patients. Neurosurg Focus. 2015;39(2):E19.
76. McCormick PC, et al. Intramedullary ependymoma of the spinal cord. J Neurosurg. 1990;72(4):523–32.
77. Mastronardi L, et al. Intradural extramedullary cavernous angioma: case report. Neurosurgery. 1991;29(6):924–6.
78. Klekamp J. Treatment of intramedullary tumors: analysis of surgical morbidity and long-term results. J Neurosurg Spine. 2013;19(1):12–26.

79. Steiger HJ, Turowski B, Hanggi D. Prognostic factors for the outcome of surgical and conservative treatment of symptomatic spinal cord cavernous malformations: a review of a series of 20 patients. Neurosurg Focus. 2010;29(3):E13.
80. Jiang L, et al. Diagnosis and treatment of vertebral hemangiomas with neurologic deficit: a report of 29 cases and literature review. Spine J. 2014;14(6):944–54.
81. Fox MW, Onofrio BM. The natural history and management of symptomatic and asymptomatic vertebral hemangiomas. J Neurosurg. 1993;78(1):36–45.
82. Slon V, et al. Vertebral hemangiomas: their demographical characteristics, location along the spine and position within the vertebral body. Eur Spine J. 2015;24(10):2189–95.
83. Gao C, et al. Spinal epidural cavernous hemangioma: a clinical series of 7 patients. World Neurosurg. 2018;111:e183–91.
84. Hemalatha AL, et al. A pure epidural spinal cavernous hemangioma - with an innocuous face but a perilous behaviour!! J Clin Diagn Res. 2013;7(7):1434–5.
85. Cossandi C, et al. Rare case of dumbbell-shaped spinal cavernous hemangioma and literature review. World Neurosurg. 2018;120:181–4.
86. Esene IN, et al. Pure spinal epidural cavernous hemangioma: a case series of seven cases. J Craniovertebr Junction Spine. 2016;7(3):176–83.
87. Jang D, et al. Pure spinal epidural cavernous hemangioma with intralesional hemorrhage: a rare cause of thoracic myelopathy. Korean J Spine. 2014;11(2):85–8.
88. Zhong W, et al. Pure spinal epidural cavernous hemangioma. Acta Neurochir. 2012;154(4):739–45.
89. Khalatbari MR, Abbassioun K, Amirjmshidi A. Solitary spinal epidural cavernous angioma: report of nine surgically treated cases and review of the literature. Eur Spine J. 2013;22(3):542–7.
90. Meng Y, Shamji MF. Solitary spinal epidural cavernous haemangiomas as a rare cause of myelopathy. BMJ Case Rep. 2015;2015:bcr2015211644.
91. Sharma MS, et al. Thoracic extraosseous, epidural, cavernous hemangioma: case report and review of literature. J Neurosci Rural Pract. 2013;4(3):309–12.
92. Alexander J, et al. Vertebral hemangioma: an important differential in the evaluation of locally aggressive spinal lesions. Spine (Phila Pa 1976). 2010;35(18):E917–20.
93. Pastushyn AI, Slin'ko EI, Mirzoyeva GM. Vertebral hemangiomas: diagnosis, management, natural history and clinicopathological correlates in 86 patients. Surg Neurol. 1998;50(6):535–47.
94. Acosta FL Jr, et al. Comprehensive management of symptomatic and aggressive vertebral hemangiomas. Neurosurg Clin N Am. 2008;19(1):17–29.
95. Kosary IZ, Shacked R. Spinal epidural hematoma due to hemangioma of vertebra. Surg Neurol. 1977;7:61–2.
96. Persaud T. The polka-dot sign. Radiology. 2008;246(3):980–1.
97. Kato S, et al. Surgical management of aggressive vertebral hemangiomas causing spinal cord compression: long-term clinical follow-up of five cases. J Orthop Sci. 2010;15(3):350–6.
98. Ogawa R, et al. Total en bloc spondylectomy for locally aggressive vertebral hemangioma causing neurological deficits. Case Rep Orthop. 2015;2015:724364.
99. Roger H, Paillas JE, Bonnal J, Vigorous M. Angiomes de la moelle et des racines. Acta Neurol Psych Belgium. 1951;7:491–5.
100. Petillon P, et al. Spinal intradural extramedullary cavernous hemangioma. Neuroradiology. 2018;60(10):1085–7.
101. Er U, et al. Spinal intradural extramedullary cavernous angioma: case report and review of the literature. Spinal Cord. 2007;45(9):632–6.
102. Kivelev J, et al. Cervical intradural extramedullary cavernoma presenting with isolated intramedullary hemorrhage. J Neurosurg Spine. 2008;8(1):88–91.
103. Sharma R, Rout D, Radhakrishnan VV. Intradural spinal cavernomas. Br J Neurosurg. 1992;6(4):351–6.

104. Katoh N, et al. Spinal intradural extramedullary cavernous angioma presenting with super-ficial siderosis and hydrocephalus: a case report and review of the literature. Intern Med. 2014;53(16):1863–7.
105. Abdullah DC, et al. Thoracic intradural extramedullary capillary hemangioma. AJNR Am J Neuroradiol. 2004;25(7):1294–6.
106. Mataliotakis G, et al. Intradural extramedullary cavernoma of a lumbar nerve root mim-icking neurofibroma. A report of a rare case and the differential diagnosis. Spine J. 2014;14(12):e1–7.
107. Rachinger J, et al. Intradural-extramedullary cavernous hemangioma of the left motor root C7--case report and update of the literature. Zentralbl Neurochir. 2006;67(3):144–8.
108. Yasargil MG. Microsurgery; cavernous and occult angiomas. Stuttgart: Georg Thieme Verlag; 1988. p. 415–72.

# Chapter 15
# Intraorbital Cavernous Malformations

David Netuka

## 15.1 Introduction

There is considerable histological variability of intraorbital lesions. Vasculogenic lesions represent 17% of all orbital lesions while fibrocytic lesions represent only 1–2% [1].

According to Günalp et al. [2] cavernomas are the most common orbital vascular tumours.

Typical symptoms represent: exophtalmus, retroorbital pain, visual field deficit, diplopia. There is a significant number of cases where a suspected cavernous malformations is asymptomatic or minimally symptomatic. In these cases watch and wait strategy should be adopted. Only symptomatic lesions should be considered for a treatment. Surgery is the only reasonable treatment modality if active approach is indicated.

Numerous approaches have been described for orbital cavernomas. Schick et al. [3] published one of the largest series of orbital cavernomas. They tailored the approach according to location of the cavernoma in the orbit. The following approaches were used: lateral orbitotomy, transconjuctival, ipsilateral intradural, ipsilateral extradural, supraorbital and contralateral pterional. They used a contralateral pterional approach for lesions in medial posterior intraconal space.

Brusati et al. [4] published a report of their experiences with 19 orbital cavernomas. Lateral orbitotomy combined with an anterior medial approach to gain access to retrobulbar space was used in seven cavernomas located medially to the optic nerve in the posterior half of the orbit.

The choice of the approach also depends on the surgeon's specialty.

The contralateral pterional approach may be considered suitable for lesions located medially and inferiorly to the optic nerve in posterior intraconal space [5].

D. Netuka (✉)
Department of Neurosurgery and Neurooncology, First Medical Faculty, Military University Hospital and Charles University, Prague, Czech Republic

© Springer Nature Switzerland AG 2020
O. Bradáč, V. Beneš (eds.), *Cavernomas of the CNS*,
https://doi.org/10.1007/978-3-030-49406-3_15

This approach leads along the sphenoid wing to the planum sphenoidale from the contralateral side. The dura is opened and the ethmoid and sphenoid sinus is entered. Afterwards, the orbit is opened.

The different approach for medial posterior extraconal cavernoma represent combined lateral orbitotomy with inferior transconjuctival incision. The globe is displaced laterally, medial rectus muscle is retracted inferiorly and superior rectus muscle superiorly [4].

The first cases of endonasal approach to orbital apex was described by Sethi et al. [6] They performed six biopsies. Otolaryngologists were the first to adopt and practise endonasal surgery for orbital lesions. Mir-Salim et al. [7] described the endonasal, microsurgical approach to the retrobulbar region. They performed ethmoidectomy after septal mobilisation, identifying the optic nerve in the wall of the sphenoid sinus. Then they resected the lamina papyracea between the sphenoid sinus wall, skull base and ethmoid. The medial rectus muscle was mobilised and the cavernoma was removed under microscopic control.

In the past years case reports of the endoscopic approach for orbital apex lesions have appeared in the literature. The first transnasal endoscopic removal of an orbital cavernoma was described in 1999 by Herman et al. [8].

Later on, Yoshimura et al. [9] published a case of cavernoma that was found to extend from the orbital apex to the pterygopalatine fossa. They performed wide sphenoidotomy, resected superior turbinate and identified opticocarotid recess. Further on, posterior and anterior ethmoidectomy was performed. They continued with medial and posterior maxillectomy in order to expose the pterygopalatine fossa.

Another technique represent combined endoscopic endonasal approach with anterior orbitotomy via a transcaruncular approach described by Campbell et al. [10].

Murchison et al. [11] presented a series of an endoscopic technique for 18 orbital apex and periorbital skull base lesions. In two cases, cavernoma was resected.

Our team described endoscopic endonasal resection of the orbital cavernous malformations with application of intraoperative MRI. Intraoperative MRI was valuable in a case of intraconal cavernous malformation which was not easy to find deep to occular muscles. Netuka et al. [12]

Zolli et al. [13] presented series of 23 patients with intraorbital lesions. They treated five cavernous hemangioma. Exophthalmos was the most common symptom. They applied endonasal endoscopic approach in 16 cases, endoscopic transpalpebral approach in seven cases. In 13% of cases temporary diplopied developed.

We believe that cavernous malformation located medially to optic nerve and especially the onces located mediocaudally to optic nerve are the best candidates for endonasal resection.

Cavernous malformation may be located extraconally, i.e. outside to ocular muscles. These lesions are much easier for endonasal resection (case 1).

More complex cases represent intraconal location of cavernous malformations where the dissection between ocular muscles is mandatory (case 2).

## 15.2    General Description of Surgical Technique

The endonasal approach is mononostril in these cases. Therefore we resect the middle turbinate on the side of the lesion in order to get a wider exposure. Then, the sphenoid sinus is opened and then the posterior ethmoid sinuses are entered. Next, anterior ethmoidectomy and antrostomy is performed. Based on exact location of cavernous malformation in anterioposterior plane the optic canal is drilled out. Optic canal opening is not needed in cavernomas located more ventrally. The lamina papyracea is partially removed, the extend is tailored according to size and location of the cavernous malformation. Afterwards the sharp opening of the periorbita is performed. Frameless navigation is used repeatedly during the procedure. The cavernoma is disected within periorbital fat in case of extraconal cavernoma location (case 1). Manipulation with ocular muscles is needed in intraconal cavernomas (case 2). Typically, the medial and inferior rectus are disected and cavernoma is inspected. Cavernoma is circumferentially dissected and removed in one peace. The optic nerve is decompressed and haemostasis checked. The opening of the orbit is usually limited and therefore no bone reconstruction is needed. The periorbita is covered with mucosa only.

## 15.3    Conclusions

Endoscopic endonasal technique is an excellent approach for lesions in the medial retrobulbar space and in orbital apex medial to the optic nerve. Neuronavigation is mandatory for these cases. Intraconal cavernous malformations are more challenging lesions while dissection between ocular muscles is needed.

**Key Points**
- Intraorbotal cavernous malformations are but may cause significant ocular symptoms
- Only symptomatic lesions should be considered for a treatment
- Surgery is the only reasonable treatment modality in these cases
- Endoscopic endonasal approach is best suited for leasions medial or inferiomedial to optic nerve
- Cavernous malformations located intraconally are more surgically challenging than extraconal lesions

**Case 1**
A 60 years old lady with retroorbital pain, partial visual field deficit on the left eye (Figs. 15.1 and 15.2).

**Case 2**
A 35 years old lady with headaches and partial visual deficit. MRI disclosed intraconal cavernous malformation. Surgery was uneventful, cavernous malformation was resected. No postoperative eye movement was observed (Figs. 15.3 and 15.4).

**Fig. 15.1** Preoperative MRI, T2-weighted image, coronal plane showing hyperintense lesion in the orbital apex, in extraconal space

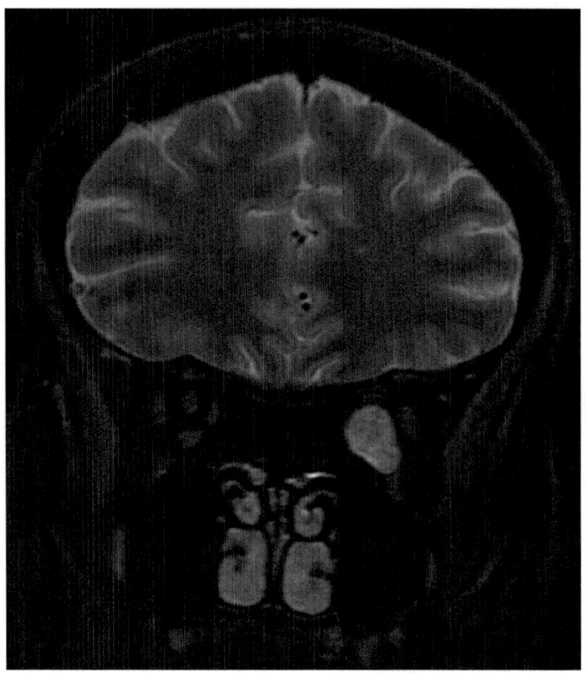

**Fig. 15.2** MRI 10 years after surgery, FSPGR, coronal plane, radical resection of cavernoma, optic nerve decompressed. All the symptoms completelly resolved within 4 weeks after surgery. No signs of recurrent disease

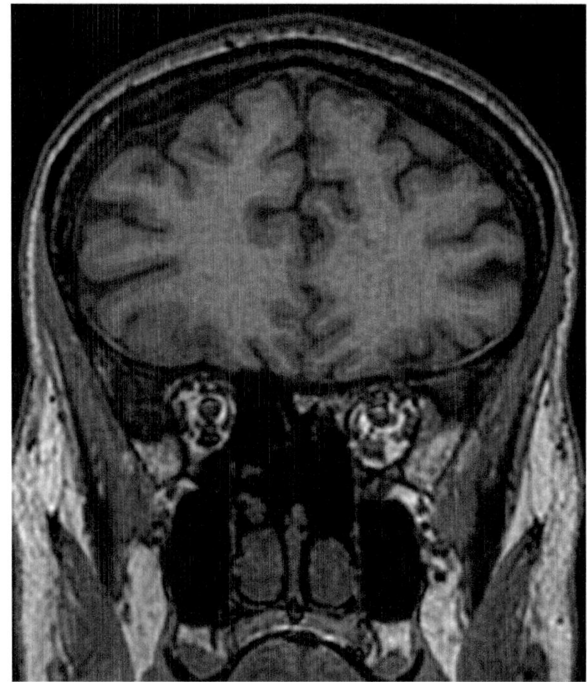

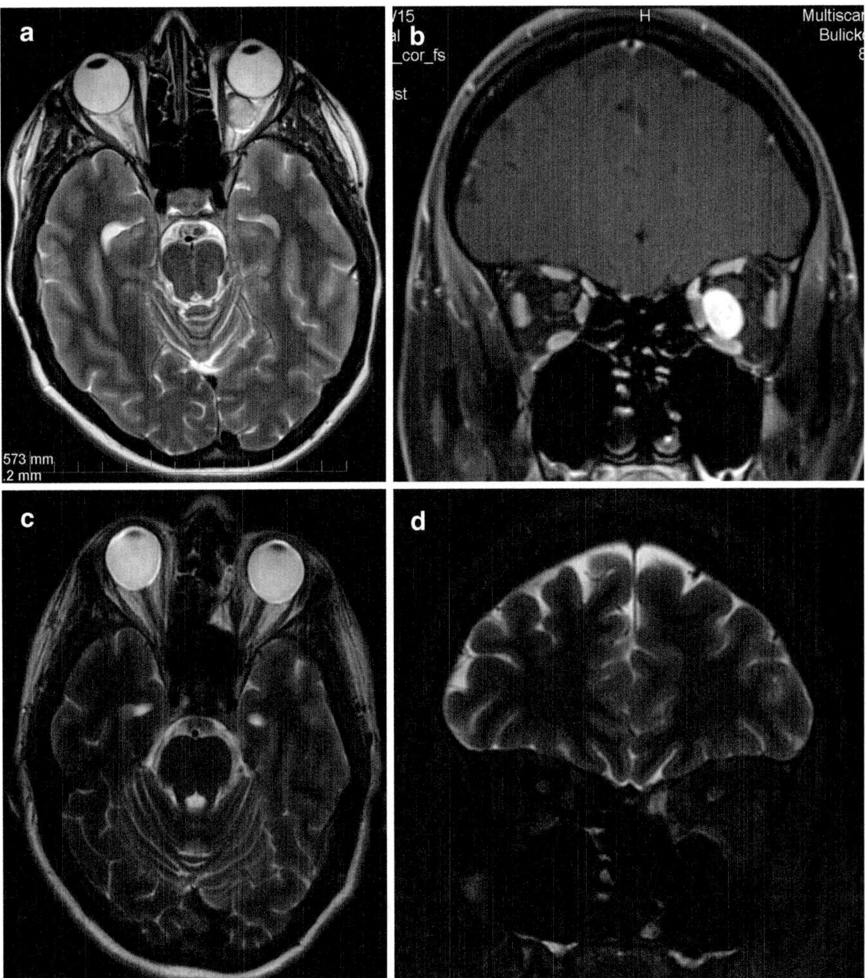

**Fig. 15.3** (**a**) Preoperative MRI, axial plane, T2-weighted image showing lesion medially to medial rectus muscle, ie. lesion in intraconal space, (**b**) preoperative MRI, coronal plane, T1-weighted image with Gadolinium, lesion is highly contrast enhancing, (**c**) postoperative MRI, axial plane, T2-weighted image showing decompressed optic nerve an no signs of cavernoma, (**d**) postoperative MRI, coronal plane, T2-weighted image

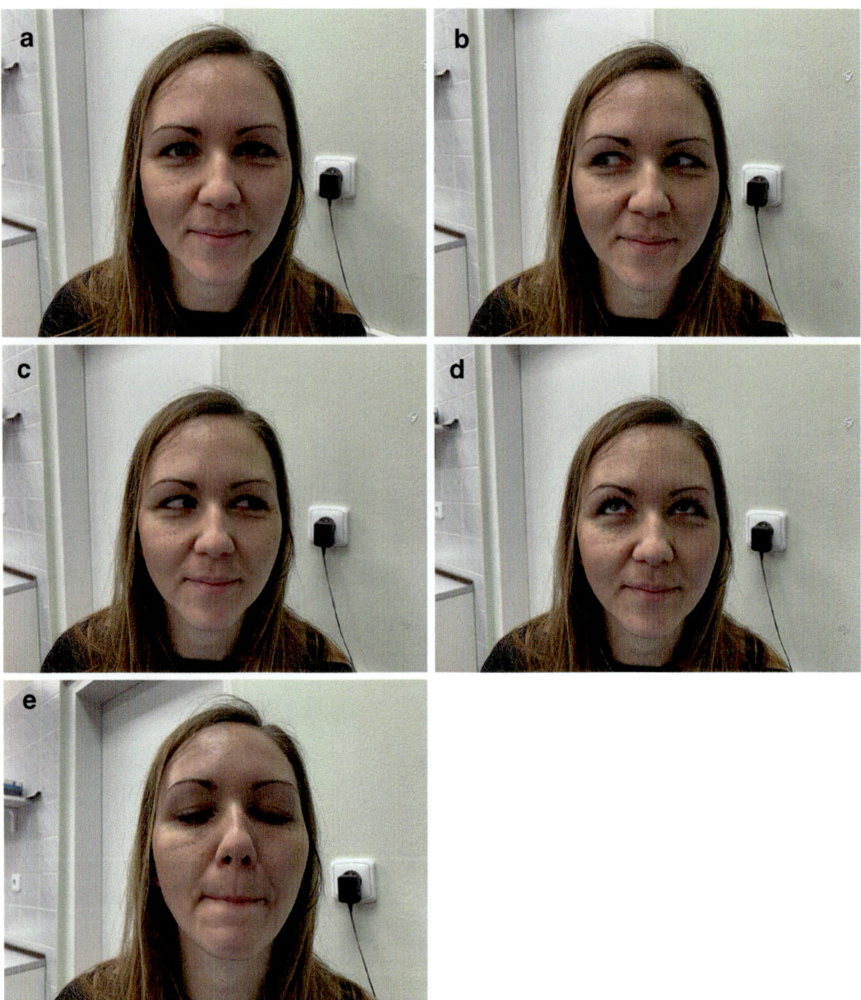

**Fig. 15.4** Patient suffered temporary postoperative diplopia which resolved withind 6 weeks. (**a–e**) no restriction in eye movements

**Acknowledgement** Supported by MO 1012 and Q 27.

# References


1. Shields JA, Shields CL, Scartozzi R. Survey of 1264 patients with orbital tumors and simulating lesions: The 2002 Montgomery Lecture, Part 1. Ophthalmology. 2004;111(5):997–1008.
2. Günalp I, Gündüz K. Vascular tumors of the orbit. Doc Ophthalmol. 1995;89(4):337–45.
3. Schick U, Dott U, Hassler W. Surgical treatment of orbital cavernomas. Surg Neurol. 2003 Sep;60(3):234–44.

4. Brusati R, Goisis M, Biglioli F, et al. Surgical approaches to cavernous haemangiomas of the orbit. Br J Oral Maxillofac Surg. 2007;45(6):457–62.
5. Hassler WE, Meyer B, Rohde V, Unsöld R. Pterional approach to the contralateral orbit. Neurosurgery. 1994;34(3):552–4.
6. Sethi DS, Lau DP. Endoscopic management of orbital apex lesions. Am J Rhinol. 1997;11(6):449–55.
7. Mir-Salim PA, Berghaus A. Endonasal, microsurgical approach to the retrobulbar region exemplified by intraconal hemangioma. HNO. 1999;47(3):192–5.
8. Herman P, Lot G, Silhouette B, et al. Transnasal endoscopic removal of an orbital cavernoma. Ann Otol Rhinol Laryngol. 1999;108(2):147–50.
9. Yoshimura K, Kubo S, Yoneda H, Hasegawa H, Tominaga S, Yoshimine T. Removal of a cavernous hemangioma in the orbital apex via the endoscopic transnasal approach: a case report. Minim Invasive Neurosurg. 2010;53(2):77–9.
10. Campbell PG, Yadla S, Rosen M, Bilyk JR, Murchison AP, Evans JJ. Endoscopic transnasal cryo-assisted removal of an orbital cavernous hemangioma: a technical note. Minim Invasive Neurosurg. 2011;54(1):41–3.
11. Murchison AP, Rosen MR, Evans JJ, Bilyk JR. Endoscopic approach to the orbital apex and periorbital skull base. Laryngoscope. 2011;121(3):463–7.
12. Netuka D, Masopust V, Belšán T, Profantová N, Beneš V. Endoscopic endonasal resection of medial orbital lesions with intraoperative MRI. Acta Neurochir. 2013 Mar;155(3):455–61. https://doi.org/10.1007/s00701-012-1585-9.
13. Zoli M, Sollini G, Milanese L, La Corte E, Rustici A, Guaraldi F, Asioli S, Cirillo L, Pasquini E, Mazzatenta D. Endoscopic approaches to orbital lesions: case series and systematic literature review. J Neurosurg. 2020;3:1–13. https://doi.org/10.3171/2019.10.JNS192138.